The Angel of Bethesda

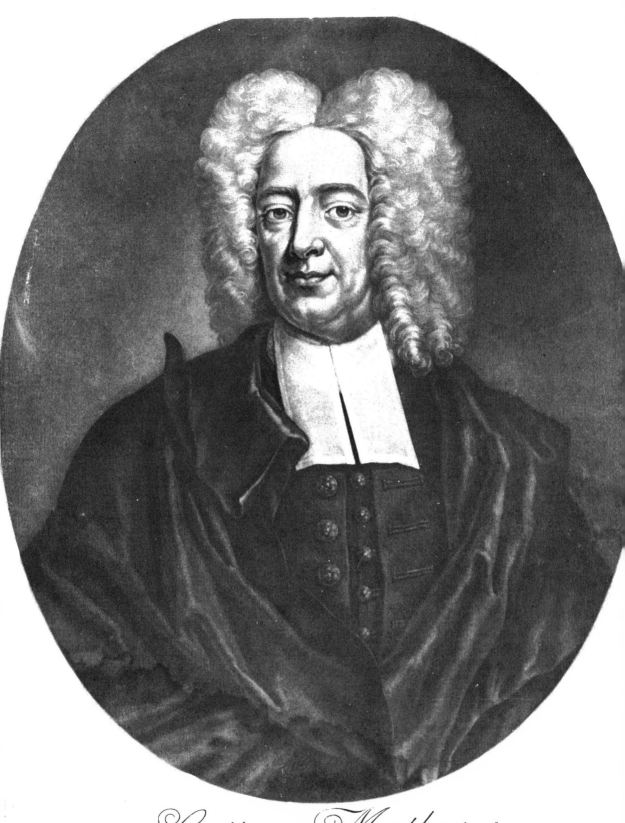

Cottonus Matherus

S. Theologiæ Doctor. Regiæ Societatis Londinensis Socius et Ecclesiæ apud Bostonum Nov-Anglorum nuper Præpositus

Ætatis Suæ LXV, MDCCXXVII.

The Angel of Bethesda

BY

COTTON MATHER

Edited, with Introduction and Notes, by

GORDON W. JONES, M.D., F.A.C.S.

American Antiquarian Society

AND

Barre Publishers

Barre, Massachusetts, 1972

Contents

Preface and Acknowledgements

AFTER a quarter of a millennium Cotton Mather's manuscript *Angel of Bethesda* is being published. We hope that it will appeal to a varied audience: theologians, American historians, medical historians, and also everyday "history buffs." My editorial policy has been aimed at this diverse readership. Parts of the brief introduction will seem elementary to some, a worthwhile review to others. The same is true of the footnotes. Some are perhaps obvious to most persons living today. However, since this old work is only now seeing print, it is unlikely to be reprinted for several generations, if ever. With the total change from old educational curricula, from the change from a rural to an urban society, in another few decades many terms familiar to us may become obscure.

In preparing this work I have had much help from friends. Those at the American Antiquarian Society have been most cooperative in furnishing me advice and materials. Mr. Clifford Shipton revised and partly rewrote my brief biography of Mather. Drs. Owsei Temkin and John B. Blake reviewed and corrected my essays on world medicine and medicine in Massachusetts. My good friend and Greek scholar, Mr. Dudley Sherwood, has helped me who knows no Greek, with the problems Mather's few Greek references involved. Dr. Daniel Woodward of the Mary Washington College Library and Father William Monihan, librarian of the University of San Francisco have been helpful. I wish to thank all these good people.

Christopher and Micheline Jedrey deserve particular acknowledgement for their painstaking review and editing of the final typescript.

Introduction

PART I

COTTON MATHER (1663–1728) represents a landmark in the development of the American mind, the first long step in the series from Benjamin Franklin (whose boyhood studies he encouraged) and Thomas Jefferson to Robert McCormick and Henry Ford. His background was essence of English Puritan. One grandfather was the Reverend John Cotton (1584–1652) of the First Church of Boston, and the other was Richard Mather (1596–1669) of the First Church of Dorchester, Massachusetts. His father, Increase Mather (1596–1669), was minister of the Second Church of Boston, president of Harvard from 1685 to 1701, the author of 175 published works, and, having been sent to England by an alarmed Colony, the political agent who obtained the Second Charter which carried Massachusetts over the shoals between colony and province times.

These Puritans did not share the medieval belief that this world does not matter. They were insatiably curious about it and they gave science a long start in both England and America. Cotton Mather was a climax in this development and the great popularizer in New England of the new discoveries being made in Europe. Among the nearly 500 books which he published was *The Christian Philosopher* (London, 1721), which provided a "new science for the millions" and proposed to show that "Philosophy is . . . a mighty . . . incentive to religion." More interesting has been the discovery over the last century that his experiments and speculations which appeared first in letters to correspondents in England have great significance. More than two centuries after his death, the 1936 *Year Book of the United States Department of Agriculture* carried his portrait and a discussion of him as the first observer of natural hybridization in plants. He was far ahead of the body of medical science in thinking that diseases might be seperate ills, that they might be caused by the living "animalcula" which he saw in his microscope. No one else in America commented on this possibility, in print, until John Crawford did so in 1811, nearly a century later. One is still discovering his footprints in the most unexpected places.[1]

The impact of his advanced thinking on his fellow colonials

was probably not great. In part this may have been caused by the considerable personal unpopularity which he endured during his lifetime. This was due largely to the way in which he identified himself with the causes and interests of his father (whom he survived by only five years), but also in part to his own volatile temper and occasional imperiousness. In 1688 Increase Mather was chosen by the churches to carry to England the colonists' plea for the restoration of the Old Charter, abrogated by Charles II in 1684, under which the colony had been practically an independent state. Two years later the General Court, ignoring the Puritan axiom that the clergy must never hold political office, appointed him official agent. As such he obtained the New Charter of 1692. For this the Mathers were never forgiven by the very orthodox, by the popular politicians, and by the isolationists. Yet, their unpopularity was far from total. Remember the fact that in small Boston their congregation at the Second Church numbered 1500 souls.

Religion played small part in the differences which Cotton Mather had with his contemporaries. They all lived in a world of profound religiosity, a world about half way between that of the sailors of Columbus and ours. They saw themselves as a part of a generalized European Protestantism with minor local differences. Increase, when in the old country, attended services of the Church of England, and Cotton recorded with pleasure the day when members of five different denominations took communion at his hands. The Mathers were Calvinists in that they accepted the doctrines of Original Sin, Predestination, and Eternal Damnation. The Mathers preferred not to preach on these subjects, but like all of their contemporaries they lived under the shadow of death, particularly that of the terrible infant mortality. Thus great emphasis was laid on the preparations for holy dying, and some children were so well trained that they actually welcomed death as an early progress to Jesus.

The Angel of Bethesda cannot be understood if not read with this religious orientation in view. Cotton Mather constantly sought communion with God. He found fasting a good means, and during his life he spent hundreds of days in this manner. While fasting he spent much of his time praying or singing psalms in the privacy of his study or library. Sometimes he prayed on his knees, and sometimes he lay prone for hours mortifying his flesh on the hard floor, often dampening the boards with his tears as he prayed.

Next to fasting and prayer came doing good deeds, daily if possible. One sees here a reaction gainst Calvin's Grace versus Works. His pastoral visits were inexorable. Indeed, he is credited with having been the originator of this ministerial duty. He began, or joined, more than a dozen religious societies created for the better instruction of both youth and elders, for the wealthy and for black slaves. Among the many resolutions for good deeds in his diary is this, "I would alwayes have about me some little Matters, (as Pennies, or Fruits, or Paints) proper to be bestow'd on little children."

A personal Devil was an essential to all of the Christianity of these centuries, a Devil working ceaselessly in many forms to foil God. Mather's contemporary and correspondent, the great English scientist, Robert Boyle, sent a circular letter to the miners of England asking them to describe the devils whom they encountered in the underground works. And, of course, cooperating with the Devil was witchcraft. In the next generation Chief Justice Sir James Mansfield and the Wesleys declared that to deny the reality of witchcraft is to deny the reality of God.

Cotton Mather believed in witchcraft, and he gathered records of it as he did of the aurora borealis, two-headed snakes, and the like. In 1688 he took charge of two Boston girls who could produce the most amazing parapsychological phenomena seen in his region from that day to this. He described the phenomena as aspects of witchcraft, treated the girls as ill, and cured them. In most parts of the civilized world they would have gone directly to the stake. There is not the slightest evidence that he ever preached a sermon or did anything else to bring on or promote the Salem outbreak of 1692, but after it he took up his pen to vindicate the judges. The popular party coupled this with its attacks on the New Charter and distorted his writings on witchcraft into a weapon with which to beat the establishment. Their side of the story prevailed in history for two centuries, obscuring his sincerity and integrity, his gentle private life, and his passion to do good. They did not need to exaggerate his hot temper, his own over-estimation of his great intelligence, and his sometimes unfortunate attitude toward lesser men.

Without his religiosity Mather could not have come well through his unhappy life. His sickly childhood foretold his neurotic adulthood. A child prodigy, he was fitted for college by his father in the fine family library and by some private schooling. At the age of twelve he entered on the four-year Harvard course with the class of 1678, one of a total enrollment of twenty-three. It may well be true that he was a very unpopular undergraduate, but the usual evidence cited to prove this point simply is not pertinent.

In his years at Harvard he studied arithmetic, geometry, logic, ethics, politics, astronomy, Greek, and Hebrew. Apparently he gained a reading knowledge of French, Spanish, German, Italian, and good knowledge of at least one American Indian language privately, then or later. Science at Harvard was only encouraged after Increase Mather assumed control of the college. Of Mather's college contemporaries, a majority entered the ministry. A few graduates became physicians. Some of the presidents were medical men. Perhaps this only emphasizes the close relationship between medicine and the clergy in early America. In the Harvard Library catalog of 1723 (few books had been added after 1701 when Increase lost the presidency) there were about 2200 theological works listed and only about 200 medical and scientific ones. We shall examine the list a little more thoroughly later.

Despite his preparation for the ministry, Cotton Mather's dearest ambition to follow his father into that field promised to be frustrated by a stammer which he had had since childhood. The question might be asked if this psychological problem might have been due to the dominance of a strong father. At any rate, he did manage to overcome this disability "through prayer" and diligent practice so that he could be ordained in 1685. He developed into an effective preacher.

During the time that he was combating his stammer he turned to the study of medicine as a possible alternative calling. Evidently this took the form of reading. No mention is made in the sources of any apprentice training, which was the usual avenue to medical practice. Indeed, in his diary he only mentions one of the many medical books in his father's library, William Salmon's *Pharmacopeia*. He never lost his interest in medicine and science which was aroused in these months of study.

Unlike many New England preachers, Cotton Mather never practiced medicine despite his extensive bookish knowledge of it. When in trouble he usually called the physician. In this he was unlike his contemporary, William Byrd II of Virginia. That medically well-read gentleman little trusted medical practitioners. Mather's great interest appears in many of his writings. There are medical notes all through his diary. In many of his sermons he mentioned medical matters. In his huge unpublished *Biblia Americana* he tried to diagnose the diseases of the Ancients. Like many, then and now, who read medicine, Mather was an intense neurotic. He had many minor illnesses and constantly, year after year, sensed the approach of death. Only after sixty-five years of living was he correct.

Well he might worry. He certainly knew first-hand much about illness and death. Thirteen of his fifteen children pre-deceased him. It is not certain what killed them all. A son, Joseph, died shortly after his birth because of an imperforate anus. Cotton reported the autopsy in his diary. A daughter died suddenly in its nurse's arms. Another son died after many "fits." Three children died of measles, one of tuberculosis, one in childbed. Another son drowned at sea.

Not only children but wives died. The first died in 1702, probably of cancer of the breast. The second wife died of measles. His third wife became so mentally deranged as to be a torment the rest of his life.

Despite his troubles he retained always his intense interest in all things: one of the marks of a genius. He wrote much and well. In 1712 he resolved to write "a book a month" for publication. He read very widely. He corresponded with the Royal Society, sending it eighty-two letters between 1712 and 1724 concerning his scientific observations. In 1713 he believed that he was elected a Fellow of that Society, to the disgust of some in Boston.[2] Partly from reading accounts in the *Transactions of the Royal Society* he learned of smallpox inoculation, the more dangerous fore-runner of vaccination. When a smallpox epidemic threatened Boston he proposed to the local physicians that they practice the method and save the town. Only one, Zabdiel Boylston, to his undying fame, agreed to try. The only man in town with a medical degree, Dr. William Douglas, was much opposed. There was also violent opposition on the part of the laity, largely because it was a method learned from the heathen Turks and pagan Negroes and not fit to be used on Christians bent on salvation. Mather gives a graphic description of his troubles in Chapter XX of *The Angel of Bethesda*.[3] This episode and the various disappointments of his life, including failure of election as president of Harvard to succeed his father, embittered him against his city and he finally called Boston "a miserable and detestable town." It was the only town he knew. He had hardly traveled more than twenty miles from it in his entire lifetime, despite the fact that he took an active interest in all New England. Yale College greatly interested him.

In his last years this man who had seen the deaths of so many loved ones, who had struggled so fiercely for what he considered in his somewhat autocratic way the best, had worked so hard, had seen so much disappointment, had felt the malice of so many, often noted in his diary that he welcomed death. But he kept on writing. He finished his *Angel* in 1724. This remarkably well-written book shows no diminution of powers, shows an advanced and liberal mind.

A friend of Baptists and Quakers, he deprecated the controversies of his father's generation, and although he could not agree with the Brattle Street reformers, he held the normal theological position of a New Englander of his age. His theological contribution was nil. The great interest of his mind to us lies in its explorations of science, including its speculations upon the still unseen world.

Introduction
PART II

World Medicine in the Time of Mather

ONE of the striking impressions which one gets from the reading of Mather's *Angel of Bethesda* is of the wealth of contemporary, and ancient, medical literature available to him in Boston. He, and undoubtedly a number of his friends, were both aware of and greatly interested in medical science as it was evolving in the old world. This interest in the new is markedly reflected in the *Angel* as well as in *The Christian Philosopher*. Thus, a cursory view of medicine in Mather's day will form, for some at least, an important background for an appreciation of his book. In such a short essay as this errors of interpretation of such a huge and varied subject may be inevitable. Many scholars have produced an enormous literature concerning the medical history of this period. Naturally, they often differ somewhat in viewpoint, but all seem to agree in placing the rather tenuous base of our medicine in the changes of view and in the experiences of the seventeenth century. That century saw something of a struggle between those who favored the teachings of the score or so of Ancients and those who espoused new ideas. The ancient reputations of Galen and Aristotle suffered, especially late in the century. Some men spun arm-chair theories and proved them in their own minds, but not by experiment. Others ridiculed them. A few conceived correct ideas, as proven two hundred years later, for the wrong reasons. Others who criticised their ideas for the right reasons were eventually proven wrong. But out of all the disputation, often acrimonious, there did come forth some light. As Lester King wrote recently, the most significant feature of the medical advance of the seventeenth century was "the growth in critical acumen rather than the accumulation of facts."[1] Our well-being today is based on that.

Cotton Mather showed occasional flashes of it; he also spun arm-chair theories (see his Chapter V). He was born and reared in the seventeenth and died in the eighteenth centuries. He remained in many respects a seventeenth-century man. He is recognizable as such in both his portrait and in his handwriting. But he showed many signs of an ability to grow, a characteristic of the intellectual elite of that century. His fervent Calvinism was tempered by a gentleness in his personal life, by a perhaps non-Calvinist desire to "do a good deed daily." This led to his interest in German pietism, an eighteenth-century development. However, the liberal swing of New England religion after his death probably would have annoyed him. He seems to have felt that the fact of the existence of the Devil and of his assistants, the witches, was biblically and "scientifically" proven. In this belief he was of the century of his birth. Yet, in the non-religious field he was able to grasp and push ideas not at all in vogue. He expressed very well the idea of the germ theory of disease.[2]

Doubtless his convictions about the animalicular cause of disease made him intellectually capable of his passionate, and wonderfully correct, advocacy of inoculation for smallpox prevention. Certainly the well-received report of the Boston experiment, given by Zabdiel Boylston in London, was one of the several important contemporary contributions which prepared the world for the fairly prompt acceptance of Jenner's far safer vaccination discovery late in the eighteenth century (1798).[3] And Boylston would never have dared try the experiment without the suggestion and backing of Mather. This was enough advanced thinking, apparently. Except for his Chapter VII and the appendix of his Chapter XX, *The Angel of Bethesda* presents only a fascinating summary of the medical practice, beliefs, and theory of the seventeenth century.

That century was one of the most stirring in history. For England it was the century of the Stuart romance and the Civil War, of the "martyrdom" of Sir Walter Raleigh, of the defeat of the doctrine of the divine right of kings, of the last days of Shakespeare, of Ben Jonson, of Milton, of Inigo Jones and the new architecture, of Bacon, Harvey, Boyle, Newton, Sydenham, Locke, Willis. And continental Europe, in the midst of its misery, knew Louis XIV, but also Molière, Malpighi, Galileo, Spinoza, Rembrandt, Leeuwenhoek, Racine, Descartes. It was the century of the discovery of cinchona. That alone would have made it distinguished.

It was not a comfortable century. There was peace in all Europe in only two years of the hundred. Religious strife was the rule. Witches were still being burned in Europe and hanged in New England. Care of the sick was poor. Molière does not let us forget that. Disease was as terrible as it had been in previous centuries.

Life was short. The people of Europe were just as wretched and devoid of hope as the pathetic citizens of today's most deprived nations. But it was a century of great minds who began building the scientific base upon which our marvellous health structure is built. It is not necessary that misery and poverty stifle intellectualism. Some of the fine minds came from poor families. Even the very rich did not approach in luxury the lower middle class Americans of today.

The sixteenth century had seen the beginning of modern anatomy. This science of gross anatomy really flowered in the seventeenth century. A great number of individuals made many discoveries. Physiology began in the seventeenth century: Sanctorius created the study of metabolism in 1614, Harvey published the proof of the fact that the blood circulates in 1628. Mather spends little time on such basic science in his *Angel,* since that is, after all, largely a text of the practice of medine. However, as proven by his statements in *The Christian philosopher* (London 1721), he was cognizant of the new science of his age. He was the first American to discuss it.[4]

The seventeenth century has always been viewed as the century of the rebirth of science in general. It had been more or less dormant since the time of Galen (c.130–200 A.D.). Francis Bacon first urged the study of science. Collect facts, he said, and from these facts assembled you can create scientific truths. This inductive method was rather less popular than the deductive one of arguing from the general to the particular. Bacon first outlined his scientific proposals in his *The Twoo Bookes . . . of the Proficience and Advancement of Learning* (London, 1605). His last book, *Sylva Sylvarum* (London, 1627), was a vast collection of facts, observed facts and facts determined by experiment. His most famous experiment was his last. With his bare hands he packed a freshly dressed fowl with snow to see if the meat would be preserved by the cold. He died a few days later of pneumonia.

Bacon apparently made no great impression on his contemporaries but he did influence Robert Boyle (1627–1691), the "father of modern chemistry," who won perhaps the greatest reputation of the century. Independently wealthy, he spent his days in chemical experimentation and in dabbling in medical practice. His *Skeptical Chymist* (London 1661) is an intellectual landmark, but most readers of the day missed the point. It was bought by Virginians, for instance, seeking the practical advice it might yield in their efforts to exploit their natural resources.[5] Mather was apparently much more interested in his *Medicinal Experiments* (London, 1692), a little book full of "receits," an uncritical collection of ancient popular remedies. It is hardly a work which one would expect from the pen that wrote the *Skeptical Chymist* and *Of the Reconcileableness of Specific Medicines to the Corpuscular Philosophy* (London, 1685).[6] But that is the contradiction of the century. Great men had a few advanced ideas, but the firm grip of early religious training and the heritage of centuries of medieval lore and tradition even influenced a Boyle. This was found in Cotton Mather, too. He could grasp the essentials of the germ theory of disease, could introduce inoculation, and at the same time believe in witches.

Isaac Newton (1642–1727) was just as deeply religious as Boyle. Both wrote much on biblical subjects. Newton, unlike Boyle, had no direct influence on medicine, but his mathematical and physical discoveries helped create the fundamental scientific substratum upon which scientific medicine is based.

Galileo Galilei (1564–1642), who died in the infancy of Newton after having partially anticipated some of the latter's discoveries is not considered a medical man either, though the study of medicine was his first ambition before mathematics, physics, and astronomy captured his imagination. We physicians are indebted to him for his introduction of mathematics as one of the fundamental tools of science and for his contributions to the development of the microscope, an instrument apparently first invented by the Dutchman Zacharias Jenssen in 1590.

That instrument, so precious to medicine, was eagerly developed during the century. Some of the finest models were made by Anton Leeuwenhoek (1632–1724) of Delft, largely as a hobby. The lenses which he ground were marvellous and he must have attained magnifications of 300–500X. He was quite secretive and only a handful of the hundreds of microscopes he made are extant. He used these in furthering his studies of "animalcules" (bacteria and protozoa), muscle fibres, nerves, blood vessels, etc. His reports of his findings endeared him to the Royal Society of London, which published many of them. Cotton Mather was well aware of these studies. They may have influenced the formulation of his ideas about the cause and dissemination of disease. He owned a microscope.

Another notable figure of the century, the Frenchman René Descartes (1596–1650), also contributed a little to the development of the microscope. His book *De Homine,* published posthumously in 1662, has been called the first textbook of physiology. In it he established the iatrophysical or iatromechanical school of thought. He looked upon the body as a machine, divinely created to be the habitation of the soul. At the same time he was sufficiently cognizant of the chemical processes in the body to have been respected by the group called iatro-chemists who looked upon the body as a mass of chemical processes rather than a machine. We shall notice these two ideas again later.

The upsurge of interest in science during the seventeenth century stimulated the development of several scientific societies. First in the century was the Accademia dei Lincei of Rome (1603), which is still in existence. There followed the Accademia del Cimento in Florence in 1657, the Academie des Sciences in 1665, and the German Academia Caesarea-Leopoldina which began publishing its *Epheme-rides* in 1670. Mather had access to this publication. All of these seem to have been inspired by the "secret academy" of Porta, started in Naples in 1560. Directly descended from the last was the "invisible college" founded by Robert Boyle and others in 1645 at Oxford. In 1662 this became, by grace of Charles II, the world famous Royal Society of London. Its *Philosophical Transactions* became so prestigious that it published many of the important scientific works of the century. It was widely read in the colonies. Mather sent many contributions, a few of which were published. One was on rattlesnakes. Another was concerned with the effect of lightning on the compass of a ship at sea. Many of the men quoted by Mather in his *Angel* published articles in the *Transactions*.

The members of these societies were the first internationally minded scientists. By correspondence as well as by their publications they shared eagerly their observations of natural phenomena, medical affairs, mathematics, etc. The correspondence of Henry Oldenburg, secretary of the Royal Society, was so voluminous, in fact, that he came under a cloud: the government suspected that he was a spy. Despite science's findings, gropings, and slow building of the scientific base, it was not until the nineteenth century that people began to glimpse the possible wonders of scientific medicine in actual practice.

Most of us tend to remember first the builders of the base, Bacon, Galileo, Boyle, Newton, and so on. But there were great physicians in the seventeenth century also. The greatest of them, and one of the greatest base-builders too, was William Harvey (1578–1657) who died only a few years before Mather's birth. He was a practitioner, a teacher of anatomy in London, and an active research scientist. He established experimentally the fact that the blood circulates, pumped about the body by the force of the heart. His *Exercitatio Anatomica de Motu Cordis et Sanguinis* (Frankfort, 1628) is one of the half dozen great books in medicine if not in all world history. It made possible all future advances in physiology by proving the basic fact of the circulation. His teaching was not accepted at once. When Mather mentions the circulation of the blood in a matter-of-fact way we should remember that it had been generally accepted as fact amongst a conservative profession hardly more than a decade before his birth.

No such experimenter was Thomas Sydenham (1624–1684), the "English Hippocrates," who must be considered one of the founders of modern clinical medicine. He was a great observer. He was not much impressed by "science." He believed that the important advances in medicine could only come through the careful studies of sick people at the bedside. He considered each disease an entity. He discarded the vague notion, prevalent then and for some time in the future, that disease is really all one condition, the result of an improper bodily function, which is merely manifested in different ways. After Sydenham the realization grew that just as there are many different kinds of plants, so there are many different diseases.

Almost as great a clinical observer as Sydenham was Thomas Willis (1621–1675). He is often credited with having discovered the sweetness of diabetic urine. The ancient Hindus, however, wrote of it as "honey urine." He first described the conditions which we know as myasthenia gravis, puerperal fever, and typhoid fever as found in troops. Unlike Sydenham he was an anatomist and a fair neurophysiologist. Both of these men left books important to their fellows and to posterity.

The seventeenth century was a time of many medical theories. For an appreciation of Mather's medicine it is important to recognize some of them. The idea of the body as a machine seemed to appeal to him. Thus, he might be labeled an iatromechanist. Adherents of this "school" or theory delighted in rather futile theoretical exercises in comparison. Georgio Baglivi (1668–1706) of Ragusa, well thought of in England, liked to compare the teeth to scissors, the lungs to bellows, and so on. This man whom Mather often quotes, did not, however, let these fancies interfere with his being a shrewd bedside clinician. Perhaps anticipating this iatromechanical group was the founder of the science of metabolism, Santorio Santorio (1561–1636), known as Sanctorius, a professor at the University of

Padua. He spent a lifetime measuring the results of all bodily processes. He often slept, ate, and rested on a steelyard and recorded all observations and variations.

Distinguished from these were the adherents of the iatrochemical school. This originated with Jean Baptista van Helmont (1577–1644), a Belgian, who believed that all bodily processes are chemical in nature, and that each such process is controlled by its special archeus. This notion he probably got from the writings of Paracelsus (1493–1541), the part quack, part mystic, part true medical reformer of Swiss birth, with whose work Mather was acquainted. Van Helmont believed that the whole organism is presided over by a sensory-motive soul.

Georg Ernst Stahl (1660–1734) of Germany extended Helmont's ideas. He felt that the body is a machine activated by a soul which directs all the processes. He believed that when the soul is improperly channeled disease develops. If we wish to be charitable we may say that his system is an ancestor of our field of psychosomatic medicine. His idea was perhaps the forerunner of eighteenth-century vitalism which maintained that all depends on the impulse of living things to grow and to reproduce. Stahl's view seems to be rather like Mather's, although the latter does not mention Stahl. See Chapter V of the *Angel,* where Mather discusses his Nishmath-Chajim, or Breath of Life. All these theorizers owed something to the ancient metaphysical theory or concept of the pneuma or universal spirit.

Accepted without real question by most theorists were the likewise ancient doctrines of the humours and qualities. One does get the impression that frequently 'humours' was used as an abstract term rather than one referring to the classical four. These were phlegm, blood, black bile, and yellow bile. Phlegm, or pituita, was supposed to drip down from the brain via the pituitary gland. This notion was attacked by van Helmont and later disproved by Konrad Schneider (1610–1680) in his publication *De Catarrhis* (Wittenberg, 1660). These attacks were long ignored by practitioners. The origin of the blood is obvious. Black bile was thought to arise in the spleen; an excess caused melancholy. Yellow bile had its origin in the liver; an excess caused jaundice.

The qualities were hot and cold, dry and moist. Each organ and each plant of pharmacological significance was noted for a combination of these qualities. The stomach, they said, is cold and moist. Mint is warm and dry. Mint, quite logically, soothes the stomach.

The elements of the ancients were also four: air, earth, fire, and water. Paracelsus had tried to discard these and proposed three: sulfur (it burns), mercury (it volatilizes), and salt (it stays as a residue in all chemical processes). Boyle, and others, of the seventeenth century harked back to the fifth century B.C. Democritos of Abdera and began the trend of believing that matter is composed of corpuscles, approximately our atoms and molecules, in motion.

No matter what the theory or notion or archaic beliefs they held, all practitioners used practically the same treatments. And those treatments were generally more or less adhered to until fairly late in the nineteenth century when more rational methods of treatment, based on science, came to the fore.

Treatment was all worked out logically and systematically, with faithful reference to theories and humoral doctrines.[7] Most believed that disease is characterized by a change in the quality, quantity, and motion of the humours. Thus, cure must be based on evacuating some of the abnormal quantity, altering the quality, and moderating the motion. The first was treated with evacuant methods, the second with alterants, the third with moderants. Seemingly less complicated was the treatment scheme of those who adhered to the belief of the "Methodists" of ancient times that there are only two states of disease, tension and relaxation. But the evacuants cured the former and the alterants and moderants the latter. So, I repeat, physicians tended to come up with the same prescriptions for the same conditions for different reasons.

Evacuant methods were the most abundant and widely used. They were relaxant also, even to the point of shock, I might add. The means was either surgical or medical, or both for that matter. Among the surgical, venesection comes first to mind. Even slashing of arteries was sometimes employed. As late as our Civil War venesection was still occasionally done. To us it is incredible how extensively the method was used. But before we criticize too harshly we must realize that even today there is an occasional justification. When the pressure in the great central veins of the body is high, as determined by a rather delicate test perfected only relatively recently, the patient is in some danger. Recently, a bled-out accident patient was over-transfused. As a result of too much blood volume she developed pulmonary and cerebral edema. Her central venous pressure was 35 instead of 6–10. She made a rapid recovery (48 hours) after the removal of somewhat less than a pint of blood. This accounts for the temporary relief venesection gives to patients in heart failure. It lowers the central venous pressure for a while. We know that the older doctors were keen observers. Their practice depended on their senses, not on the laboratory tests. When a man like Dr. Thomas Watson claimed speedy relief when a patient in the early stages of pneumonia was bled, we cannot doubt him.[8] Perhaps there had been an element of heart failure in his observed cases. Most of the older experienced doctors had seen a few dramatic benefits from venesection, or at least had been told about them by their preceptors. If a given treatment works in a few cases it should work in all. Such would be the reason-if a knowledge of basic physiology and hemodynamics is a science of the future. Physicians of old treated symptoms and hoped to cure disease. We more generally treat the disease and trust that the symptoms will disappear. We must always remember to judge physicians of other times by how well they used or advanced the use of tools then available, and not exercise our twentieth-century amused superiority.

Blood was let in other ways, by scarification, by cupping, by leeches. Cupping involved setting fire to a little alcohol in the bottom of a cup and slapping the cup mouth against the skin. This raised a blister which made the method a counter-irritant or tonic treatment. If the bluster was then lanced a fair amount of blood might flow. This made the method evacuant. Leeches as blood-letters were applied until recently at least in France.

"Issues," consisting of serum and sero-purulent material, were encouraged by means of setons. A piece of skin was raised with a knife and kept raised with a thread left in place. Issues were also caused by means of a moxa. Here, tow was allowed to burn down onto the skin over an affected part. This was a Japanese invention. Western observers have marveled at but have been unable to reproduce the benefits claimed for it in arthritis. Faith! Edematous legs were lanced to let the water out. Mather mentions all these methods. Trephination of the skull was done rarely. Paracentesis and thoracentesis were performed on appropriate occasions.

Medical evacuant methods were used with great enthusiasm. Mather constantly notes them in chapter after chapter. Emetics and cathartics were the favorites. Drugs thought to produce sweating and increased production of urine were tried. Irritants like cinnamon or snuff might be placed in the nose or on the gums to produce an increase in the production of "phlegm." Salivation by means of mercury was tried in the seventeenth century in the treatment of syphilis and was used as the generations went by with increasing enthusiasm for many conditions.[9] We still use expectorants in cough medications. This, again, may be a matter of persistent faith. The promotion of natural bleeding was considered wise in many cases. Such drugs as black hellibore were thought to be effective in increasing menstrual flow. Violent laxatives often promoted the benign development of bleeding hemorrhoids.

Some alterants thickened too-fluid humours, others thinned too thick ones. The physician decided according to his experience or imagination. Correctives were used to reform peccant or bad humours. Constrictives corrected relaxation, relaxants corrected too much constriction. As examples we may mention the use of figs and well-cooked bread in thickening humours. Rhubarb powder and nasturtium leaves thinned thick humours. Mercury compounds reformed. Rhubarb and mercurials also relaxed constrictions. They are laxative. Fruits promoted the constriction of too-relaxed tissues. All this is confusing simply because it is so foreign to present-day training.

On the basis of these ideas complicated prescriptions composed of several different herbs were compounded for each indication. Sydenham liked very complicated prescriptions, especially when he thought the patient's condition was "mixed," as when there might be peccant humours in the presence of thick ones. Most physicians thought likewise. In practice, the physician had to rely on his observation and experience to determine which of the many vague and varied conditions were present. He might get a consultation with another physician and have a great wrangle. Then he would choose several out of hundreds of possible pharmacological preparations. Mather mentions more than 175 such. Of these only a few are still used in some form or other, cinchona (quinine), senna for instance. We are fortunate in that it is much easier to practice using experimentally proven facts instead of imagination and 'impression."

This polypharmacy was blessed by antiquity. From quack to physician, all used it. Ingenious men of that century did try to think up new treatments. The first tentative experiments in intravenous therapy were made. Dr. Richard Lower was apparently the first to transfuse blood from one animal to another.[10] He transfused blood from dog to dog, from calf to sheep, from a wether to a horse, all without notable ill effects. He transfused the blood of a sheep into a man, again without mortality. However, about this time the same procedure tried in Paris led, predictably, to disastrous results. At once transfusions were outlawed and not attempted again on human subjects until the nineteenth century.

Various substances injected into the veins of dogs usually killed the animals.[11] Nevertheless, one "Dr. Fabritius" of Danzig injected a small amount of laxative medicine into a man "heavily infected" with venereal disease. There was considerable pain, but in about five hours the man began to have many stools. The observer thought that the patient had been improved.[12] Other such injections were occasionally mortal in their effect. The method was dropped. It is only in this century of ours that transfusions and infusions have become safe and widely used.

Two great new treatments did arise in Mather's lifetime. With one of them, inoculation for smallpox, Mather was greatly involved, as we have seen. The other benison was the introduction of cinchona bark or Jesuit's bark, under somewhat mysterious circumstances, from Peru. From ancient times malaria has been a terrible scourge, causing death and debility to countless millions, rendering great districts uninhabitable. We are now relatively safe because of quinine, and mosquito control. Cinchona bark was the first great specific. It cures malaria and nothing else. It became generally recognized as such a cure in the last third of the seventeenth century. It is significant as a great drug but also as the very proof that disease is not all one great vague condition of ill-health. Cinchona cures one disease and one only. Thus, there must be distinct diseases with distinct characteristics and different causes. That was a very important concept to establish. It was thought in the early years of its use that the bitterness (qualities, again) of the drug was the essential element in effecting the cure, and some time was wasted trying "the bark" for other conditions in the hope that the famous bitterness would be of avail there too.

General medical practice, then, saw two great advances in the century. That was praiseworthy, but advances did not accelerate. Just as importantly for the future was that basic medical science, including chemistry, got its essential start. Harvey proved the circulation of the blood. The Dutch Leeuwenhoek, the Italian Marcello Malpighi (1628–1694), and the English Robert Hooke (1635–1703) established microscopy. The scientific societies began.

Nothing new and brilliant happened in surgery. Boils were lanced, bones were set, and dislocations were reduced as in previous millennia. Surgeons treated wounds, usually with ointments and washes. In a pre-antiseptic era wound, healing was necessarily usually by second intention. Scars were ugly. Skilled men cut quickly for stone while the patient was being held securely by strong assistants. Breasts were amputated for cancer. Ligatures were not used. Bleeding from such major work as breast surgery was stopped by means of the cautery. "I secured the artery by the touch of the hot iron," reported Richard Wiseman (1622–1676), the greatest English surgeon of the period.

In obstetrics, François Mauriceau (1637–1709) knew fame and did much good with his great treatise *Des Maladies des Femmes Grosses* (Paris 1668). However, it was not he but Pierre Chamberlen (1601–1683) who made one of the three or four greatest discoveries in the history of obstetrics, the forceps. The knowledge of it was retained in his family for several generations, but once the secret was well out (about 1732) it became a boon to millions. Mather's New England did not know it. Retention of secret remedies was not considered unethical then. Now a doctor with a new idea rushes into print sometimes too quickly out of a fear that someone will beat him to the credit. The Chamberlens retained their secret for at least six decades. It took Harvey many years to put in print his revolutionary *De Motu Cordis*.

The sources of care, the administrators of these methods of cure were varied and of different rank in London. At the top of the list were the well-educated physicians who had much more professional and social prestige than did the surgeons who ranked next. Then came the apothecaries, the compounders of medicine, who practised on the side, rather to the dismay of the physicians, and who finally in the nineteenth century became the general practitioners of England today. Outside London this hierarchy was by no means rigid; the same man might combine all three functions. Especially in the provinces of England there were the "empyricks" as Boyle called them. There were the only source of help for the sick in a great many communities. They administered whatever drugs they or their preceptors had unscientifically observed to help. They were often wisewomen or midwives. These empirics can be thanked for foxglove and its digitalis. But it was a physician named William Withering (1741–1799) who was shrewd enough to pay attention and educated enough to study scientifically the drug and promote it. We learned about ergot from the midwives who did most of the obstetrics. But foxglove and ergot were not seventeenth-century victories. Lastly there were the quacks, the anathema of all physicians. They were incredibly numerous in the seventeenth century. Ben Jonson in his *Volpone* gave a splendid portrayal of the quack or mountebank of his day. Undoubtedly the quacks of that long past day did some good. They sold drugs cheaply to folk who could not afford the prices of the apothecaries, often the very same drugs, admittedly ineffectual. It was a quack, Robert Talbor, who introduced Jesuit's bark to England secretly. There was a prejudice against anything discovered by the Jesuits and so no one else had used it. He even denied it himself, to protect his secret. He became rich despite the opposition of the physicians. He even cured King Charles II of malaria. For this he was knighted. He was not the only quack knighted in our period. Queen Anne thus favored William Read, a quack oculist who pleased her. About 1704 he wrote a little tract about his "famous receipts."[13]

These, then, were the people who treated the incredible amount of illness which afflicted the folk of the seventeenth century. Age-old methods had to suffice for the treatment of all diseases except malaria. Prevention of smallpox became possible, but the treatment was, and is still, unsatisfactory. It was both endemic and epidemic in Europe where it carried a mortality of fifteen or twenty per cent. In America it appeared in epidemics whenever a sufficient number of non-immunes developed. Among the Indians its mortality approached one hundred per cent. It was most disfiguring. President John Adams once called it the King of Terrors. We know it not. Malaria still made parts of Europe desert. Typhus was rife. Typhoid ignored all social barriers. It killed the most promising of the Stuarts, Prince Henry. His case was well described by Sir Theodore de Mayerne (1573–1655) whom Mather quotes frequently. There were all the diseases of filth, malnutrition, and of tainted unrefrigerated food. Worm infestation was common. Tuberculosis was everywhere. Bubonic plague was endemic and occasionally terribly epidemic. Many died of it each year in the London slums. Only when the whole city was affected did people flee in terror, as during the great plague of 1665.

With death on every side life was held cheap, as cheap as in the Orient today. Wars showed the ultimate in personal brutality. Whole provinces were rendered deserts. With poverty so widespread the laws against crime were especially savage. A nursing mother might be hanged for the theft of a loaf of bread.

All this misery was endured by a people who seem, perhaps out of desperation, to have been ready to believe anything. Thousands sincerely believed in the efficacy of the King's touch in the cure of scrofula. Mary Toft of Surrey, England, had no difficulty in persuading her neighbors and much of her nation that she was having a glorious and fascinating time giving birth to rabbits. What bothered the one astute observer was the fact that there were hay and corn in the digestive tracts of the dead-born rabbits which he autopsied. He pricked the bubble. This was in 1726. Few doubted the marvelous then. Yet, may I add, less than twenty years ago I was asked by an apparently intelligent young woman if it was true that a college girl had given birth to a puppy at the hospital recently.

Few doubted, less few dared express doubts about, religion. Wars were fought over the interpretation of the Bible but not over the fact of God and Christ. An intense religiosity was perhaps the sole recourse of a people beset with the misery of war, hunger, poverty, dreadful diseases, and early death. The Bible is the word of God. And no one believing this statement could doubt the existence of an anti-Christ, the Devil. And if you believed in the Devil you had to believe that the Devil had servants, the witches. People died for the offense of witchcraft all over Europe, not just in Salem, Massachusetts. The great champions of these poor victims, Reginald Scot (1538–1599) and Johann Weyer (1515–1588), who showed to the satisfaction of nearly none of their contemporaries that the witches were merely mad, did not actually deny the existence of the Devil. Perhaps they dared not. As it was, poor Scot received a stern "counterblast" from his king, later James I of England. The Mathers were in good company, though, if I may repeat, they opposed the harsh penalties the witches received.

Introduction
PART III

Medicine in Massachusetts in the Time of Cotton Mather

THE same people with many of the same problems, the same fears, the same diseases, and the same beliefs, lived in Massachusetts. Due to their isolation the great infectious diseases tended to be epidemic rather than endemic, and probably were rather little in evidence in the earlier years. Thus, a large population of susceptible people was built up. Smallpox, measles, or diphtheria might arrive with devastating effects and then disappear for years until a large enough body of non-immunes had been developed. No one has explained why bubonic plague was apparently totally absent from the American colonies at a time when it was both epidemic and endemic in London. It is to be found in rodents over much of western America because of imports from the Orient before or about 1900. But the rodents of eastern America are still free of it.

The first reported New England "plague" had decimated the Indians a few years before Plymouth was settled. Mather noted that this had largely emptied the country and had made the settlement of it much easier for the English.[1] Undoubtedly the Indians had contracted it from white traders or fishermen who had frequented the coasts for years. There had been small trading posts in Maine and New Hampshire. Most white man's diseases sorely afflicted the Indians. Smallpox had a nearly total mortality and measles was often about as bad a scourge. No one has proven what this first epidemic could have been. Our only clue lies in the report that dying Indians were turned yellow. The disease could have been influenza which in some epidemics has caused jaundice.[2] Infectious hepatitis is a disease which ordinarily has a low mortality though a high misery rate. As a disease new to the Indians it may have been fatal. And the virulence of most diseases seems to vary from century to century. Weil's disease and relapsing fever seem perhaps less likely possibilities.

Whatever disease it was, from that time onward for many generations terrible diseases, infectious, and other, were the lot of both the Indian and the white man. For two centuries the medical story of our land was one of a high birth rate fighting a high death rate and winning only slowly until relatively recently. Remember, Cotton Mather was survived by only two of his fifteen children.

Scurvy and exposure are blamed for most of the many deaths during the first Plymouth Colony winter of 1620. If scurvy was present so most certainly also were the other avitaminoses. Beriberi was present among the Newfoundland fishermen.

Since typhoid fever was rife in the earlier Virginia Colony,[3] it was certainly sooner or later a factor in the health picture of Massachusetts. Dysentery was common late in the seventeenth century and probably earlier.[4] As Mather reports in his Chapter XLIV of the *Angel,* intestinal parasites were a problem. Even one of his own children when ill vomited and passed worms. Probably, however, the cold climate made the incidence of worms less than the astonishing prevalence in colonial Virginia.[5]

Measles was a terrible scourge, being far more deadly then than now. Mather's wife, three children, and a maid died of it in one epidemic. Tuberculosis, including the scrofula seldom seen today, was common. Mather saw it frequently among his flock. The cold of New England, which of course encouraged influenza[6] and pneumonia, was not enough to prevent a small epidemic of yellow fever in Boston in 1693, during which several people died. Mather only escaped it, he thought, because illness prevented his making a pastoral visit to the afflicted ship anchored in the harbor. As usual, he recognized the handiwork of God in sparing him.

When we reflect upon the known prevalence in Mather's day of infectious diseases and diseases recognized as due to poor sanitation and upon the probable prevalence of nutritional ailments, we realize that the conditions in Massachusetts were very like the terrible ones in such underdeveloped modern states as Nepal.

Cancer was present. Mather feared it. He reported its presence in both Indians and white persons. His first wife probably died of cancer of the breast. And people had sudden cardiac deaths then, too.[7]

Undoubtedly mental illness was as common then as now. Mather's third wife was evidently a manic depressive. For others, alcoholism was a disturbing problem. Hysterical illness was common. Stress has been present in every period of history and there have always been some unable to cope with it. Mather himself had many psychosomatic illnesses. Psychoses and neuroses were all treated in the home. There were no mental hospitals in Massachusetts in Mather's day. Mather treated at least two disturbed girls in his home. Others may have been brutal but Mather was far in advance of his time in urging gentleness.

Who treated all these illnesses? Except in Boston the physician-patient ratio was unfavorable indeed. Most people had to rely on midwives and wise women who knew a little about herbs, but more about how to comfort the ill. Likely their patients did about as well as those in Boston since their treatments were surely less heroic. Boston did have many practitioners. Not all were affluent. Mather pitied one physician named John Perkins who was imprisoned for debt. But, judging from their numbers in town, they must have done well enough in general.

The rigid London structure of separation of physician, surgeon and apothecary was necessarily non-existent both in the "provinces" of England and in the colonies. The frontier situation of America and the horse-back distances of rural England made essential the general practitioner who also dispensed medicines. In Boston, there were apothecary shops, selling nostrums as well as prescriptions. Even so, Sylvester Gardner (b. 1706), for instance, though he became a prominent apothecary, was also an active physician and a surgeon who even cut for stone.[8] Perforce, these men in America did as extensive work as their English contemporaries. Mather mentioned in a rather matter-of-fact way a child who had to have an operation for stone.

In Mather's Boston there was only one physician who was able to claim a degree of M.D. This was William Douglass who received his degree from Utrecht in 1712. He was a Scot who had studied under Pitcairn at Edinbunrgh and under Boerhaave at Leyden. He is thought to have studied for a time at Paris. Apparently the actual taking of a degree was cheaper at Utrecht. With all this training he inevitably came to enjoy great prestige and a large practice in Boston. This professional background made him understandably intolerant of Mather's meddling in medical affairs.

The other physicians and surgeons, John Clark, Elisha Cooke, Thomas Oakes, Benjamin Bullivant, John Cutler, Zabdiel Boylston, Thomas Bulfinch, to mention a few, were all trained by the apprentice system. John Cutler taught Boylston, Boylston taught Bulfinch.[9] The apprentice read his master's books, did household jobs, helped in the office, and made patient rounds with the teacher. Such a period of training usually lasted three years. Prior education may have been minimal or may even have been at Harvard.

In New England many men were both clergymen and physicians, for it was a long and honored tradition for minister and healer to be united in the same person. Probably in the outlying districts the parson was a great source of succor, and Jared Eliot (1685–1763) of Connecticut was a famous example.[10] Many practiced medicine for fees, but it was not a lucrative business for them. Probably because there were so many physicians in Boston, Mather, despite his great interest, did not practice. He did try frequently to influence the type of treatment a doctor gave and likely this was annoying. He always called a physician when there was a serious illness in his household, though in his diary he does not name his personal physician.

It may have been Boylston since he was the only physician Mather was able to interest in practicing inoculation, at least at first. The others, even and especially Douglass, were violently opposed to the method until Boylston, with Mather's powerful backing, had gone through the veritable tornado of abuse while proving its worth. It bears repeating: the abuse came from the populace and from the other physicians, but not from the clergy who were sympathetic. This is an interesting commentary upon who were the more broad-minded men of the colony.

Medical investigative science as we know it was attempted only this one time in colonial Massachusetts. This smallpox inoculation experiment was carefully done. Boylston inoculated 247 persons and of these only six died, apparently not all of smallpox. The mortality from naturally acquired smallpox was more than fifteen per cent and was far more disfiguring. When the virus is inhaled it causes a systemic rather than a localized skin disease before the body can build up antibodies. Each of Boylston's patients was listed and the result shown. He made a classical report when, on invitation, he went to London to report his experience.[11] It was Mather's idea, but Boylston had the courage.

Basic medical science was as limited as clinical science in early America. Apparently no formal anatomical dissections were done in Massachusetts in our period.[12] But that does not imply that there was no interest in human anatomy and physiology. Mather devoted nearly sixty pages of his *Christian Philosopher* to these subjects. Probably every physician had anatomical texts at hand. Certainly, inventories of estates of Virginia physicians and non-physicians alike showed a fascination for anatomy in their libraries.[13] The same would be true for New England. Probably, as in England, intelligent practitioners developed an every-day knowledge of anatomy by performing autopsies, partly to demonstrate "no fault" to the family and partly to enhance their basic knowledge. Mather implied approval of this practice when he reported in his diary the autopsy of his son Joseph in a matter-of-fact way, as though it were a common occurrence.

Some medical printing was done in the colony. The leaders of Massachusetts Bay were a highly literate group who had brought books with them and they continued to import them. The Mathers had a great private library, but most men had many books. In Cotton Mather's time Boston became an active printing center. He himself wrote hundreds of books and tracts, mostly religious in nature, but some slightly or largely medical. A study of Guerra's bibliography shows that there were published in Boston perhaps eighteen different pieces of more-or-less medical interest by Cotton Mather. Boylston, Douglass, Thacher, and Increase Mather also published medical items, printed in Boston. The English writers Culpeper, John Smith, and Darby Dawne (Dr. Edward Baynard) were reprinted in Boston.

In sum, then, medicine in Massachusetts in Mather's day was essentially like that of one of the more remote counties of England, except that we like to think that a rural English shire was unlikely to have nurtured and retained a Cotton Mather or a Boylston.

Introduction

PART IV

THE manuscript of this, Cotton Mather's last major work, has been preserved in the library of the American Antiquarian Society since early in the nineteenth century. It was deposited there by Isaiah Thomas who had acquired it from the author's granddaughter, Mrs. Hannah (Mather) Crocker.

This is the only large inclusive medical work of the entire American colonial period. Considering its obvious importance, it is justifiable that we feel surprise at the fact that it has never been published *in toto* before. As may be seen from his tentative prospectus, Mather did try to have it published. Expense may have been the problem. His *Christian Philosopher* had not sold well. Perhaps the undoubted contemporary opposition such men as William Douglass felt toward clerics in medicine prevented immediate publication and perhaps the enmities aroused by the inoculation controversy of only a few years before were a stumbling block. In his diary Mather does not enlighten us, nor does the 1729 biography of him by his son explain the failure. In a few years its highly religious tone probably made it seem antiquated. It was finally stored away, largely forgotten, and eventually sold to Thomas along with the remnant of the Mather library.

Oliver Wendell Holmes rediscovered Mather's manuscript in 1869. In a lecture that year and in an article in 1881 he was very scornful, as he did not like the idea of clerics in medicine. He was opposed to medical writing by all non-physicians, and furthermore, modern medicine was evolving then, and practitioners of Holmes' generation felt very superior to all who had gone before. We are sufficiently secure today to be able to afford tolerant feelings toward all our forbears.

Others became interested. The manuscript was summarized by Joseph Sargent in American Antiquarian Society, *Proceedings* (April 1874), pp. 11–26. William Thayer, M.D., published a few extracts from it in the *Johns Hopkins Hospital bulletin*, XVI (1905). Worthington C. Ford was, in 1911, so much interested that he prepared an excellent typescript. However, he went no further. In

1954 Otho T. Beall, Jr. and Richard H. Shryock, Ph.D., published
unedited selections from the manuscript in their excellent work,
Cotton Mather, First Significant Figure in American Medicine
(Baltimore, 1954 and 1968, reprinted from AAS, *Proceedings,*
LXIII (1953). The reader is urged to consult it.

The existing manuscript consists of 410 pages, many of them
very closely written, especially in the numerous marginal insertions
which are to be found on nearly every page. As the years of writing
the work went by Mather expanded by means of these marginal insertions and supplied proper hatch marks to guide the printer as to
the points of introduction into the body of the text. He seldom corrected his wording. He occasionally deleted a sentence or a paragraph. In other words, this manuscript is a first draft with additions.
Time has blurred and smudged the ink to some extent. There is remarkably little evidence of damp-staining. There are a very few tears
with loss of text. For the most part, the handwriting, late seventeenth-
century in character, is quite legible and easy to read. The fact that
there are a few additions in another, typically eighteenth-century,
hand makes it evident that a hope to publish was kept alive for some
years after the author's death. I may note here that in this transcrip-
tion the spelling and punctuation of Cotton Mather have been retained except that such very commonly used contractions as &, ye,
ym, or, being merely annoying to modern readers, have been expanded.

It is evident from Mather's index of chapters that five (XV,
XVI, XVII, XVIII, and XIX) are missing. They dealt respectively
with cancer, scrofula or king's evil, fever, febrifuges, and measles.
Presumably they were written. The pagination of the extant manuscript is continuous but it is not in Mather's hand. Possibly the chapters were misplaced or removed by whoever, as noted above, added
to the manuscript later. Perhaps some member of the family removed
them for personal reasons since the first and last chapters were concerned with diseases intimately connected with the author's wives.
Cancer killed his first wife and measles his second. Thus this small
block of chapters may have been lifted because someone wished to
conceal family matters.

For the most part Mather was a lucid writer who shunned the
involved style of Boyle, Brown, and others of the seventeenth century.
It may be that he was favorably influenced by the style of Sir William Temple (1628–1699) who influenced many in England, includ-

ing Swift. Nothing in American history is more readable than Mather's *Magnalia Christi Americana* (London, 1702). His *Christian Philosopher* (London, 1721) is equally pleasant reading. This is generally true of *The Angel*. Occasionally he seems to have been more hurried or careless than in the other two works. His sermonizing may seem tedious but it was pertinent to his time. Indeed, to enjoy the entire work the reader would be wise to imagine himself a devout citizen of the more unhurried world of 1724.

Foreign language quotations are not overdone. There are none in German, French, Italian, or Spanish, all languages he knew, while many of his prospective readers did not. He used surprisingly little Hebrew and the Latin quotations, while numerous, are usually pertinent and simple. He employed a score or more Greek phrases for which he usually offered immediate translations. He used Hellenistic, not Classic, Greek words and spellings. His Greek orthography was poor. He paid little attention to breathings and accents. Some of his letters are open to question. At sixty-one years old, at least, he was not at home in Greek. But that is a trifling lapse.

In the work Mather quoted more than 250 medical writers. Perhaps twenty per cent of these are secondary quotes, but that still leaves a personal acquaintance on his part with the writings of 200 men. Some of this may have been by correspondence. His son stated that he had a busy correspondence with as many as fifty Europeans at a time. Some of his acquaintance may have been through conversation with Boston physicians. Granted all this, there remains a great body of non-theological reading that he must have done all his mature life. According to his son, the work "cost the doctor many years study to fill and embellish it." Perhaps he read and took notes with this book in mind for two decades before he finally finished it in 1724.

For this a fairly complete medical library was necessary, either his own, his friends', or at Harvard College. There is extant a presumably complete catalog of the Harvard books as of 1723.[1] Julius Herbert Tuttle assembled a list of known Mather-owned books which is certainly not complete.[2] Mather quoted far more authors than are listed in either of the above. In fact, he quoted a few books which cannot be found in any modern bibliography. More than once he noted editions which must have been earlier than any now known. In no case was the book on either the Harvard or the Tuttle list. It is often difficult to decide just what publication of a given author Mather used as authority for a statement. Whenever it has been possible to identify a book he must have owned or had at hand the fact will be noted in the footnotes. We must conclude that there was an astonishing wealth of medical books in Boston, more likely in Mather's own home.

As a bibliophile Cotton Mather rivalled William Byrd II of Virginia, if indeed he did not surpass him. His collection was of course far more heavily theological. On one occasion he happily acquired a whole 600-volume library of sermons. Mather frequently noted with satisfaction the size of his library, "the best in all this land." Even at the age of twenty-two he was thanking God for his large library. And his collection grew steadily. He owned a large brick house on Hanover Street in Boston and kept his books in the "capatious library which is three stories above my study." It may seem surprising that a minister of that time could have afforded a library of more than three thousand volumes. Some came to him from his grandfather, many from his father. The above-mentioned collection of sermons was bought with money given him for that purpose by a Boston friend. God, not the friend, got the major credit for this, of course. There were other sources of book money. Mather seems to have engaged in various business enterprises the profits of which doubtless afforded him book money. His many writings sold well. A thousand copies of his *Valley of Hinnom* (Boston, 1717), for instance, sold in five days. However, at that time authorship brought small financial reward.

The family library of the Mathers was, as noted, first begun by Richard Mather. With, I am certain, much loss, it remained in the family for two hundred years until a remnant of it was acquired by the American Antiquarian Society in 1814. Both Richard and Increase bought books, but Cotton was the bibliomaniac of the family. Apparently his son Samuel inherited the books but not the intense desire for more.

According to Tuttle's list there were about forty medical and scientific books to be found in the collection. Between the time of Mather's death and the sale of the books in 1814 to Isaiah Thomas (who gave them to the Society) many others must have been given away, loaned, or misappropriated. Among these many items would have been those considered most useful or most interesting. Mather certainly owned all the Boston medical imprints. He quotes some of the authors. He must have had Salmon's pharmacopeia and Boyle's little book of prescriptions, but neither is listed by Tuttle or by the

Harvard Catalog. Judging both from the information and from actual borrowed phrases works by Ramazzini, Benjamin Marten, and
Baglivi must have been at hand. Thomas J. Holmes[3] mentions several
items not listed by Tuttle. These are just examples. Many others can
be assumed from a study of both the *Angel* and the *Christian Philosopher.*

Tuttle's list does include many interesting books. Of anatomical
works in the Mather library we find those by du Laurens, De Graaf,
Bartholin, Riolan. General works on medical practice by Willis,
Wirtzung (Mosan translation), Sydenham, Cole, and Sennert were
there. Botany was represented by books of Parkinson and Evelyn.
Strother's pharmacopeia was present. Several of Francis Bacon's
works and five by Boyle were listed.

Seemingly the books at Harvard supplemented Mather's own.
The location of the books may not have been convenient to such a
busy man although Mather was aware of the books available there.
In March of 1716 he urged the College to buy J. Lange's *Medicina
Mentis* (London, 1716) and it did, for it is listed in the catalog with
many other worthy medical and scientific works. The remarkable
thing is how *few* of them are to be found as references in the *Angel.*
My conclusion is that he used the College library very little, but relied almost entirely on the books in his own "capatious library." The
College owned eleven volumes of the *Philosophical Transactions,* but
he must have owned it also. Considering his great interest in all things
intellectual in Germany we may say that it is just as likely that he
owned a run of the Nuremberg *Ephemerides* to rival the twenty year
run at Harvard.

capsula, I ~~[crossed out]~~

Some Remarks ~~[crossed out]~~
on The Grand CAUSE of Sickness.
~~[crossed out]~~
~~[crossed out]~~
Felix qui potuit rerum cognoscere causas.

~~Felix qui potuit rerum cognoscere causas.~~ Man
-kind has been ~~[crossed out]~~ sorely puzzled about, The
Origin of Evil. The ~~Question~~, Whence
Evil comes, has been as vexing a problem, as ever
was in ye world. The opinion of the old Magians
(Before ye Reformation of Zoroaster, in his Revived
Magianism,) ~~and~~ which was afterwards followed
by ye Manichees, as numerous a Sect of Hereticks
as ~~[crossed out]~~ almost any that ever was upon the
face of the Earth, was of old strongly imbibed
among ye Persians. But or Glorious God, speaking
about the affairs of Persia, will have Two Gods
no longer believed among them. No, He sais, Isa.
XLV. ✝. I form the Light, & create Darkness: I make
peace, & create Evil; I the Lord do all these things.
And now ~~[crossed out]~~ Glorious God, we Believe it. And
yet how the thing remains unto us Incomprehensible!

~~[crossed out]~~ If we enquire after the Origin of ~~the~~
DISEASES, we shall not enquire wrong after this
matter, if we do not find of SIN against the Holy
and Blessed ONE, to be ye ~~[crossed out]~~ Root of Bitterness, from whence they have all arisen.

~~[crossed out]~~ I will chuse to express my sentiments
of this matter, in ye Terms, which in a Trea-
-tise Entituled, mens sana in corpore sano, I
gave unto the publick about Twenty years
ago.

' Let us look upon SIN as the Cause of Sickness.
' There are it may be, Two Thousand Sicknesses:
' And indeed, any one of them able to crush us!
' But what is the cause of all. Bear in mind,
' That sin was that which first brought sickness
' upon a sinful world, and which you continue
' to sicken the world, with a world of Distempers. ✝
' Sickness is in short, Flagellum Dei, pro peccatis
' mundi.

It has been a Maxim with some, That a wise
man will be melancholy once a day. I suppose, they mean something more than, Serious, & Thoughtful. Of such a Frame as Th[is]
is to be advised for more than, once a day,
must rather say, My Son, Be thou in it all
day long. I am sure, a Dying Man, as thou
art, has Reason to be so.

But, for a Crazy Melancholy, or a froward Me-
-lancholy; For This, Once a Day, is too much.

There is a Malady, which goes by ye Name of
Melancholy. And commonly ca[lld]
This Hypocondriac Melancholy; [and for Some
& for seasons, oaks, often called, The Hypo':] &
Flatulencies in ye Region of the Hypocondr[ia]
often accompany it. And so, the poor Sple[en]
frequently, but wrongfully enough, comes to b[e]
charged with it.

None are more subject unto it than such a[s]
have had Invetorate Headaches torturing of [them.]

How ye System of ol Spirits, comes to be du[ll]
& Sowred, in this Distemper, Let them, who kn[ow]
declare; They who can only guess, will be mode[st]
& silent.

The Fancies and Whimsies of people ov[er]
-run with Melancholy are So many, & So var[ious]
& So Ridiculous, that the very Recital of the[m]
one would think, might somewhat serve as [a]
Little cure for Melancholy. The Stories might
be, what ye Titles of some Silly Books Rather b[e]
Pills to purge Melancholy. — The Truly
Cases Violations of Reason, are a Melanchol[y]
Spectacle.

These Melancholicks, do Sufficiently fr[et]
themselves, and are Enough their own Torm[en-]
-tors. As if this present Evil world, would n[ot]
Really afford Sad things enough, they [heap]

And Women,
who labour
under these
obstructions.

unto a Reasona-
ble & Religious
Beholder of ym.

Proposals

for printing a BOOK Entituled;
The Angel of Bethesda.[1]

' An ESSAY upon the *Common Maladies of Mankind*.
' Offering, first, *The Sentiments of PIETY*, whereto the
' Invalids are to be awakened in and from their *Bodily Maladies*.
' And then, a Rich Collection of *plain* but *potent* and
' *Approved* REMEDIES for the *Maladies*.
' Accompanied with many very practicable directions, for
' the PRESERVATION OF HEALTH, to such as enjoy a good
' measure of so great a Blessing.
' And many other curious, and grateful and useful entertainments,
' occasionally intermixed.
' This whole being A *Family-physician*, which every *Family*
' of any *Capacity* may find their Account in being supplied
' withal.

Tho the Title of the Book thus exhibited, may somewhat explain the Design and the value of it, yet for a further and fuller explanation, here shall be given the *contents*, and some Account of what is contained in the sixty six *Capsula's* into which it is divided. *Capsula* I. *Salvianus, or some Remarks of Piety* on the grand *Cause of* Sickness. II. *Valerianus*, or, points of *Health* to be always attended to: and famous Methods for the *Prolongation of Life proposed*. III. *Th[era]peutica Sacra*. or, The Symptoms of an *Healed Soul*, with the Methods of coming at it. IV. The *Tree of Life*. Whereto there is annexed *Panacea;* or, A proposal of an *Universal Medicine*, to them that would consult their *Health* under and against *All diseases*. V. *Nishmath Chajim*. The probable *Seat* of all Diseases, and a general *Cure* of them, further discovered; More particularly for *Splenetic* and *Hysteric* Maladies, which make so great a part of the Distempers. VI. The *Gymnastic*. or, An exposition [exercitation?] upon *exercise*. VII. *Conjecturalia*. or some Touches upon a *New Theory* of many Diseases. VIII. *Raphael*. or, Notable Cures from the *Invisible World*. IX. *Stimulator*. or, Considerations upon *pains*, Dolours, aches, in general. X. *Cephalica*. or, Cures for The *Head-ache*. And, of the *Ague in the Head*. XI. *Dentifrangibulus*. or, The Anguish and Relief of the *Tooth-ache*. XII. The *Prisoners of the Earth,* under the GOUT, with some notable and Instructive Entertainments for them. XIII. The *Gouts* younger Brother. or, A *Rheumatism,* and *Sciatica,* quieted. XIV. *Flagellum*. The *Stone;* and other Diseases of the *Kidneys* and *Bladder*. XV. *Magor-Missabib*. or, The *Cancer*. XVI. *Scrophularia*. or, The *Kings-Evil* touched upon. XVII. *Pyretologia*. or, *Fevers* extinguished. XVIII. *Febrifuga*. or, *Agues* conquered. XIX. The *Inevitable*. or, The *Measles managed*. XX. *Variolæ triumphate*. or, The *Small-pox* encountred. And, a Poem upon it, by one coming out of the Jaws of the *Destroyer*. XXI. *Kibroth Haltaavah*. or, Some clean Thoughts on the *Foul Disease*. XXII. *Malum ab Aquilone*. or, The *Scurvy* discoursed on. XXIII. *Moses*. or, one drawn out of the *Dropsy*. XXIV. *Bethlem* visited. or, The Cure of *Madness*. XXV. *De Tristibus*. or, the Cure of *Melancholy*. XXVI. *Paralyticus resuscitatus*. or, The *Palsey*-struck, *taking up his Bed and walking*. XXVII. *Attonitus*. or, The *Apoplexy* considered. XXVIII. *Caducus*. or, The *Falling-Sickness* considered; with a New Discovery of a most unfailing Remedy for all *Convulsive Diseases* in old or young. XXIX. *Vertiginosus*. or, how to steer under *Dizziness*. XXX. *Dormitantius*. or, The *Lethargy;* And other *sleepy* Diseases. XXXI. *Ephialtes*. or, the *Nightmare* beaten off. XXXII. The *Oculist;* considering Diseases of the Eye; Especially, *Blindness*. With a poem upon it. XXXIII. *Colaphizatus*. or, Diseases of the *Ear,* Especially *Deafness*. with an Appendix, of, Advice to the *Lame*. XXXIV. *Stiptica*. or, *Bleeding* at the Nose. XXXV. *Suffocatus*. or, A Sore *Throat;* and, *Quinzy*. XXXVI. *Adjutoria Catarrhi*. A *Catarrh,* And what we call, A *Cold,* how to Stop it. XXXVII. The *Breast-beater;* or, A *Cough* quieted. XXXVIII. *Breath Struggled for*. or, The *Asthma,* and *Short-windedness,* releeved. XXXIX. *Desector*. The CONSUMPTION, the grand *Mower* felt by the grass of the Field. XL. *Medicina Medicanda*. A Pause made upon the *Uncertainties* of the Physicians. XLI. *Icterus* Looked upon; or, The *Jaundice* cured. XLII. The *Main Wheel* Scour'd and Oil'd. or, Help for the *Stomach* depraved; And *Vomiting*. XLIII. *Edulcorator*. Help for the *Heart-burn*. And, *Stomach-ache*. XLIV. The *Vermine-killer;* Upon *Worms*. XLV. *Intestina Omnia Recta*. or, The Disorders of a *Flux* rectified. XLVI. *Jehoram* visited. or, The *Bloody-flux* remedied. XLVII. *Miserere Mei*. or, Compassion for the *Cholic;* and the *Dry-Belly-ache*. XLVIII. *Ashdodes*. or, The *Piles*. XLIX. *Scabiosus*. or, The *Itch* safely and quickly chas'd away. L. *Singultus finitus.* or, A Stop to the *Hiccough.* LI. *Ephphatha.* or, Some Advice to *Stammerers:* How to *get good* by, and how to *get rid* of, their grievous Infirmity. LII. *Muliebra.* or, Foeminine Diseases. LIII. Retired *Elizabeth.* A Long, tho' no very Hard, Chapter for a Woman whose *Travail* approaches; with Remedies to abate the *Sorrows of Childbearing.* LIV. Great Things done by *Small Means;* With some Remarks on a *Spring of Medicinal Waters,* which Every body is at home an owner of. LV. *Mirabilia et Parabilia.* or, more Great Friends to *Health,* very *Easy* to come at. LVI. The Eyes of poor *Hagar* opened. or, A Discovery of *Unknown Stores,* for *Cures,* which Every body is Master of. LVII. A *Physick-Garden.* or, A Consideration of the admirable Vertues of Certain *Plants* which Every *Common Garden* may be furnish'd with. LVIII. *Thaumatographia Insectorum.* or, Some Despicable *Insects* of admirable Vertues. LIX. *Infantilia.* or *Infantile* Diseases. LX. *Paralipomena.* or, Cures and Helps for a Cluster of *Lesser Inconveniences.* LXI. *Medicamenta sine quibus.* or, Certain Remedies, that People of any Condition, may always have ready at hand for themselves and their Neighbours. LXII. *Fuga Daemonum.* or, Cures by *Charms* Considered; And a *Seventh Son* Examined. LXIII. *Miso-capnus.* Taking the use of TOBACCO under Consideration. With a *Pinch* upon the *Snuff-box.* LXIV. *Restitutus.* or, A perfect Recovery, in the Wise and Good Conduct of one Recovered from a Malady. LXV. *Liberatus.* or, The Thanksgiving of one advanced in years and præserved from grievous and painful Diseases. LXVI. *Euthanasia.* or, A *Death* Happy and Easy.

You see the *Bill of Fare.* It would be too great a Reproach upon Humane Understanding to imagine, That a Treatise of *Such Intentions,* and Composed with such a Variety of *Good Things,* both for SOUL and BODY, and of such *Universal Benefit* for all Sorts of People, *Sick* or *Well, High* or *Low, Old* or *Young,* would not find a General Acceptance. What *Gentleman* would not be willing to have such a *Companion* with him! Or what *Family* would not be willing to Save *Life,* and *Health,* and *Money* too, and serve a *Greater Interest* than all of These, by having Such a *Counsellour* alwayes at hand! This Book paies all due Regards to our Skillful and Faithful *Physicians;* our *Necessary Friends.* The *Divulgation of Medicines,* is no more than has been made by Charitable *Physicians* times without Number. The Medicines in this Book are very many of them Such as the Best *Physicians* have already published. And as *They* will not be, So tis incredible that any others can be Enemies to this Publication.

The *Angel of Bethesda* is now *Lying at the Pool;* and waiting to be *called forth.*

It can't well be carried on, but in the Ordinary Way of *Subscription.*

It shall be delivered unto Subscribers, at the Price of <u>Twelve Shillings</u> the book; which is as Cheap again as a Book of the like Bulk from *Europe* is usually Sold for. And very probably it will at some time or other save the Expense of more than as many *Pounds* unto the purchaser.

He who sends in Subscriptions for *Six Books,* may Expect a *Seventh* gratis. The Subscribers also, (except any of them forbid it) may Expect their Names to be published with the Work, as tis now become Customary.

The subscriptions are taken in, by

To _____

Sir, You have here put into your hands, PROPOSALS of a Work, which you cannot but be a Well-wisher to. By procuring Such a Work to have its operation in your Neighborhood, you will very much do them an Unknown Service, both in their *Spiritual* and their *Temporal* Interests; and many will both in *Soul* and *Body* fare the better for you. Your known *Good Will towards Men,* and *Zeal to do Good,* unto men, has Encouraged the *Undertakers,* to lodge these PROPOSALS, more particularly in *your Hands,* that by *your Means* a Number of *Subscriptions* may be obtained, for the Enabling of them to go thro' the Undertaking; which is thought Necessary by,

Your Servants,

The BOOKSELLERS

Capsula I.

Some Remarks
on The Grand CAUSE of <u>Sickness</u>.

Felix qui potuit rerum cognoscere causas.[1]

MANKIND has been sadly puzzled about, *The Origin of Evil.* The question, πoθεv τo κακov, *Whence Evil Comes,* has been as *Vexing* a *problem* as ever was in the World. The Opinion of the old *Magians* (before the Reformation of *Zoroaster,* in his Revived *Magianism,*)[2] which was afterwards followed by the *Manichees,*[3] as numerous a Sect of *Hereticks,* as almost any that ever was upon the face of the Earth, was of old strongly imbibed among the *Persians.* But our Glorious God, speaking about the affairs of *Persia,* will have *Two GODS* no longer beleeved among them. No, He sais, Isa. XLV. 7. *I form the Light, create Darkness; I make Peace, and create Evil; I the Lord do all these things.* And now, *Glorious GOD, We Beleeve it: And yett the Thing remains unto us Incomprehensible!*

If we enquire after the *Origin* of DISEASES, we shall not *Enquire wisely after this Matter,* if we do not find we SIN against the Holy and Blessed ONE, to be the *Root of Bitterness,* from whence they have all arisen. I will chuse to express my Sentiments of this Matter, in the Terms, which in a Treatise entituled, <u>Mens Sana</u> in <u>Corpore Sano</u>,[4] I gave unto the public above twenty years ago.

Lett us, Look upon SIN as the *Cause* of *Sickness.*
' There are it may be, *Two Thousand Sicknesses:*
' And indeed, *any one of whom able to crush us!*
' But what is the *Cause* of all? Bear in Mind,
' That *Sin* was that which first brought *Sickness*
' upon a *Sinful World,* and which yett continues
' to *Sicken* the World, with a World of Diseases.
' Sickness is in short, *Flagellum Dei pro peccatis Mundi;*[5]

First, Remember, That the *Sin* of our *First Parents,* was the *First Parent* of all our *Sickness.*
' All our *Sicknesses* are but the Execution of that primitive Threatening in Gen. II.17. *In the Day that thou Sinnest thou shalt Surely dy.* If *Crudities,* and *Obstructions,* and *Malignities,* are the *Parents* of our *Sicknesses,* tis very sure, that *Sin* is the *Grand Parent* of them; and the Sin of our *First Parents* is the *First Parent* of them all. We read in Eccl. IX.18. of, *ONE Sinner Destroying much Good.* I find,

Some Jewish *Rabbis* take our Father *Adam,* to be meant by that *ONE Sinner.* Our *Health* is no small part of the *Good,* which has been *Destroy'd* by him. Had our *First Parents* eaten of the *Tree of Life,* doubtless a confirm'd state of *Perfect Health,* both in Themselves and their Offspring, had been the *Fruit* of it. But our *First Parents* criminally applied themselves to the forbidden *Tree of Knowledge.* This proved a *Tree of Death,* both to themselves and their Offspring; and *Sicknesses* are among the *Punishments* of that nefandous Crime. *Alas, our Father did eat soure Grapes, and our Teeth are sett on Edge.* When that Expression is used about our Lord JESUS CHRIST; [Heb. II.9.]*He TASTED Death for us;* I make no doubt, that it is an Elegant Allusion, unto the *Way* whereby *Death* at first came into the World; This was by *Tasting* the *Forbidden Fruit.* As *Death,* so *Sickness,* the Inchoation⁶ of *Death,* is but the Bitter *Taste* of that unhappy Action! Yea, The *Breath* of the *Old Serpent,* whereto Mankind in our First Parents hearkened, has *Poisoned* us all. The *Poison,* which that *Serpent* who is, *The Angel of Death,* has insinuated into us, has disturbed our *Health,* as well as depraved our *Heart. Sin, Sin,* was that which opened the Floodgates for a Flood of *Wretchedness* to rush in upon the world; And *Sickness* is one Instance of that *Wretchedness. Cursed SIN; I Indict thee this day, for murdering of the World:*

Secondly, Remember, That the *Sin* of every individual Man, does but *Repeat* and *Renew* the *Cause* of *Sickness* unto him. We are informed, in Psal. *CVII.*17. *Fools, because of their Transgression, and because of their Iniquities, are Afflicted,* with Sickness. Indeed *Sin* sometimes is *Naturally* the Cause of *Sickness.* A *Sickness* in the *Spirit* will *naturally* cause a *Sickness* in the *Body. Inordinate Passions* burn the *Thread* of Life. *Immoderate Courses* drown the *Lamp* of Life. The Wise Man sais about *Unchastity, It consumes the Body.* It has been said, *Plures occidit Crapula quam Gladius,* The *Cup* kills more than the *Canon.* And, *Multos Morbos Fercula multa faciunt.* Many *Dishes* will breed many Diseases. Alas, when will Men Beleeve it? The *Board* slayse more than the *Sword.* And one may say *By Suppers and Surfeits more have been killed than all the Physicians in the World have cured.* The Apostle sais about worldly *Griefs* and *Cares; They work Death.* We may add, *Ignavium corrumpunt otia Corpus. The* Humours of the Body Stagnate and Corrupt in *Idleness.* But *Sin* is yett oftener a *Moral Cause of Sickness.* What are *Sicknesses,* but the *Rods,* wherewith GOD corrects His own offending Children? Pious

Asa[7] takes a *wrong Step;* and he is *Diseased in his Foot* for it: God sends the *Gout* upon him. And, what are they, but the *Vindictive Strokes* of wrath, wherewith God Revenges Himself upon the Children of *Wrath?* Jehoran did a *Bloody Thing:* and, so, *his Bowels fell out by reason of his Sickness:* GOD smites him with a *Bloody Flux* for it.[8] Hence, our *Sicknesses* are in the New Testament called by a Name that hath *Scourges,* in the Signification of it. [Ponder also at Liesure, Exod. XV.26. and Deut. XXVIII.21.22. 27. 35. 60. 61. And say not, as he to whom the *Book,* of *Happiness,* was presented, *I am not at Liesure.*] Ah, *Sin;* How Mischievous art thou! A Man may say of every *Sin,* when he meets with it, *Have I found thee, O mine Enemy?* The *Soul* and the *Body* constitute *One Person;* and the *Body* is unto the *Soul,* the *Instrument* of Iniquity. Hence for the *Sins* of the one, there come *Sufferings* on the other. Syrs, Be afraid of *Sin.* I tell you Tis a very *Unwholesome Thing.* When you are gone to drink the *Stolen Waters* of *Sin, there's Death in the Pott.*

Thirdly. Hence, under *Sickness,* we should make a Solemn Enquiry after *Sin.* As upon other *Disasters,* there was that Call given; Hag. I. 5.7. *Consider your Ways:* Tis to be heard most sensibly in our *Sicknesses.* There is a *Self-examination* incumbent upon *All* Men: Upon *Sick* Men it is peculiarly incumbent. I pray, Lett our *Sickness* itself, be such an *Emetic,* as to make us *Vomit* up our *Sin,* with a poenitent *Confession* of it. A Time there was, when *Sacramental Profanations* were chastised with *Sicknesses* among the *Corinthians:* They had not come in an *orderly Manner* to the *Body* of the Lord, and GOD rebuked it with *Disorders* upon theirs. [Compare 2 Chron. XXX.20.] Now, sais the Apostle, *Judge Yourselves.* Indeed, *Sickness* does not always come to manage a *Controversy* of God with us for some *Iniquity.* A Job, that *Perfect and upright Man,* may have his *Ulcera Syrraca,*[9] [so tragically described by *Aretaeus,*[10] and admirably answering the *Diagnosticks* which the Sacred Writ has given us of *Jobs* Distemper:] To *Try* his patience. Tis said of that Man of God *Elisha.*[11] He *fell sick of the Sickness whereof he died:* It seems he had been *Sick* some times before. Our Lord may have a *Lazarus,*[12] of whom it shall be said, *One whom thou Lovest is sick.* Strange! *Diseases* may be *Love-tokens!* A *Timothy,*[13] that rare Minister, whom one of the Ancients calls *An Admirable Young Man,* may be troubled with often *Infirmities.* Our Lord JESUS CHRIST is to be *Visited* in the *Sickness* of His dearest *Brethren.* [*Lord, That ever thou shouldest call them so!*] But yett, it becomes us to be very Inquisitive and Sollicitous, lest there be *Wrath in our Sickness;* and Thoughtful, *What is the Controversy?*

Wherefore, Both under our *Sickness* and after it, we should be more concerned for being saved from *Sin* than from *Sickness.* Our *Sins,* indeed what are they, but the terrible *Sicknesses,* under which our *Souls* are fearfully Languishing and Perishing. A *Sinful Soul* is a *Sickly Soul. Original Sin* is a *Leprosy.* Every *Lust* is a *Distemper* of the *Soul.* An *unsteady Soul* has a *Palsey.* A *Wanton Soul* has a *Fever.* A *Worldly Soul* has a *Dropsy. Anger* in the *Soul* is an *Erisypelas. Envy* is a *Cancer* in the *Soul, Sloth,* a *Scurvy.* Whenever we have *Sinned,* we have cause to say, *Lord, HEAL my Soul, for I have sinned.* Now, *Sickness* is to awaken our Concern, first, for the *pardon* of the Maladies in our *Souls;* and so, for a *Power* against them all.

First; *Under Sickness,* what should be our *Chief Concern?* It should be *That;* Psal. XXV. 18 *Lord, look upon my Affliction and my Pain, and forgive all my Sin.* If it be then putt unto us, *What lies Heaviest now upon you?* Say not, *My Sickness,* but say *My Sinfulness: That I have done so little Service for my Lord JESUS CHRIST; That I have mispent so much of my precious Time; That I have made no more Provision for Eternity; And, that I am still so Sottish, and Slothful, and Sensual, and Carnal, and Alienated from the Life of God.* And for to quicken this our Concern under our *Sickness,* we are to think, *What will become of me, if I dy unpardoned; what will become of me throughout eternal Ages?*

Next, *After Sickness;* what should be our *Chief Concern?* It should be That; Psal. CIII. 3. *Bless the Lord, O my Soul, who forgiveth all thine Iniquities; who releeveth all thine Infirmities.* The *Iniquities* are to be taken away *first;* and *Then* the *Infirmities.* Lett us not count our *Sickness* well gone, except our *Sin* be gone too. But Lett us now putt this unto ourselves; *Am I now more Assured of my being pardoned, than I was before? Am I in better Terms with Heaven? Can I see and say, Tis in Love to my Soul, that God has brought me back from the pitt of Corruption?* It should now be more of our Care, That our *Sickness* be removed *in Mercy,* than ever it was, that it should be removed *at all.*

In fine; *The Sickness* that *enfeebles* us, must make us fly more *Vigorously* than ever unto the *Expiatory Sacrifice* of our Lord JESUS CHRIST, for the *Forgiveness of our Sins.* Our Sickness is utterly lost upon us, if it render not a CHRIST more *precious* unto us than ever He was, and instruct us not how to make more *Use* of Him. As the Sick in the Gospels, much cried out for, A CHRIST, So *Sickness* is to teach us, the Worth of a CHRIST, and cause us more to see, that without a CHRIST we are undone forever. There is a *Ransome* which a *Sick Man* is to be minded of; that *Ransome,* Job. XXXIII. 34. *He is Chastened with Pain upon his Bed, his Flesh is consumed away, his Soul draweth nigh to the Grave,—Then God is Gracious to Him, and Saith, Deliver Him from going down to the Pitt. I have found a Ransome.,* Syrs, when we are Sick, Lett us behold our Lord JESUS CHRIST as *going down to the Pitt* for us, and plead that *Ransome* that we may not ourselves *go down.* In the *Directories* for *Visiting the Sick,* used many Ages ago, the *Sick* were directed to say, *Lord, I place the Death of my Saviour JESUS CHRIST between Thee and my Sins.* Tis impossible to say a Better Thing than *that!*

Upon *Sickness,* our Address must be made unto our Lord JESUS CHRIST; of whom it is said, Matth. VIII. 17. *Himself bare our Sicknesses.* Indeed, we cannot say, That there were any proper[14] *Sicknesses* among the *Sufferings* of our SAVIOUR. We do not find, that he was ever properly *Sick.* His *Body* being formed by a special Efficacy of the *Holy SPIRIT,* seems to have been of so exact a *Temper,* as to be less liable to Diseases than other men. But our SAVIOUR *bore our Sicknesses,* because as tis elsewhere Said for it, *He bare our Sins,* which are the *Cause* of our *Sicknesses.* Wherefore,. In every *Sickness* lett us repair to the *Death* (of) our Lord JESUS CHRIST, and struggle with our *Unbeleef* more than our *Sickness,* until we are able to say, *Lord, My whole Dependence is on my SAVIOUR, who has made Atonement for the Sins, for which thou has made me Sick in Smiting me.*

I will recite you a Contemplation of the Blessed *Austin,*[15] which under *Sickness* may be the sweetest *Anodyne*[16] of our uneasy Minds. "There lay Extended over the whole World a great Instance of *Sickness;* That is to say, All *Mankind,* Subject unto many *Diseases* both of *Soul* and *Body.* And therefore there is come into the world that great Physician, by whose *Wounds we are Healed.* Indeed, we see that the *Soul* of Man labours under the Numberless *Diseases* which are its *Vices.* And the *Body* of Man Suffers more *Diseases,* than any other Creature. But O Admirable and Amiable Matter! and a Thing full of Compassionate Goodness! [*Fusus est sanguis Medici, et factum est medicamentum phrenetici:*] The *Blood* of the *Physician* being shed, becomes the *Cure* of the *Distempered*.

In fine, There were *malignant Ulcers*, which *Galen*[17] sais, the Greeks called *Chironian*,[18] because none but *Chiron* could cure them. The *Malignant Mischiefs* which our *Sin* has brought upon us, we are sure, are such that *None but CHRIST can cure them!*

It was a mistake in some of the Ancients to make JESUS a Greek Name, carrying of *Healing* with it. But it will be no mistake in us to look on our JESUS, as, *The Lord our Healer.*

The Design of all this Essay, is to Lead the Reader unto HIM. And therewithal to prosecute that grand Maxim, The Cure of a *Sin-Sick SOUL*, is what all Invalids ought to reckon their Grand *Concern.* I will express it in the Words of *Rhegius*[19] translated from the High-Dutch by *Lorrichini,* in a Treatise Entituled, *Psychopharmacon. Adversa Valetudo, membrorumque intentus, ac Mors, Terribilis quodem judicatur: Sed omnium quae accidere poterunt homini rerum est horrendissima aegritudo et Exitium Animarum. Quod si Membris Languentibus et infirmo Corpori Salubria Medicamenta Studio diligentiore quaerimus, Cur non Cura Majore, quae sanant atque vivificant Animos ad Laboramus indigate!*[20]
And We will upbraid many *Christian People* with the Words of an *Heathen Poet,*

> *Ut corpus redimas, ferrum patiens, et ignes;*
> *Arida nec Sitiens Ora Lavavis Aqua.*
> *Ut Valeas Animo, quic quam tolerare negabis!*
> *At praemium pars haec Corpore majus habet.*

Thus Englished.

> To save your Bodies Cutts and Burns you'l chuse;
> And you're *parch'd,* to quench your *Thirst* refuse:
> Your *Soul* to keep in Health bear any Thing!
> For this a greater Happiness will bring.[21]

It is a Thing strongly pressed by the Noble *Morney,*[22] that *Julian*[23] himself beleeved *Æsculapius*[24] the son of *Jupiter* to have descended from Heaven, to be *Incarnate,* and have appeared among Men as a *Man,* in order to the Restitution both of their Spirits and of their Bodies, to their pristine Perfection. O *Invalids,* I am leading you to your true *Æsculapius!*

CAP. II.

Points of HEALTH,
to be always attended.

non est Vivere; sed Valere, Vita[1]

VERY Emphatical are the Words of the Apostle *John,* unto his Good-Spirited *Gaius.* III. Epist. 2. *I wish above all things, that thou mayst prosper, and be in Health, Even as thy SOUL prospereth.* A Good Wish! And yett at Good as it is, it would be no better than a direful *Curse,* if the most of Men had it applied unto them. If the most of Men were to have the Measures of their *temporal Prosperity* taken from their *Spiritual Prosperity,* then Men would be *undone* for Both Worlds, and beyond all Expession miserable. Should the most of Men *Prosper and be in Health,* but as *their Soul prospers,* we should see the Men *Bereaved of all that is Good;* lying with the *Needy on the Dunghil;* their *Bodies* become a meer *Hospital* of all the *Diseases* imaginable. *But* now and then, *But* here and there, such a Saint is to be mett withal, as may with *Safety* and unspeakable *Comfort,* have this *Prayer* putt up on his behalf; *mayst thou prosper and be in Health, even as thy Soul prospers.* And such an one was our *Gaius.*

Yett this *Godly* Man seems to have been a *Sickly* Man. One whom our SAVIOUR does *love,* yett may be *Sick.* Tho' PIETY be naturally as well as morally, an Help unto our *Health,* and the Maxims of the Gospel are always *Wholesome* Words: yett the Children of *God* may be chastened with *Sickness.* The Apostles of our LORD, who frequently dispensed *Miraculous Cures,* yett had not the *Gift of Healing* at their own Dispose: they could not cure when and whom they pleased. A *Languishing Body* and a *Prospering Soul* may dwell together. Yea, Tis no Irrational or Improbable Conjecture, that the *Prosperity* found in the *Soul* of this Excellent Man, might be very much owing to his feeble and crazy constitution. Verily, the *Maladies* of the *Body,* frequently prove the *Medicines* of the *Soul.* O *Invalid,* Mayst thou in thy Experience find it so.

All *Prosperity* is to be wished. But it seems, *Above all things,* This, *That thou mayst be in Health.* That is to say, *Above all* the Blessings of a *Temporal Prosperity. To be in Health,* is a very considerable Article of our *Temporal Prosperity.* Indeed our *Temporal*

Prosperity is all pall'd, and Spoil'd, and lost, if *Health* be wanting. As to all the *Blessings* of *this Life,* a Man must be *in Health,* or he can have no Relish of them: *Valeat possessor oportet.* What would a *Slipper* set with *Diamonds* be to a *Foot* under the Tortures of the *Gout?* Yea, what would a *Diadem* itself signify to an *Head* that were always *Aking? Grievous Diseases* (like the *Death* in which they terminate) make the Difference between *Monarchs* and *Beggars* to cease. Most certainly, our *Health* is not so Thankfully acknowledged as it ought to be: The *God of our Health* is never praised with the Acknowledgments that are due unto Him. Nor indeed has the Skilful *Physician* always the *Esteem* and *Reward* that he deserves. He that appears like an *Angel* while the Cure is yett expected, appears in quite another Shape after it is accomplished. *Praemia cum possit medicus!*[2]

But, syrs; tis the *Health of the SOUL,* that is most of all to be wish'd for. It is a *Soul in Health* which is the *Prospering Soul.* Now, The *Healing of the Soul* is brought about in its *Conversion* unto *God.* So we read, Isa. VI. 10. *They Convert and are Healed.* This *Healed Soul,* confirmed in its Turn to God, and in all the Inclinations of PIETY, becomes an *Healthy Soul.* Well; But what is to be done for this *Prosperity of the Soul?*

Be sure, this First Thing we have to do, that our SOUL may *Prosper and be in Health,* is, To repair unto our SAVIOUR, for the *Healing* of all that is Amiss in our SOUL. O *disordered SOUL,* Thy first Work must be to Look unto a SAVIOUR who So calls upon us; Isa. XLV. 22. *Look unto me, and be ye Saved.* When He appeared Incarnate among us, with amazing *Miracles* He *healed all manner of Sickness and all manner of Disease among the People,* as well as *went about preaching the Gospel* unto them. Truly, those *Healing Miracles* of our SAVIOUR had this *Gospel* in them; *Repair to your SAVIOUR, that He may bestow the Blessings of an Healed Soul upon you.* Concerning our SAVIOUR, it is declared unto us, Mal. IV. 2. *The Sun of Righteousness shall arise with Healing in His Wings.* It is reported, That in the Eastern World, it has been a Custom among the Pagans; When they had ineffectually tried all ordinary Means for the Releef of their *Sick,* they would Expose them abroad unto the *Sun,* Expecting the *Sun-beams* to perform the *Cure,* which was by no other Means to be attained. But, *O SOUL ruined by Sin;* Tis by *Beams* falling from thy SAVIOUR upon thee, that thou shalt have the *Cure* of all the Ruines, which thy *Sin* has brought upon thee.

But then, observe, Syrs, what you *have* to do and what you *use* to do, for the *Health* of your *Body;* Lett the SOUL have done for it, the Things that are like to these. All that have any Sense in them, *Shun* many things, *Do* many things, that their *Bodily Health* may not be impaired. But now, from your own Conduct about the *Health* of a *Body,* Learn what your Conduct must be that a SOUL may *Prosper and be in Health.* If you *Spiritualize* your Care about your *Bodily Health,* you will see how careful you ought to be that your *Spiritual Health* may be provided for.

Be attentive to some Notable Instances. Most Certainly they that would have an *Healthy SOUL,* must avoid Every Thing that would endanger the *Health* of the SOUL: All *Company* that has *Contagion* in it; All *Business* that brings a *Cold* upon Good Affections; All that *Leads into Temptation;* yea, *All Appearance of Evil.*

Yett more particularly, an Ingenious Person takes notice of it, That the *Conscience* is to the SOUL, what the *Stomach* is to the *Body.* Be it so! There is no point of *Health* more to be regarded than this; To take nothing into the *Stomach* that may be offensive to it. But then, O Man, If thou wouldst have thy SOUL to *Prosper and be in Health,* take heed of Every thing that will offend thy *Conscience.* Do nothing that shall be contrary to, and condemned by, the *Light of God* in thy SOUL. Keep *a Conscience Void of offence towards God and towards Man.*

Again; Wouldest thou have an *Healthy* SOUL? Then, lett thy SOUL not want a proper *Food,* a wholesome *Food;* and this in the due *Season* of it. The *Word* of God is that *Food. O Find it, and Eat it, and Lett it be the Rejoicing of thy Heart.* Be able to say, *Lord, I esteem the Word of thy Mouth more than my Necessary Food.*

But is not *Physick* required for our *Health,* as well as *Food?* There are *Mortifications* of *Repentance,* which will be a *Physick* for thee. *Whole Days* ought sometimes to be sett apart for them, if thou wouldest have an *Healthy Soul.* Yea, when Heaven administers *Physick* to thee, in the *Calamities* which it inflicts upon thee, do what thou canst, that they may *Work Well,* and thy *Iniquity* be *purged,* and the *Fruit* be to *take away* thy Sin.

Yett more, The *Health* will be Injured, if the *Cloathing* be neglected. That thou mayst have an *Healthy* SOUL, the Advice must be, *putt on the Lord JESUS CHRIST.* Appear in the *Durable Cloathing* of His *Righteousness.* And be *cloathed with Humility, cloathed* with the Holy SPIRIT, and with all conspicuous and observable *Goodness.*

But more than this. *Health* has not a greater Friend than *Exercise;* A Regular and moderate *Exercise* will do Strange Things: the *Gymnastic* will do what Nothing else will do. But then, to gett an *Healthy* SOUL, *Exercise thyself unto Godliness.* There are the *Devotions* of Christianity: *Exercise* thyself in those Things; Take Pains, and Rowse up all the Spirits and Powers of thy SOUL in these *Devotions.*

May not this be also offered? For an Healthy SOUL, there are those *Medicines* to be taken, of which there are the dispensations in the *Ordinances* of thy SAVIOUR. In the *Institutions*[3] of thy SAVIOUR, what sovereign *Medicines* are to be mett withal! What *Coolers*[4] of our Intemperate Passions! What *Correctors*[5] of our sharp Humours![6] What *Anodynes* for our uneasy Minds! What *Cordials*[7] for Hearts fainting and *stouping with Heaviness!* What *Rectifiers*[8] of all that may be out of order within us! Visit the *Institutions* of thy SAVIOUR, for those Intentions. For their *Health* People sometimes *go to the Waters.* Thy call in the Institutions of thy SAVIOUR, is in those Terms, *Come unto the Waters.*

The SOUL will certainly *prosper and be in Health,* if it be thus cared for.

Appendix.
Famous Methods for the PROLONGATION of LIFE, proposed.

A Famous Physician has an Observation, worthy to be engraved on Tables of Brass, worthy to be registered in Letters of *Gold:* "The infinitely wise *Author* of *Nature* hath so contrived things, that the most remarkable RULES of preserving LIFE and HEALTH are *Moral Duties* commanded us. So true it is, that *Godliness has the Promise of this Life, as well as of that to come."*

The learnedest Man *Then* [or, for ought I know, *Ever*] in the World, more than an hundred Years ago Remarked it, That all the *Rules* for the *Conservation of Health,* were comprised in those Words of *Cicero,*[9] a Gentleman who was more of an *Orator* than of a *Physician:* But how happily would he answer *Both Characters,* if he could *Effectually Perswade* us to the Practice of them! *Sustentatur Valetudo, Notitia Sui Corporis, Et Observatione earum rerum quae res aut prodesse Soleant, aut Obesse: et Continentia in Victu omni atque Cultu Corporis tuendi causa, et praetermittendis Voluptatibus.* In short; my Friend, Know and Mind thy own *Constitution,* taking thy *Measures from it;* Observe what proves most *Healthful,* and what most *Hurtful* to thee; Be moderate in Feeding and in Trimming thy *Body:* and be *Temperate* in the Use of *Bodily Pleasures.* Good Counsel from a *Roman;* And such as a *Christian* might not be ashamed of. Follow it, and thy *Soul* as well as thy *Flesh,* will fare the better for it.

The most consummate Physicians will tell us, That for the Prevention of Sickness, the Grand Secret is Only [*Sustine* et *Abstine,*] to *Bear* and *Forbear.*

Indeed, for the *Conservation of Health,* and so for the *Prolongation of Life,* the *Chief* of all Rules, yea, the *Sum* of all, is, TEMPERANCE. It is an incontestible Maxim, *Ingluvies omnium morborum mortisque Causa.*[10] The *Hippemolgians*[11] in *Homer,* owe their *Long Life* to their *Simple-Diet.* And the Custome of living on *Milk* is to this Day præserved by the *Tartars,* who inhabit the Same Country and *Live* like their Ancestors.

The famous *Cornaro,*[12] after a Sickly youth, lived in good Health to about one Hundred Years of Age. In his Book, *De Vita Sobria,* we find his Rule was, Twelve Ounces of *Meat,* and Fourteen Ounces of *Drink,* in four and twenty Hours. Towards the Period of his life, he lived by very near starving of himself. A *Single Egg* would serve him two or three Days. But as he *lived Pleasantly,* so he *died Easily.*

Democritus[13] arriving to a very great Age, reported the Rules of his Conduct, in these two Words: *Intus Melle, Extus Oleo. Honey* within, *Oil* without.

It has been the Remark of Great Men that *Evening Dews,* and *Nocturnal Studies,* and *Unseasonable Watchings* cannot be too much avoided, by them that would live *long* and *well,* in the World.

The memorable Sir *Theodore Mayern*[14] on his Death-bed, gave this Advice to a noble Friend, who demanded his Advice for the praeservation of Health: *Be Moderate in your Diet; Use much Exercise, and little Physic.*

Take the Advice, and *exercise thyself to Piety* with it. Both Inward and Outward Man in Health, will be the Consequence.

Galen, tho' a weakly Gentleman, lived unto Seventy. And *Sepontinus,*[15] that wrote his Life, mentions three Maxims, constantly observed with him: *To Eat and Drink very Moderately;* Never coming Full from the Table; And, To *Swallow nothing Raw;* And, *To have Sweet Scents about him, always refreshing of him.*

Celsus,[16] in his first Book, observes, that *Homer* mentions no sort of *Diseases*, in the old Heroic Times, but what were immediately *Inflicted by Heaven:* As if their *Temperance* and *Exercise* praeserved them from all besides.

One of the learned *Hoffmans*,[17] has written several curious Dissertations: Whereof one is *Des Moyens de Vivre Longtemps*, or, *The Wayes to Live Long*. He shows, There is nothing so considerable in this regard, as *Temperance:* unto which he adds, *Tranquillity of Mind*. For this Cause, he says, it is, That God promises *Long Life* to them that walk in the Ways with the Frames of PIETY: And we read, *The Fear of the Lord tendeth to Life*.

One of the *Bartholinus's* relates concerning his learned Grandfather *Finckius*,[18] That after a *Sickly Youth* he lived unto near an Hundred, a lively and an Healthy Man. And of the old Gentleman, he gives this Description: *Coercuit Luxuriam*,—He restrained his *Appetites;* He despised *Riches;* He maintained *Frugality;* He governed his *Passions:* He was easy under *Adversity;* and tho' he saw many Funerals of his dearest *Relatives*, he bore all with Patience and Constancy; He never wept, but upon mentioning the Death of his *Lady*, and the Burning of his *Library*.

Nicolas Leonicenus,[19] a Physician, lived Ninety Six Years. He was, they report, *Cibi et Vini Maxime abstinens, Somnique Minimi, praesertim vero Veneris continentissimus:—Nec unquam de Fortuna quereretur.*[20]

Manlius[21] lays mighty stress on *going Early to Bed*. He says also, *Ego multos periculosos morbos ac miserias hujus corpusculi mei vito, hac unica ratione, quod semper utor ista diligentia, cito eundi cubitum.*[22] This is very sure, *sitting up late* is Bad for the *Body*, and *Lying abed late* is not Good for the *Soul!*[23]

There is *Virtue* as well as *Humour* consulted in the old Epigram,
> *Si tibi deficiant Medici, Medici tibi fiant*
> *Haec Tria, Mens laeta, Requies, Moderata Diaeta.*[24]

When all Physicians fail, call Dr. *Quiet*,
With Dr. *Merry-man*, and Dr. *Diet*.

Some insist much on this as a most important Maxim, *Sint Tempestivae Caenae, laetaeque, Brevesque.*[25]

What if we should add an observation of that Great Man, The Lord *Verulam: Nihil magis conducit ad Sanitatem et longaevitatem quam, crebrae et domesticae purgamines. A Family Purge* now and then taken, præserves *Health*, and prolongs *Life*, to Admiration![26]

Monsr *Galland*[27] has a pretty Story, in his Collection of *Orientalisms*. A King of *Persia* sent a Physician to *Mahomet*, who staid some years in *Arabia*, without any Practice. The Physician at length made a Sad Complaint, That Nobody had made any Use of him; whereto *Mahomet* answered: *I don't know what's the Matter, but its the Custome of our Country never to eat but when we are Hungry, and always wrise with an Appetite.* The Physician replied, *Nay then, good Syr, lett me be gone. Your people will never have any Need of a Doctor.* So he took his leave, and returned for *Persia*.

We will clinch all with a Stroke of Dr. *Cheyne*,[28] in the Conclusion of his *Essay of Health and Long Life*. The *Grand Secret*, and *Sole Method* for *Long Life*, is, To keep the Blood and Juices, in a due State of *Fluidity*.[29] In spite of all we can do, Time and Age will *Stiffen* them.

It is a Mistake, that *Thin Blood* is *Poor Blood*.

There is nothing under the Sun, that can render the Blood and Juices, *Thin*, and *Sweet*, and *Right*, and constantly in a Flowing State, but keeping to a *Spare, Lean, Fluid* sort of a *Diet*.

No *Voluptuous* Person, and one abandoned unto *Laziness*, is a *Long Liver;* Except he has an original Constitution of *Brass*. And Even *Then*, his Life has more Misery in it, than ever any *Sober Galley-slave* endured; and at last he dies on the *Rack*, in all the *Sufferings*, but without the *Comforts*, of a *Martyr*.

All who have *Lived Long* and without much Pain, have *Lived Abstemiously;* and in their latter days done little Short of *Starving*. Hereby they have a little weakened their Natural Strength, and qualified the Fire of their Spirits; But they have preserved their *Senses*, prevented their *Griefs*, prolonged their *Days*, and procured themselves a gentle and easy passage through the *Valley of Death*.

Gentle Domestic *Purges* frequently repeated, and moderate *Exercise*, will mightily contribute unto this Happiness; But, as my Doctor says, *The Ground-work, must be laid, carried on, and Finished, in ABSTEMIOUSNESS*.

I will conclude with a Note of Dr. *Morgan*.[30] "The *best Rule* that I know for Health, is to observe strictly *no particular Rule* at all; but upon the general principle of MODERATION to follow the Dictates of *Sober Nature*." Eating and Drinking exactly by *Weight* and *Measure*, he explodes as a *Cook-pedantry*, and a most

Ridiculous as well as pernicious *Regularity*. Such an *Oeconomist* (he says) might as well impose upon himself to stand or sitt always in the *Same Place*, ly in the *Same Bed*, wear exactly the *Same Weight* of Clothes, Ride or Walk every Day præcisely the *Same Number* of Inches. Nay, he must compound with Providence for the same Immutable *Weather* too. For the Changes of *That*, require sometimes *Larger* and sometimes *Lesser Meals*, and the *occasional use* of stronger or weaker Liquors.

The *Vita tuta ad Vitam Longam*,[31] has been thus laid out by the *Wise Men of Enquiry*. The *Natural Means* for the *Prolongation of Life*, hitherto proposed, have many of them something of *Morality* in them. Those that are more purely *Moral* ones, ought also to come into Consideration with us.

R. *Nechonia*,[32] a long-lived Jew, being asked on his Death-bed, *How he came to live so long?* Answered; *I never sought my own Honour by the Disgrace of another Man. I never Injured my Neighbour. And I liberally dispensed my Wealth to them that wanted it.* It was thought he had in his Eye, the *Twelfth* and *Thirteenth* Verses of the *Thirty fourth Psalm*.[33]

It has been often observed, That very *Liberal Men*, are very *Long-Lived Men*: And so, *After many Days* they reap the *Harvest* of the *Seed Corn Cast into the Moist Ground* by their Bounties.

The *Fifth-Commandment* has a well-known *Promise* annexed unto it.

But One very Notable Way to *Live Long*, is to *Dy daily;* or, to *Live* in a Daily Expectation of *Death*.

One writes thus, "Men have a great many good Rules; As, *Too much Oil putts out the Lamp*. And, *Spare Diet is the greatest Cordial of Nature*. And, *Discreet Fasting is the best Physick*. But they have one Rule, which spoils all; *Temperance must needs prolong our Time: The Moderate Man shall have many Days*. The *over-ruling* providence of God, must not be *overlooked*."

The promise of *Long Life*, and of *Terrestrial Blessings*, will be sufficiently, yea, and in the very *Letter*, fulfilled in what *our God* will do for us in the *World to come*. The Beleever will very patiently consent unto it, that his *Harvest* be deferr'd unto the *Life that is to come*.

The *Expectation of Death*, in one who *So Numbers his Days, as to apply his Heart unto Wisdome*, will putt him upon those Things, that will certainly secure a Long Life unto him: that is to say, To

Redeem the Time, and *Live Long in a Little Time.*

Concerning the Children of Men, who *spend their Days in Vanity,* we read, *They are as a Sleep;* that is, They Spend their *Days* [their *Nights,* I should say; for they are always *in the Dark!*] like People that are *Asleep.* They neither mind how the *Time* goes, nor think why the *Time* is allow'd unto them. *One Third* of our *Time,* we ly *Dead,* in regard of the *Sleep* which *Nature* calls for. *The Rest* of our *Time,* if it be not wisely Employ'd, is a *Sleep,* wherin we are *Dead while we live.* An Impious Thing, whom we may call *A Sinner an hundred years old,* must yett have that *Epitaph* upon him; *Diu fuit, Sed parum Vixit.*[34] And how justly may *the Days of the Wicked be shortened!* if God will not lett them *Live,* who know not how to *Live!*

CHRISTIAN, Fill thy *Life* with most explicit *Acknowledgments* of the Glorious God, and acts of *Obedience* to Him: Lett even the whole Business of thy *Temporal Calling,* be explicitly designed for an *Obedience* to God. At the same time, fill thy Life, with *Good Offices* to Mankind, and with *Actions* that shall be *Blessings* (and make the *Doer* a Rich one) unto thy Neighbours. This will be *Living. Caetera Mortis erunt.*[35] The man who has done the most of these Things, is the *Longest Liver.* In Three Sevens of years, one who *Lives* at this rate, may have a *Longer Life* than a drowsy, and a thoughtless wretch, that should gett along to *Nine hundred and sixty nine.* I may make the more free with the Number in my Expression on this Occasion. Because the Jewish Rabbis venture to tell us, That the Time lost by *Methuselah* in impertinent Things being defalk'd from his *Nine hundred and Sixty nine* years, he will have no more than Ten years of *True Life* left unto him.

An Old Man, who began to Turn and Live unto God but *three years before* his Expiration, ordered these Emphatical Words for his Gravestone; Here Lies an Old Man, that lived but Three years in the World.

It is a Maxim of Truth, *Non Annis Sed Factis Vivunt Mortales.*[36] And, *They have Lived Longest in the World, who have done most good in the World.*

Come then, *Awake, and Live, ye who dwell in the Dust!* Measure your *Lives,* not by your *Almanack,* but by your *Conscience* and your *Usefulness.* *Live* to God, and for the Good of Men; and Remember,

Vita, Si Scias uti, Longa est.[37]

CAP. III. *Therapeutica Sacra.*

or,

The Symptoms of an HEALED SOUL,
With the Methods of coming at it.

Melius est audire Socratem *de Moribus, quam*
Hippocratem *de Humoribus disputantem.*[1]

The most *Illustrious,* and the most *Comprehensive* of all Blessings, we have now in Prosecution. We will in the most *Affectuous* as well as in the most *Compendious* manner that may be, prosecute it. It shall be done, by an Exhibition of a *Contemplation* formed by One, who was thus *Taught by the Thorns and Briars of the Wilderness.*

Of the ancient *Essenes,* there was one Sort, called *Therapeutae,*[2] or *Physicians;* Not from their studying *Physick,* but because the *Health* of the Soul, and a Care to come at the Blessings of an *Healed Soul,* was the chief of their Studies. Reader, a *Therapeuta* is now addressing of thee.

It is a notable Expression of *Salvian, Sancti Viri infirmi; quia si fortes fuerint, sancti esse vix possint.*[3]

I have known a Servant of God under Languishments and Confinements, often make this an *Episode* in the *Hymns,* of the *Nightingale.*

My Glorious Healer, Now Restore
My Health, and make me whole.
But this is what I most implore:
Oh! for an HEALED SOUL!

"Upon the Occasion of SICKNESS on myself and others, I sett myself to consider PIETY, and the Effects of it, under the Notion of *An HEALED SOUL.*

That I might have the Symptoms and the Comforts of, *An Healed Soul,* I proposed these Attainments.

First: Lett me come to entertain the *Right Thoughts of the Righteous,* concerning the Infinite God; and therewithal, by *Faith* in the *Sacrifice* of my SAVIOUR become *Reconciled* unto Him.

Secondly: Lett me come to make it the *Chief End* of all my *Actions,* That God may be gratified and glorified in the *Acknowledgments* which He sees we pay unto Him.

Thirdly: Lett me come to make it the *Main Sweet* of all my

Enjoyments, That I may See God in all my *Enjoyments,* and *Serve* Him with them.

Fourthly: Lett me still have my Eye to God, in all my *Expectations,* and look upon all *Second Causes* as no more than Such.

Fifthly: Lett me have my *Will* entirely swallowed up in the *Will* of God.

And finally: Lett me be full of *Benignity* towards my *Neighbour;* and make it my Continual Study *To do as I would be done unto.*

Now have I an HEALED SOUL. And now no *Events* can come amiss unto me.

The *Cure* of what I feel at any time amiss in my Condition, lies *Within.* My Appetites *Within,* which give me all my Disturbance when any Thing seems amiss, these are now happily cured.

Such a Soul will be able to take the *Bitterest Cup* which the *Heavenly Father* shall appoint for its Portion, and find a *Sweetness* in it.

Yea, I have God now *Reigning* in my Soul. There is a Return of God unto His *Throne* in my Soul, upon this *Healing* of it. And will God so *disgrace the Throne of His Glory,* as to condemn it unto the Flames; or, a *Palace* which the Holy SPIRIT of God has prepared and Adorned for Him, Will He throw it among the *Dunghils* of the Earth, and make it the *Fuel* of His Indignation? It were an *Impiety* to imagine it.

The *Healing* of my Soul, takes away from it those *Maladies* of a *Carnal Mind,* which unfitt me for an Admission into that City of God, where *Nothing which defiles may Enter.* Nay, my *Healed Soul* will have God forever *dwelling* in it: It Adheres to God; It Conforms to God; It Rejoices in God at such a Rate, that it has *Heaven* itself, after some Sort, inwrought into the very Temper of it. Were it possible for such a Soul to be thrown down into the *Place of Dragons,* it would carry *Heaven* thither with it. O *Soul sure of Heaven!* As fast as thou art *Healing,* so fast art thou *Ripening* for *Heaven:* So fast *Heaven* is *Descending* to thee: Verily, Thou *hast Everlasting Life.*

Now, that I may come at the *Blessings* of such *An Healed Soul,* my Course must be to Repair unto a Glorious CHRIST continually, A Glorious CHRIST who is, *The Lord my Healer,* And, the *Sun of Righteousness* from whose *Wings* alone, *Healing* is to be looked for.

And among other *Methods* of applying to my SAVIOUR, there are Especially *Two,* that I must make a *Daily Improvement* of.

There is, first, the *Blood* of my SAVIOUR: O marvellous Word! The *Blood* of my *Physician:* A Sovereign *Balsam* for all the *Distempers* of my Soul. I am to plead it with the great God; *Lord, The Blood of my SAVIOUR has purchased for me the Happiness of an healed Soul; For the Sake of that Blood, Oh, Lett me have an happy and an healed Soul.* Upon Every *Malady* in my Soul, and upon every fresh Commission of *observable Sin,* which is an out-breaking of a *Malady* there, oh! lett me make a *New Flight* unto the *Blood* of my SAVIOUR.

But then, secondly, I must *Meditate* much on my SAVIOUR: and especially employ serious and Frequent *Meditation* on the *Pattern* of my SAVIOUR. This will be the *Changing* of my Soul, *into His Image from Glory to Glory.* A Soul *Full* of a CHRIST, and *Like* to a CHRIST, is an *Healed Soul.* That I may come at this, I must be much in *Beholding the Glory of the Lord.* Especially, Lett me *Behold* Him, as *Glorious in Holiness,* and *Behold* Him in the *Exemple* of all *Goodness* which He has given me. For the Cure of my *Slothfulness* in and *Backwardness* to, the *Service* of God, Lett me behold my diligent SAVIOUR, *Eaten up with the Zeal of God.* For the Cure of my Inclinations to *Sensual Pleasures,* Lett me Behold my Self-Denying SAVIOUR, a *Man of Sorrows and Acquainted with Griefs.* For the Cure of my Disposition to *Anger* and *Revenge,* Lett me behold my SAVIOUR, the *Lamb of God,* Oppressed and injured, and *not opening His Mouth.* For the Cure of Every *Envious* or *Evil* Frame towards my Neighbour, Lett me behold my SAVIOUR *moved with Compassion for the Multitude.* For the Cure of a Mind sett upon *Earthly Enjoyments,* lett me behold my SAVIOUR willing to be among the *Poor of this World.* For the Cure of my *Pride,* Lett me behold my SAVIOUR, *Humbling Himself,* becoming *of no Reputation,* Willing to be *Despised and Rejected of Men.*

In this Way the Blessings of <u>An Healed Soul</u> are to be waited for."

I will add a Passage of One, upon that Praise of *Wisdome;* "It shall be Health to all the Flesh [Prov. IV.22.] *All the Flesh* of Man, is not his Body. There is a *Fleshly Part* of the Soul, and a *Sickly Part* it is. To *This* there is an *Health* derived, by the Maxims of *Wisdome.*"

As a *Succedaneum* to these Meditations, I will transcribe a Passage or two from the Life of the famous Dr. *Henry More.*[4]

He made this Remark upon himself; *That the more he applied himself to* Piety, *he found his very Body the better for it.*

An Eminent Lady having Long Languished under a Chronical Malady, he advised her *To betake herself wholly to* God, and make that noble Experiment, Whether the *Consummate Health of her Soul,* would not recover also in due time the *Health of her Body.*

In his Illustrations on Daniel (Ch. 5. Ver. 13, 14) he has this passage, *"Temperance* and *Devotion* and a *Cheerful Dependence on God's Blessing,* even with *Mean Diet,* must contribute much to *Health* and *Beauty,* and a quick and delicate Air in the Countenance. This is what the *Pythagoreans*[5] call *Philosophical Temperance,* the Mother of that *Wisdome* which *makes the Face to shine,* and nourishes the *Luciform Vehicle* of the Soul."

Allow me also to transcribe another passage from Dr. *Cheyne,* "The *Love of God,* as it is the Sovereign Remedy of *all Miseries,* so, in particular, it *Prevents* all the *Bodily Disorders* the *Passions* introduce; by keeping the *Passions* themselves within due Bounds; and by the unspeakable *Joy,* and perfect *Calm,* Serenity and Tranquility it gives the Mind, it becomes the most powerful of all the Means of *Health* and *Long Life."*

CAP. IV. The *Tree of Life.*

with a
Mantissa[1] of a *Panacaea.*

THE Blessings of, *An Healed SOUL,* are what we have in prosecution. We read of a glorious *Tree* to be seen upon the *Earth* when the Holy City of God shall *come down out of Heaven,* and be *near* to it, and be *seen* by it, and make it a *Paradise* by its Blessed Influences: Rev. XXII.2. *The Leaves of The Tree are for the Healing of the Nations.* In the mean time, why should not our *Bible* be such a *Tree of Life* unto us? Most certainly, *The Leaves* of this Tree will do wonders *for the Healing of the Nations!* I have read of a *Rabbi* among the ancient Hebrews, who putting himself into the Habit of a Travelling Physician, gave out, that he had a Sovereign *Remedy,* which would be no less than a *Water of Life* unto as many as used it. People repairing to him for his *Remedy,* he produced the Bible unto them; This, he told them, was the *Fountain of Life:* and he assured them, that the Oracles of Heaven in this Book well-employ'd, and well-observ'd, would help them who *desired Life,* to obtain the Answer of their Desires. I am now going to do the part of the *Hebrew Rabbi*. Attend then unto a PROPOSAL of PIETY, which will be followed with Happy and mighty Consequences.

The *Holy Men of God* who wrote the SCRIPTURE, were *moved by His Holy SPIRIT*, in and for the Writing of it; and the *Spirit of Holiness* at the Time of the Inspiration made suitable *Impressions* on the *Affections* of His Faithful Servants. When the Holy SPIRIT with His *Afflations*, disposed them to write what we have in our Hands, He doubtless produced in their *Hearth*, those *Motions of Piety* which were agreeable and answerable to the *Matter* then flowing from their Pens. In what they have written there is very legible, and a very ordinary Capacity may see, A *Confession* of Divine *Truths*, with an Heart *Beleeving* of them, *Consenting* to them : A *Desire* of promised *Blessings*, with a *Value* for them ; A *Love* to God, and His People ; A *Zeal* for His *Kingdome*, and His *Word*, and *House*, and *Ordinances;* a *Faith* in God, and our SAVIOUR, and His *Promises* with a *Joy* in Him, and a Rapturous *Admiration* of him, and of His *Works*, both in *Creation* and in *Providence;* an *Horror* of *Sin*, and a *Sorrow* for it; and a *Fear* of the *Judgments* threatened unto it; with an *Abhorrence* of, and yett *Compassion* for, them that Committ and Follow it; a *Resolution* for the Service of God ; and a *Retreat* unto Him under Difficulties, with a *Despair* to find Releef in Creatures ; And other *Motions of Piety* which belong to the *Life of God* in the Soul. All true PIETY which lies in *An Healed SOUL*, is begun by the Enkindling of such *Affections* in the Soul; and it prospers as these *Affections* improve in Vigour there. *O Lord, By these Things men Live, and in all these things is the Life of my Spirit: So wilt thou Recover me, and make me to live.*

Now, my Friend, Lay one *Sentence,* and then another, and so a Third, of thy Bible before thee. Find out, which of these *Affections* is most Obvious and Evident, in the *Sentence* under thy Consideration. Try, Strive, do thy best, that the Same *Affections* may stir, yea, flame in thy Soul. Be restless till thou find thy Soul Harmonizing and Symphonizing with what the Holy SPIRIT of God raised in His *Amanuensis* at the Time of His writing. Be not at Rest until thou feel thy Heart-strings quaver, at the Touch upon the Heart of the Writer, as being brought into an *Unison* with it, and the *Two Souls* go up in a flame together. When thou wouldest bring thyself into the *Best Frame* that can be wished for, Take a short Paragraph of the

Word by which Men live, and with humble Addresses unto Heaven, pertinent unto the Occasion, *Consider* What *Affections of Piety* are plainly discernible in the *Word* now before thee; And then with a Soul turning to the Lord, essay to utter the Language of the like *Affections.* Ere thou art aware, thou will be *caught up to Paradise.* Thou wilt *mount up as with the Wings of Eagles.*

Nothing would contribute more unto the *Health of the Soul,* than such an *Exercise!* In some countries they have a fond and vain Superstition: to *fan the Face of the Sick with Leaves of the Bible;* Which they imagine to Contribute unto the Health of the Patient. *My Friend,* it will be no superstitious, but an highly serviceable and profitable Thing for thee to gett thy Soul *fanned* with *Afflations* of such Things as are to be found in the *Leaves* of thy Bible; it will contribute unto thy *Health* exceedingly.

Yea, if thou art languishing under *Sickness,* but capable of hearing thy *Bible* read unto thee, Call for as much of it, as thou shalt be able to bear. I have read of a famous Divine, that while he was under the Languor of the Sickness whereof he died, he would often call for *More Julip!*[2] *More Julip!* He meant more *Scripture;* the *Promises* whereof gave him *Hope in his Death,* and were *Life* to him in a *dying* Hour. This *Julip* never comes out of Season. It will *do good like a Medicine.*

The *Egyptians* kept in their Temples with much Care, a *Book* (or more) which was doubtless the same that is by *Diodorus*[3] called, *The Sacred Book:* And the *Physicians* were to regulate their practice by it. Observing the praecepts of that *Book,* they were justified, tho' their Patients died; but if they deviated from it, they were upon the Death of their Patients punished as *Murderers.*

Christian, Thy BIBLE being with thee, thou now hast in thy Hands, a Book much more worthy to be kept unto.

In a Coin of the Emperour *Aurelius Antoninus,*[4] there is a Woman presenting a little *Cake,* before the Altar of *Salus:*[5] [perhaps for the *Health* of the Empire then grievously afflicted with contagious Diseases;] And we are told, That this little *Cake,* which was called, *Sanitas,* being putt into the *Hands* of the Idol, and then taken out again, was accounted a *Sovereign Remedy* for numberless Diseases. But how infinitely short in its Vertues, were that little *Cake,* of this glorious *Book,* which comes out of the *Hands* of God our SAVIOUR unto us!

A *Mantissa*

of a <u>Panacaea</u>; or, A Proposal of an UNIVERSAL
MEDICINE, to them that would Consult their
Health, under and against *All Diseases.*

To propose an *Universal Medicine,* of the *Natural* Sort, and in the
Natural Way, which is commonly talk'd of, is a thing, which the
wiser Physicians do more generally blush to talk of. To seek for
such a Thing is to seek for the *Philosopher's Stone.*[6]

But lett us now speak *Morally;* and see what we may attain to.

It was a Message brought from Heaven, by an ANGEL, to a
Man who *feared God;* Act. X.4. *Thy PRAYERS and thy ALMS are
come up for a Memorial before God.* But What shall we say, if there
are *Prayers* in our *Alms?* As tis a Maxim of *Goodness* in general, *Qui
bene Vivit Semper Orat;*[7] All the *Acts* of it, have so many *Prayers*
in them, and potently utter that Petition, *O do Good unto them that
are Good!* So, it is very particularly to be observed, That our *Alms*
have the Efficacy of powerful *Prayers* in them; and there are passages
in the Divine Oracles which intimate, That *with the Merciful* our
God *will shew Himself merciful,* and, that what we *do for the Poor,*
we *do to Ourselves.*

It must be forever Confessed, That there is no *Merit* in our *Alms.*
No, Nor would there be any *Merit* in it, if we should *Bestow all our
Goods to feed the Poor.* A *Dream* of *Merit,* in *unprofitable Servants*
doing but their *Duty;* O Man, Away with such a *Vanity!* Lett thy
Soul Abhor the least Approaches to it!

Our *Faith* shall also carry the matter thus far. If our *Alms* never
have any Recompences in *This Life,* but while we are abounding
in them, and always *Devising Liberal Things,* we shall still be the
Afflicted, all whose *Days are Evil,* and have all Sorts of Calamities
lying upon us, there shall not be the least Murmur in us, as if the
Promises were not fulfilled, or as if our God *Suffered His Faithfull-
ness to fail.* We will cheerfully adjourn the promised Recompences
unto a *Life to come;* and wait for the *Harvest* of the *Light Sown for
the Righteous,* until we have our *Bodies* laid under the *Clods,* and our
Spirits received into the *Everlasting Habitations.*

Nevertheless, in ALMS liberally dispensed, there are those
Exercises and Expressions of our *Obedience* unto God, which do
præpare us for His Favours; and when a God, who *Waits that He may
be gracious,* beholds us arrived unto those Dispositions, which will

assure His *Praises* from the Favours which He bestows upon us, we shall soon see, what it will be His Pleasure to do for us.

It is a thing to be more thought upon; our God is to us, what *we* are to *One another:* only that *He* infinitely *Exceeds,* infinitely *Transcends,* in His Goodness, All that we can be to *One another.* Our SAVIOUR has intimated it unto us, That because we would have our *Heavenly Father give Good Things unto us,* THEREFORE all *things whatsoever that we would have Men do to us, we should even so do to them.* And in the *Platform of Prayer* which our SAVIOUR has given us, that Clause *Forgive as we Forgive,* tho' it be placed where it is, because it is of all the most uneasy to be attended *There,* yett it is to be understood that the *Like* is to be annexed unto the *Rest:* As, *give us this Day our daily Bread, as we do what we can to help others unto their daily Bread;* And, *Lead us not into Temptation, as we do what we can to keep others out of Temptation.* And, *Deliver us from the Evil, as we do what we can, that others may be Delivered from the Evil.* Thus, when we pray, *Lord, Bestow Health upon us:* Oh! That we might be able to add this Clause unto it,—*As we do what we can, that Others may Enjoy the Health which is to be desired for them!*

Now, in the Pursuance of this PIETY, how can we forgett that Word! Psal. XLI. 1,2,3. *Blessed is he that considers the Poor; The Lord will deliver him in the Time of Trouble; The Lord will preserve him and keep him alive; The Lord will Strengthen him on the Bed of Languishing; Thou wilt make all his Bed in his Sickness.* That Word! Isa. LVIII.10, 11. *If thou draw out thy Soul to the Hungry, and Satisfy the Afflicted Soul, the Lord shall satisfy thy Soul in Drought, and make fatt thy Bones, and thou shalt be like a watered Garden.* It will not be at all improper for an *Angel of Bethesda* now to address an *Invalid* with such a PROPOSAL as this. When you have *any Distemper* lying upon you, Look out for some very *poor Patient* that is Languishing under *the Same Distemper,* and either undertake to *pay for their Cure,* or at least, Send them *Something* to Releeve them, and comfort them under their Adversity.

Or, if you can't hear of any *Needy Object* under *the Same Distemper,* then find out One under some *Other Sickness,* and cause them to taste the *Cordials* of your *Bounties.*

If they are the *Children of God,* and such as know what it is to *Pray* unto Him, then very particularly and importunately Entreat them to *Pray* for you. Such *Purchased Prayers,* who can tell, how far they may be *Prevailing* ones!

I have known Some Servants of God, who have not been under the Actual Arrest of *Grievous Diseases,* but only *Afraid* of them; to exert a singular Charity, to such as were Labouring under those *Grievous Diseases.*

Be sure, *God is well-pleased with Such Sacrifices,* when a CHRIST is not forgotten in them.

Efficacissima Deprecatio in Eleemosynis,—Et velociter ad Divinas Aures Conscendit talibus Oratio Elevata Suffragiis.[8]

CAP. V. *Nishmath-Chajim.*
The probable SEAT of all Diseases,
and a general CURE for them,
further discovered.
More particularly for *Splenetic*
and *Hysteric* Maladies, which make so great a part
of our Distempers.

I.   THERE is *a Spirit in Man;* A Wonderful Spirit, which from very good Authority may be called *NISHMATH-CHAJIM;* [or, *The Breath of Life:*] And which may be of a *Middle Nature,* between the *Rational Soul,* and the *Corporeal Mass;* But may be the *Medium of Communication,* by which they work upon One another. It wonderfully receives also *Impressions* from *Both* of them. And perhaps it is the *Vital Ty* between them. The Scriptural Anatomy of *Man,* into *Spirit,* and *Soul,* and *Body,* seems to favour and invite the Apprehensions, which we are now proceeding to. When our SAVIOUR so excused His drowsy Disciples, *The Spirit is willing, but the Flesh is Weak;* Doubtless, By *the Spirit,* he means, what His Apostle afterwards called *The Mind,* and *The Spirit of the Mind,* and, *The Inner-Man.* But there being also in Man, that which is called, *The Soul,* or, *The Heart,* or that Principle and Passion, which is concerned most immediately for the Præservation of the *Life,* and of the Comforts that may sweeten it. This Principle is called *The Flesh.* The *Flesh* of the Disciples here, which now so rebelled against the Spirit, was not the Lust of *Pleasures* and *Riches* and the Like; But it was that most *Natural Affection* of the *Soul* which lay in a Desire to shun *Death* and *Grief*. And this *Flesh* here is called *Weak*, not because it wanted *Strength*, for it was in Truth, too *Strong:* But because it wanted *Health;* it was out of order. For the *Health* of the *Soul*, it lies in its *Obeying* and not *Opposing* the empire of the *Mind*.

II.   The *Great God who formed all things*, and who after a Singular Manner *forms the Spirit of Man within him*, has embued this *Nishmath-Chajim*, with marvellous *Faculties;* which yett are all of them short of those *Powers*, which enable the *Rational Soul*, to Penetrate into the *Causes of Things:* to do Curious and Exquisite Things in the *Mathematical Sciences*. And above all, To act upon a principle of *Love to God*, and with the *Views* of *Another World*.

III.   Some *Rays of Light* concerning this *Nishmath-Chajim*, have been darted into the Minds of many Learned Men, who have yett after all remained very much in the *Dark* about it.

Famous have been the Sentiments of *Helmont*[1] (and some other *Masters of Obscurities*) about it; Who would Exhibit it under the Name of the *Archaeus;* and with much of Reason press, that in the *Cure of Diseases*, there may be more of Regard paid unto it.

According to *Grembs*[2] (writing, *De Ortu Rerum*) it is, *Medium quid inter Vitam et Corpus, et veluti Aura nitens Splendensque.* A Sort of *Luminous Air*, Which is of a *Middle Nature*, betwixt Spirituous and Corporeous.

It has the Denomination of The Aerial Spirit, with some Philosophers, who trouble the Stars, more than there is any Need for.

Even the *Galenists* themselves, have not been without some *Suspicions*, yea, Some *Acknowledgments*, of our *Nishmath-Chajim*. and have given very *Broad Hints* concerning it. And no doubt, they may thank the old *Platonists*[3] for instructing of them. The great *Fernelius*,[4] One of the most Illustrious Men that ever shone among them, (writing, *De Abditis rerum Causis*) gives a very lively Description of it. Yea, He finds it in the τὸ ενορμων or, *Inciter*,[5] of *Hippocrates;* and having a great *Power of Incursion*, like the *Wind*, he allows it some Affinity with the Nature of *Body;* But inasmuch as it is *Invisible*, it must also have some Affinity with what is *Incorporeal:* So, he will have it of a *Middle Nature* between *Both*. But he supposes it the *Vehicle*, and proper Seat of the *Soul*, and all its Faculties; and if we call it, their *Body*, we shall have his permission for it.

And indeed, the old *Platonists* had a Notion, of a certain Excellent *Body*, Pellucid and Ethereal, Subservient unto the Faculties of the *Soul*, and uniting it unto the more Terrestrial *Body*.

Heurnius,[6] whom some reckon and value next unto *Fernelius,* (in his *Institutions*) describes it as, *A Kind of Ethereal Spirit, Elaborated out of the purest Part of the Blood, and changed into the Substance of a very Subtil Air; and the prime Instrument of the Soul for the Performance of its Functions.*

IV. Our *Nishmath-Chajim* seems to be commensurate unto our Bodies; and our *Bodies* are conformable to the Shape which God our Maker gives to that *plastic Spirit,* (if we may call it so.) But by what *Principle* the Particles of it, which may be finer than those of the *Light* itself, are kept in their *Cohæsion* to one another, is a Thing yett unknown unto us.

V. And how it fares in the case of *Amputations* on our *Bodies;* Whether like a Flame violently Struck off, what is so, may not nimbly, as by a sort of *Magnetism,* Reunite with what it belongs unto: But then, how far it becomes for the present folded up into it: Or, whether it be not entirely lost, but what remains, may have the power to produce a Recruit, when there shall be a Lodging again provided for it; this also is yett unknown unto us.

VI. The *Nishmath-Chajim* is the *Spirit* of the Several *Parts,* Where it has a Residence; and it is the *Life* by which the Several Parts have their *Faculties* maintained in Exercise. *This* tis, that *Sees,* that *Hears,* that *Feels;* and performs the *Several Digestions* in the *Body.* And the *Animal World,* having *Animam Pro Sale,* if it were not for *This,* would quickly putrify.

VII. We have sometimes been led by our *Microscopes,* into some Apprehensions,[7] That our *Bodies* are Originally folded up, in inconceivably minute *Corpusculicumcules;*[8] and that *Generation* is nothing but the *Evolution* of the *Stamina* so involved: Which Operation is carried on, by *filling them up* with a Matter agreeable to them, till they have an Augmentation to the utmost extent of the Dimensions, that they can reach unto: *And* that the *Resurrection of the Dead,* which is in the Sacred Scriptures called, a *Filling of the Dead Bodies,* will find out the old *Stamina* of the Forsaken Body, again Shrunk up into its first Parvity, and Replenish it with a more *Ethereal Matter,* fitt for the Coelestial Employments and Enjoyments intended for it. But this Hypothesis is Encumbred with Difficulties which drive us into a *Nishmath-Chajim,* either to support and perfect the Hypothesis, or to yeeld us a Better upon the failing of it.

VIII. The *Nishmath-Chajim* is indeed, *Generationis Faber ac Rector:* and as it Leads to the Acts requisite in *Generation,* without any further *Instructor,* So it is the *Spirit,* whose *Way we know not, for shaping the Bones,* and other Parts, *in the Womb of her that is with Child.*

IX. There are indeed many Things in the Humane Body, that cannot be solved by the Rules of *Mechanism.*[9] Our *Nishmath-Chajim* will go very far to help us, in the Solution of them. Indeed we can scarce well Subsist without it.

X. There is an astonishing Operation, and indeed some Illustration and Explanation, of the *Nishmath-Chajim,* in *prægnant Women;* whose Imagination frequently makes Impressions on the *unborn Infants,*[10] that would Exceed all Beleef, if we had them not Continually in View before our Eyes. The Instances are so Numerous and So Various, that one might compile a large Volume of them; and almost ask a *Palæphatus*[11] to afford a Title for it. But in what other Way to be accounted for?

XI. For the *Nishmath-Chajim* we may safely be *Traducians.*[12] It is a Flame Enkindled in, and so derived from, the *Parent.* And this *Traduction,* (which is *Luminis e Lumine*) may help us Considerably, in our Enquiries, *How the Dispositions of our Original Sin are Convey'd and Infus'd into us?*

XII. It was of old, yea, it is at this day, a prevailing Opinion, among the Strangers to the *glorious Gospel of the Blessed God,* That the *Manes,* which remain after *Death,* have still an *Humane Shape,* and all the Parts both External and Internal, which there were in the *Body* that is now deserted: yea, That there is a *Food* which this *Departed Spirit* Craves for and Lives on. *Homer* inflicts punishments on the Wicked after *Death,* which there must be a Sort of *Bodies* to be the Subjects of. And *Plato* Speaks of those that are punished in *Hell,* as having such *Members* and Faces as they had once upon the Earth. Indeed *Justin Martyr*[13] argues from it that these old Gentlemen must needs have some Knowledge and Beleef of our Doctrine of, *The Resurrection of the Dead.* But what shall we say, when our Glorious LORD-REDEEMER, in His *Parable* of *The Rich Man,* Supposes his *Body* in the *Grave,* and yett, being in *Hell,* he cries out of a *Body,* and particularly, of a *Tongue,* that is tormented there? Many of the Ancients thought there was much of a Real *History* in the *Parable;* and their Opinion was, That there is, Διαφορα κατα τας μορφας *A Distinction* (and so a Resemblance,) *of men as to their Shapes after Death.* We find This was the Opinion of *Irenæus;*[14] who proves, From what our SAVIOUR speaks of the *Dead Man,* that the Souls which have putt off their *Bodies,* do yett *Characterem Corporum Custodire,* preserve the *Shapes* of the Bodies, to which they were united. And from the same Speech of our SAVIOUR, *Tertullian*[15] does infer; *Effigiem Animae et Corporales Lineas,* the *Shape* and *Corporeal Lineaments* of the Soul. I will say nothing of what *Thespesius*[16] returning to Life reported about the, τὰ των ψυχων χρώματα *The Colours of Souls* and the *Ulcers* by their *Passions* Left upon them.

On this Occasion the Words of M. Dacier,[17] in her Notes upon Homer's Odysses, are not unworthy to be considered: which give us the Observation, That a fine Subtil Sort of *Body,* accompanied the *Intellect* after the Separation of the *Soul* by Death from the grosser *Body.*

XIII.   The *Nishmath-Chajim* is much like the *Soul* which animates the *Brutal World:* Even that *Spirit of the Beast, Which goeth downward unto the Earth;* but is by the Hand of the Glorious Creator impregnated with a *Capacity* and *Inclination,* for those Actions, Which are necessary for the *Præservation* of themselves, and the *Propagation* of their *Species.* The *Nidification* of *Birds,* the *Mellification* of *Bees,* and a thousand Such Things, how Surprising Works done in the Brutal World, Without any *Rational Projection* for them! And hence, there are also many Actions done by us, that have a Tendency to our Safety and Welfare, Which are not the Effects of any *Rational Projection;* but such as we do by what we call, *A Meer Instinct of Nature,* fall into. The *Sucking Infant,* yea, and the *Nursing Mother,* too do Very Needful and Proper Things, without Consulting of *Reason* for the doing of them.

It is a thing which who can observe without Astonishment? In Every other *Machin,* if anything be out of Order, it will remain so till Some Hand from Abroad shall rectify it; It can do nothing for itself. But the *Humane Body* is a *Machin,* wherein, if anything be out of Order, presently the *Whole Engine,* as under an Alarum, is awakened for the helping of what is amiss, and other Parts of the Engine Strangely putt themselves out of their Way that they may send in Help unto it. Whence can this proceed but from a *Nishmath-Chajim* in us, with such *Faculties* and such *Tendencies* from God imprinted on it?

XIV.   Having at some time or other felt a Considerable *Smart,* or been considerably *Sick,* from something that we have mett withal, we have an *Abiding Horror* for that thing perhaps all our Days. Tho' we *Certainly Know* that the Thing will now do us *No Hurt;*

but rather do us *Much Good,* yett no Conviction of *Reason* will over-come our *Abiding Horror.* We cannot Swallow the *Pill,* or take the *Meat* or the *Drink,* and do an hundred Things, which we have here-tofore been horribly frighted at. Our *Nishmath-Chajim* has an *Incurable Aversion* for them.

XV. Tis the *Nishmath-Chajim,* that is the *Strength* of Every Part in our Body, and that gives *Motion* to it. Here perhaps the Origin of *Muscular Motion* may be a little accounted for. And this is the *Spirit,* and the *Balsams,* and One might almost say, the *Keeper,* of Each Part, which is occupied and befriended with it. Yea, What Construction shall we make of it, When People have lived without any *Brains* in their *Heads,* and after the Destruction of almost all the *Bowels* in their *Bodies?* We are Supplied and Surprised with many most credible Relations of such Things. And I quæstion, Whether anything will do so well, or go so far, as our *Nishmath-Chajim,* to account for them.

XVI. The principal Wheel in the *Animal Oeconomy,* is the *Stom-ach.* And we shall now find that which above all things the *Digestion* there, is to be ascribed unto. Dispute, *O Philosophers, and Physicians,* How *Digestion* is performed in the *Stomach.* Tis the *Nishmath-Cha-jim* after all, that is above all, the *Main Digester.* Else, how could a *Stomach* that is actually *Cold,*[18] and has in it no very *Tastable* or *Notable* Humour for this Purpose, *Digest* the very *Stones* that are taken down into it?

The taking of Some *Repast,* is in our Sacred Scripture Sometimes called, *The Establishing of the Heart.* The *Heart,* is not Seldome, a term for our *Nishmath-Chajim.*

XVII. It is the *Nishmath-Chajim,* that is more Eminently the *Seat* of our *Diseases,* or the *Source* of them. To pass by what they quote of *Herophilus,*[19] we find *Plato* eloquently demonstrating, That all *Dis-eases* have their Origin in the *Soul.* Yea, as long ago as the Days of *Hippocrates,*[20] the *Essentials* of *Diseases* began to be discovered; and the Pacifying and Rectifying of the *Enforcing Spirit* was proposed as the most ready way to cure them.

Quaere: How far the Decays of *Old Age* are to be found in the Circumstances of the *Nishmath-Chajim* falling under Impairments? And whence it came to pass that when *Moses* was very old, yett *his Eye was not dim, nor his Natural Force abated?*

Is not this the true, *Humidum Radicale,*[21] they use to talk of? And is not this the *Microcosmic Air,* whereto *Tachenius*[22] ascribes the Cure of the *Gout* by a Strong Perturbation of the mind; upon which he concludes it animated?

XVIII.   It is probable, that when we dy, the *Nishmath-Chajim* goes away, as a Vehicle to the *Rational Soul;* and continues unto it an Instrument of many Operations. Here we have Some Solution for the Difficulties, about *Place,* and the *Change* of it, for such an *Immaterial Spirit* as the *Rational Soul:* And some Account for *Apparitions* of the *Dead:* the *Spectres,* which are called both *Spirits,* and *Phantasms,* in our *Gospel.* Yea, We are certain of it That Persons before they have *Died,* upon Strong Desires to Visit and Behold Some Objects at a Distance from the *Place* to which they were now confined, have been thrown into a *Trance,* wherein they have lain some considerable while without *Sense* or *Breath;* and then Returning, have reported what they have Seen. But incontestible Witnesses have deposed that *in This Time,* they were actually Seen at the *Place,* which they affirmed they had gone unto.

   And here also we do a little understand how our Apostle in the Raptures (which the Scoffing *Lucian*[23] derides him for) wherein he supposes he might be *Out of the Body,* yett he *heard Words:* he was yett *Sensible* of Occurrences.

   In reading of *Homer,* (as has been already in part observed) we find his Notion to be the same with what was in the *Egyptian* Philosophy; which Supposed that Man was compounded of Three Parts; An Intelligent Mind, called, φρήν, or, ψυχη. A Vehicle, called, ειδωλον The *Image,* or the *Soul.* And a Gross *Body,* called, εωμα The *Soul,* in which they look'd on the *Mind* as Lodged they Supposed Exactly to resemble the *Body* in Shape, and Bulk, and Features; being in the Body as the Statue in the Mould; and so after its Departure keeping the *Image* of the *Body.*

   Plutarch very distinctly delivers this Doctrine; and sais, when the *Soul* is compounded with the *Understanding,* it makes *Reason:* and when compounded with the *Body,* it makes *Passion.* The one Composition is the Principle of *Pleasure* and *Pain;* the other of *Vertue* and *Vice.* He adds, Man dies two Deaths: The *first Death* makes him Two of Three; the *Second* makes him One of Two.

XIX.   In the Indisputable and Indubitable Occurrences of *Witchcrafts* (and *Possessions*) there are many things, which, because they are *Hard to be understood,* the *Epicurean Sadducees*[24] content themselves, in their Swinish Manner, only to Laugh at. But the *Nishmath-Chajim* well understood, would give us a Marvellous Key to lett us into the Philosophy of them.

XX. And now, for Some Important Consequences.

*M*ost certainly, the Physician that can find out Remedies (particularly in the *Mineral* or *Vegetable* Kingdome) that shall have a more Immediate Efficacy to Brighten, and Strengthen, and Comfort, the *Nishmath-Chajim,* will be the most Successful Physician in the World. Especially, if he can Irradiate the Spirit in the *Stomach,* he will do *wonderfully*.

The things also, which Fortify the *Blood,* and restore a *Volatil Ferment,* in the Vapid and Languid *Blood,* will do wonders for us. It is impossible to kill a Man, (the *Nishmath-Chajim* will never leave him), till the Circulation of his *Blood* be ruined.[25]

He who will best keep in Heart the *Nishmath-Chajim,* will be, ΙΗΤΡΟΣ ΑΝΗΡ ΠΟΛΛΩΝ ΑΝΤΑΞΙΟΣ ΑΛΛΩΝ.[26]

XXI. We read, *Heaviness in the Heart of Man makes it Stoup, but a Good Word makes it glad.* We read, *A cheerful Heart does good like a Medicine, but a broken Spirit dries the Bones.* The Invigoration, or the Debilitation of the *Nishmath-Chajim,* is that wherein those ancient Observations are accomplished. Dr. *Aurbachius,* after Forty years Practice, made this Declaration, *Reipsa Comperi plures homines moestitia ac Dolore Animi mori, quam Violenta Morte.*[27] It is a Remark of *Baglivi,*[28] but it may have been made by Ten Thousand more; "That a great part of our *Diseases,* either do Rise from, or are Fed by, a Weight of *Cares,* Lying on the Minds of Men. *Diseases* that seem Incureable, are easily cured by agreeable *Conversation.* Disorders of the *Mind* first bring Diseases on the *Stomach;* and so the whole Mass of *Blood* gradually becomes infected. And as long as the *Passions of the Mind* continue, the Diseases may indeed change their *Forms;* but they rarely quitt the Patients." A *Bonifacius*[29] heretofore address'd the Physicians on this Occasion, in such Terms as these. *"Tranquility of Mind,* will do strange Things towards the Releef of *Bodily Maladies.* Tis not without Reason, that *Hofman* in his Dissertation *Des Moyens de Vivre Longtems,* does insist on *Tranquillity of Mind* as the Chief among the *Ways to Live Long;* And that this is the Cause why we read, *The Fear of the Lord tendeth to Life.* They that have practised, *The Art of Curing by Expectation,* have made an Experiment of what the *Mind* will do towards the Cure of the *Body.* By practising, *The Art of Curing by Consolation,* you may carry on the Experiment. I propound then: Lett the *Physician* with all possible Ingenuity of *Conversation,* find out, what matter of *Anxiety* there may have been upon the Mind of the *Patient;* what there is that has made his Life *uneasy* to him. Having discovered the

Burden, Lett him use all the ways he can devise, to take it off. Offer him such *Thoughts* as may be the *best Anodynes* for his Distressed Mind; especially the *right Thoughts of the Righteous,* and the Ways to a Composure upon *Religious Principles.* Give him a Prospect, if you can, of sound *Deliverance* from his Distresses, or some *Abatement* of them. Raise in him as *Bright Thoughts* as may be; and Scatter the *Clouds,* remove the *Loads,* which his Mind is perplexed withal; especially, by Representing and Magnifying the *Mercy* of God in CHRIST unto him."

XXII.   It is well known, that if *One Third* of our *Diseases,* be those which we call, *Chronical,* more than *One Half* of this Third, will be those, which in *Men* go under the Name of *Splenetic,* and in *Women* go under the Name of *Hysteric;* the *Spleen* and the *Womb*[30] are often enough unjustly accused in these Denominations. It is marvellous to see, in how many *Forms* we undergo *Splenetic* and *Hysteric* Maladies; The very *Toothache* itself often belongs unto them: And marvellous will be the *Success,* marvellous the *Esteem,* of the Physician that can Discover them and Encounter them.

The Sagacious Dr. *Sydenham,*[31] seems to have the Scent of our *Nishmath-Chajim,* when he tells us, That as the *Outward Man* is framed with parts, obvious to *Sense,* thus the *Inward Man* does consist of a due *Series,* and as it were a *Fabric* of *Spirits,* to be view'd only by the Eye of Reason: And as this is united with the Constitution of the *Body,* so the *Frame* of it is more or less Easily Disordered, by how much the *Constitution of the Spirits* is more or less Firm within us. And that the Origin of the *Splenetic* and *Hysteric* Ataxy in the *Body* is a *Feeble Constitution* of the *Spirits,* and the breaking of their *System,* so that they are Easily Dissipated, or have an unæqual Distribution.

These Maladies have many Symptoms, which may serve as *Diagnosticks* for them; Especially these Two: That the *Urine* is Clear, Limpid, and Copious; And, That the Patient is *chiefly affected* with his Indispositions, when he has just had his *Mind* under some Disturbance and Affliction.

It is plain, that these Diseases are not mainly in the *Humours:* inasmuch as *Evacuations* do not releeve, but fearfully Produce and Increase the Diseases. Only indeed, when the Ataxy of the *Spirits,* has by its Continuance at last considerably vitiated the *Humours,—then* a little *Purging* and *Bleeding* may be allowed of.

The Cure is: First, *Quiet* the *Spirits* with proper *Anodynes.*

Then bring them to Rights, and Revive them and Refresh them, and bring a *New Strength* into them. In short, *Confirm the System.* *Chalybeates*[32] do wonders this way; And usually the *Steel* in Substance, more than many of the Common Preparations. *Corroborating Plants,*[33] infused in generous Wine, or a Tea of them, have also done wondrously, yea, *Venice-Treacle*[34] alone (our *Sydenham* sais) as Contemptible as it may seem, yett if often used, and a Long While, it is a great Remedy in This, as well as very many other Diseases, and perhaps *the most Effectual that has hitherto been known in the World.*

The Force of the *Peruvian Bark*[35] Regularly administered, for giving a Vigour to the *Blood,* and so to the *Spirits,* has also been very Surprising, and for the Recovering of people to an Healthy Constitution out of *Splenetic* and *Hysteric* Diseases.

But there is nothing like the Exercise of *Riding on Horse-back* Every Day, when the Weather will allow it; and increasing the Journey by Degrees, till one comes in a Score of Miles in a Day.

XXIII. Upon the Whole;

Of all the Remedies under Heaven, for the Conquering of *Distempers,* and for the Præservation of *Health,* and Prolongation of *Life,* there will now be found none like Serious PIETY. *Many* Remedies *have done Virtuously,* (and had their Virtues) *but thou Excellest them all.* The *Rational Soul* in its Reflections has Powerful and Wonderful Influences on the *Nishmath-Chajim.* Now, in the Methods of PIETY, gett a *Soul* into the *Peace of God,* with Assurance of a *Reconciliation* to Him; and *Walk in the Fear of God,* and the *Comfort of the Holy Spirit;* keeping always in, and Filled always with, His *Love;* and indulge none of those *Lusts,* which render *the Wicked like the Troubled Sea.* Keep a *Conscience,* which in a *Continual Aim* at what is Right shall make a *Continual Feast.* Be not Anxious about *Futurities,* nor Disturbed upon *Provocations;* But lett the *Strong Faith* of a Faithful SAVIOUR *Performing the Thing that is appointed for us* in all that happens, produce a perpetual Tranquillity and Serenity in the Soul. Go on *Singing in the Ways of the Lord,* and Casting all *Burdens* on Him, and, *Rejoicing in the Hope of the Glory of God.* Thus, *I show you a most Excellent Way.*

XXIV. Lett this be Remembred: Moderate *Abstinence,* and Convenient *Exercise;* and Some Guard against injurious *Changes of the Weather,* with an HOLY and EASY MIND, will go as far, in carrying us with *undecay'd garments* thro' the *Wilderness,* to the *Promis'd* and *Pleasant Land,* which we are bound unto, as all the *Præscriptions* with which all the *Physicians* under Heaven, have ever yett obliged us.

CAP. VI. The *Gymnastick.*

or

An Exercitation upon EXERCISE.

WHY should we think of nothing but the *Drug,* When the *Design of Healing* is to be prosecuted? I will beg the Patience that will bestow a perusal upon what I have to offer of another *Proposal.* The Thing to be proposed is, EXERCISE.

When *Herodicus*[1] first brought up the *Gymnastic Physic,* it is a little diverting to see how strongly *Plato*[2] inveigh'd against it. And indeed if the *Gymnastic Rules* obliged people to spend such a vast Portion of their Lives in observing of them, as the Invectives do pretend (or, to live like *Spurinna*[3] long after mentioned by *Pliny,*[4] or even as *Pliny* did himself,) we may allow *Plato* to ridicule them. However, the matter must not go over so.

Whoever it were, that first brought the *Gymnastic,* to make a Figure among the Methods of Cure, *Hippocrates* would fain challenge the Honour of bringing it unto Perfection. How many *Exercises* does he Distinguish and Recommend; and on how many *Occasions?* His Præscription of it, for the Diseases usually ascribed unto the *Spleen,* will certainly be approved of and complied with, and go down more easily, than the Diet he præscribes with it, a Diet of *Dogs-Flesh;* he præscribes the *Cutting of Wood. Hippocrates* is followed by *Galen* in This as well as other things; who wrote a whole Book, *De Parva Pila,*[5] besides what he says of the *Strigil.*[6] It would even tire one to *Tell,* and much more, to *Use,* the various *Exercises* which, *Mercurialis*[7] alone will inform us, were used among the Ancients; and the *Expences* they were at in building of *Places* for them. In the Collections of *Oribasius,*[8] we have some Account of what the *Greek* Writers have upon them. Among the *Latins,* who rather Exceeded the *Greeks* in the *Gymnastic,* we know how much *Exercises* were brought into Request by *Asclepiades,*[9] who called them, *The Common Aids of Physic;* and among whose other Inventions were the *Ludi pensiles,*[10] which were afterwards carried unto a Strange

Degree of Costly Luxury. From *Celsus,* and the rest of the *Latin* Writers, we may learn Abundance to this Purpose. And among other Instances we have *Tully;*[11] of whom it is reported by *Plutarch,*[12] that he was recovered out of desperate Infirmities by some *Exercises;* which he himself also has reported in his *Brutus, Seu De Claris Oratoribus.* It is indeed a Subject not unworthy to be treated by the *Clari Oratores;* who might be very Eloquent and Copious upon it.

It is very Certain, That Convenient EXERCISE, does wonderfully Conduce, not only to the *Præservation* of *Health,* but also to the *Recovery* of it, by Refreshing the *Faculties,* by promoting the *Digestions,* by quickening the *Glands* in making their *Secretions,* and many other Ways too long to be at large described. Sometimes *Exercise alone* will work marvellous Cures, and sometimes in Conjunction with *other Medicines,* it will obtain what the *Medicines alone* would never have reach'd unto. Indeed there is this astonishing Difference, between such a *Divine* Peece of Mechanism as the *Body of Man,* and all *Humane Productions;* that while these are *the Worse for Wearing,* our *Body* is the better for *Exercise:* Agreeable *Motion* Strengthens it, Recruits it, gives a Longer Duration to it. How happily does a convenient *Exercise* operate, both on the *Fluids* and on the *Solids* of the *Body!* The Thoughts of Mr. *Francis Fuller,*[13] in his *Medicina Gymnastica,* have cultivated this Theme with a very notable Ingenuity. Particularly, in that famous Disease, which carries off so many of our English People, The *Consumption;* (whereof Dr. *Benet,*[14] in his *Theatrum Tabidorum,* observes, *Tacita Vi Obrepens Anglis infestissimus est, et nisi Primis Obediens Remedijs (quod rarissime evenit Funestus:)* the Success of *Exercise* begun Seasonably and held on Pertinaciously, has been incredible. Our *Fuller* does insist more particularly on what he calls *an Habit of Riding;* and writes in such Terms as these, "He that in this Distemper above all others, Rides for his Health, must be like a *Tartar,* in a Manner always on *Horseback;* and then from a weak Constitution he may come to the Strength of a *Tartar.* He that would have his *Life for a Prey,* must *hunt* after it; and when once he finds his Enemy give Way, must not leave off, but follow his Blow, till he Subdue him beyond all Possibility of a Return. He that carries this Resolution with him, will, I doubt not, Experience the Happy Effects of the good old Direction, *Recipe Caballum;*[15] He will find that the *English Pad* is the most Noble Medium to be made use of, for a Recovery from a Distemper, which we of this Nation have but too much Reason by way of Eminency to style, *The English.*" In a *Dropsy* of the *Anasarcous*[16] kind, accompanied with *Asthmatic* Distresses, the Benefit of *Exercise,* has been found inexpressible. Δει ταλαιπωρειν, *you must Labour, you must Labour;* This was the old *Coan*[17] Admonition often inculcated, when there was no other Way to dislodge Viscous and Vitious Concretions, but by applying of *Muscular Force* unto them. And particularly in a *Dropsy,* as our Exciter Expresses it, the Patient ought to be alarmed, and look upon himself as in something the like Case with those Criminals, whom the *Dutch,* upon their refusing to work, do Confine unto a Cellar, and lett the Water in upon them, that they may be in a Necessity either of pumping or of Drowning. In those which we call *Splenetic* and *Hysteric* Distempers (and which make up so great a part of our *Chronical* Maladies) there is nothing like a Resolute Course of *Exercise.* In a *Scorbutic Rheumatism* it has done Marvellous Things. In a *Nervous Atrophy*[18] it has done more than could have been Expected from a whole Dispensatory. And in the *Decay of Nature,* which is caused by the Passions and Anguishes of a too Thoughtful Mind, *This* has brought an Alacrity beyond any Cordials.

In short, There never was any Remedy in the World, that came so near to the Claim of a *Catholicon,* as, EXERCISE.

There are Many Sorts of *Exercise,* Whereof they that are Invalids, or fear to be so, may take their Choice; and indeed, an *Adaptation* to special Circumstances may be well considered and endeavoured. But no more than Three shall here be spoken of.

There is first that of Chafing. The Use of the *Flesh-brush* was prodigiously admired by the people of old Time, and employed as an *Engine of Health* which hardly could have its Equal: But it is unaccountably laid aside in *our Dayes,* tho' it appears more Commended and Enforced than ever, by our *Modern* Discoveries that the daily Evacuations made by *Insensible Perspiration* do by many ounces Exceed all the rest; and yett if any one of the rest be stopp'd, what Mischiefs Ensue upon it! It seems, people are Impatient of doing any thing, but what will make them feel an *Immediate Alteration.*

Then there is that of Walking. A little of This now and then, especially for them that lead *Sedentary Lives,* would have a Surprizing Efficacy to Quicken the *Stomach,* and *Bowels,* in their work; and keep off numberless miseries. Yea, it has restored the Limbs of those, whom the tremendous *Dry Belly-ache* has deprived of them, and Creeples[19] have, according to the Maxim, *Use Legs and have Legs,* been Strangely Invigorated from it. It would be a fine thing if we could always find a Truth in that Aphorism. *Animae Confert Deambutio* Deambu[ea]tio. *O Peripatetic,* The Employment of thy *Mind,* at the Time of the Exercise may help to make it so.[20]

But the most Noble and the most Potent of all *Exercises,* is that of Riding. It is hardly possible to Enumerate all the Advantages of the *Agitations* which this *Exercise* gives to almost Every Part of the Body. This *Exercise* indeed was not in so much Request among the Ancients; because they *Rode without Stirrups,* and with Inconveniences, which *Weak Persons* Could not well Encounter. And yett one of the Ancients, in a Chapter, *De Equitatione,*[21] after he has complained how tiresome a Slow Riding is, (for the reason mentioned,) adds upon it; *Si Vehementer impellatur* (Equus) *quamvis totum Corpus Laboriose Concurriat, tamen aliquid Utilitatis affert; Siquidem magis quam Omnes aliae Exercitationes, Corpus et Praesertim Stomachum firmat, et Sensuum Instrumenta purgat, Eaque reddit acutiora.*[22] No *Exercise* in the World, according to this Gentleman, will bring Such a Strength to the *Stomach,* or do so much to cleanse and rescue and sharpen all the *Instruments* of our *Senses.* The *Horse,* a Creature so Singularly formed for the Use of Man, Will not be a *Vain Thing for Safety,* O feeble Man, if He that made him for thee, give His Blessing to and in the Use of him. In *Splenetic* and *Hysteric* Disorders, the *Exercise of Riding* will often do, Things that one would hardly have imagined; And indeed the Cases wherein its Vertues will be admired can scarce be numbered. People hearing this Council from a Physician, *Gett on Horseback,* are prone to despise him, as if he were Entirely at a Loss, what he should say to them. They take him (if not for an *Ass*) yet for no better than an *Horse-Doctor* at the best, who shall propound an *Horse* unto them. Whereas, an *Horse* may do for them, what no *Doctor* could. Yea, a *Baglivi* will tell, what the ugly Trott of an *Ass* has done for wondrous Cures, in *Italy,* where an *Horse* is not so usual as he is with us. But above all, a *Moderate Riding* is to be advised unto *Consumptive People:* who (if they be not gone too far in the *Road of Death*) should at first Ride a Mile or two; and keeping at it every day as the Weather will permitt, should increase their Journeys, as they find their Forces increasing, until they can reach to twenty or thirty Miles in a day, and give not over till they have Rid first and last some Hundreds of Miles. How many did our celebrated *Sydenham*[23] Cure of *Consumptions,* by advising them to this *Exercise? Cum* (sais he) *certo Sciam me, vel*

Medicamentis quantivis pretii, aut alia Methodo, quaecumque de-
mum ea fuerit, nihil magis iisdem proficere potuisse, quam si multis
Verbis hortatus fueram ut recte Valerent: When all other Methods
or Medicines, would have Signified no more than a long Exhortation
to them, *Not to be Sick.* In short, The *Saddle* is the *Seat of Health.*
And our *Sydenham* observes more particularly in the *Gout,* as well as
in most other chronical Distempers; *If a man knew, and could keep to*
himself, any Remedy æqual to that of a Course of *Riding, Opes ille*
Exinde amplissimas facile accumulare posset,[24] he might soon come to
keep *a Coach,* and know the English of *Dat Galenus opes.*[25]

I hope, the *Rider* in the meantime, won't be unmindful of *Darby*
Dawn's[26] Caution.

> *But lett the Rider take a Care,*
> *Lest from a Stumbling Horse or Mare*
> *He don't take Earth instead of Air.*

And lett it be remembred, That there are Some Cases, (Especially where the Blood may be too attenuated, and easily raised into
Fermentations, and more particularly, in some *Feminine* difficulties,)
Wherein *Riding* should not be præscribed. I leave it unto a *Strother*[27]
to Enumerate them, who Observes on this Occasion, That the pegging
of *Encomiums* too high is a custome, that in Physic should be more
guarded against than it is.

But I shall not Keep Touch with my *Main Intention,* if I dis-
miss this Matter, without making this Reflection.

An Apostle of God has remarked, *Bodily Exercise profiteth a*
little: [Tis *Good* for Something; The *Health* is befriended by it:]
But PIETY is profitable for all things. There are certain EXER-
CISES of PIETY, Which will befriend the *Health of the Soul*
exceedingly; yea, without them, the Soul will *Pine away in its*
Iniquities. It is thro' the Neglect of the Christian Asceticks,[28] which
were much maintained in the days of *Primitive Christianity,* that the
Power of Godliness is now almost lost in the World: The *Astraea*[29] is
gone out of the World.

Christian; Often go through a *Process of Repentance.*

Not only be much in *Prayer;* but also sett apart *Whole Days* for
Supplication, and *Whole Days* for *Thanksgiving,* in the *Religion of*
the Closett.

Accustome thyself to *Meditation;* and often *Retire* to *Meditate*
on some Divine *Truths,* first *Informing* thy Mind about them, then
Affecting thy Heart upon them, and so coming to some agreeable
Resolutions.

Often Renew a *Self-Examination;* and in *Examining* what thy Attainments are, at the Moment with repeted Acts of Devotion so come *Now* unto them, as to assure thy having of them.

Do the part of an Holy *Sacrificer;* and with the most Humble Resignation, turn all thy Enjoyments into *Sacrifices.*

By abounding in such *Exercises;* all the Blessings and Comforts of an *Healthy Soul* will be arriv'd unto.

CAP. VII. *Conjecturalies.*
or, Some Touches upon,
A *New Theory* of many *Diseases.*

Faelix qui potuit Rerum cognoscere causas![1]

OF a *Distemper* we commonly say, *To know the Cause, is Half the Cure.* But, alas, how little Progress is there yett made in that *Knowledge! Physicians* talk about the *Causes* of *Diseases.* But their Talk is very *Conjectural,* very *Uncertain,* very *Ambiguous;* and oftentimes a meer *Jargon;* and in it, they are full of *Contradiction* to One another. It may be, One of the truest Maxims ever yett advanced by any of the Gentlemen, has been That: *Ventriculus malis Effectus est Origo omnium Morborum.* A *distempered Stomach* is the Origin of all *Diseases.* I am sure Tis as useful a Caution as ever they gave; and it is the very Sum of all *Prophylactic Physick.* But, Syrs, whence is it, that the *Stomach* is *distempered?*—

Since we are upon *Conjectures,* I pray lett us allow some room, to those of Dr. *Marten*[2] and Company.

Every Part of Matter is *Peopled.* Every *Green Leaf* swarms with *Inhabitants.* The Surfaces of Animals are covered with other *Animals.* Yea, the most Solid *Bodies,* even *Marble* itself, have innumerable Cells,[3] which are crouded with imperceptible Inmates. As there are Infinite Numbers of these, which the *Microscopes* bring to our View, so there may be inconceivable Myriads yett Smaller than these, which no glasses have yett reach'd unto. The *Animals* that are much *more* than Thousands of times *Less* than the finest Grain of Sand, have their *Motions;* and so, their Muscles, their Tendons, their Fibres, their Blood, and the *Eggs* wherein their Propagation is carried on. The Eggs of these Insects (and why not the *living Insects* too!) may insinuate themselves by the *Air,* and with our *Ailments,* yea, thro' the Pores of our skin; and soon gett into the Juices of our Bodies. They

may be convey'd into our Fluids, with the Nourishment which we received, even before we were born; and may ly dormant until the
Vessels are grown more capable of bringing them into their Figure
and Vigour for Operations. Thus may Diseases be convey'd from
the Parents unto their Children, before they are born into the world.[4]
As the *Eggs* whereof *Cheese-mites* are produced, were either in the
Milk before it came from the Cow, or at least the *Runnet* with which
the Cheese was coagulated. If they meet with a *Proper Nest* in any of
our Numberless Vessels, they soon multiply prodigiously; and may
have a *greater Share in producing many of our Diseases than is commonly imagined.* Being brought into Life, then either by their Spontaneous Run, or by their disagreeable Shape, they may destroy the
Texture of the Blood, and other Juices: or they may Gnaw and
Wound the Tender Vessels. It may be so, that one Species of these
Animals may offend in one Way, and another in another; and the
Various Parts may be *Variously* offended: From whence may flow
a Variety of Diseases. And Vast Numbers of these Animals keeping
together, may at once make such Invasions, as to render Diseases
Epidemical; which those particularly are, that are called, *Pestilential.*
Epidemical and almost universal *Coughs,* may by this *Theory* be also
accounted for.

Strange *Murrains*[5] on Cattel seem to have been sometimes of this
Original. Dr. Slare[6] observes, of the famous one that passed from
Switzerland thro' *Germany* to *Poland,* that in its Progress, it Spred
still Two *German* Miles in Twenty four Hours; and he Sais, *"It were
worth Considering,* whether this Infection is not carried on by some
Volatil Insect, that is able to make only such Short Flights as may
amount to such Computations."[7]

As for the Distempers in Humane Bodies, *Kircher*[8] and *Hauptman*[9] assert, That *Malignant Fevers* never proceed from any other
Cause than *Little Animals. Blancard*[10] affirms, That the *Microscope*
discovers the *Blood* in *Fevers* to be full of *Animals.*

Ettmuller[11] sais, Unwonted Swarms of *Insects* resorting to a
Countrey, foretell a *Plague* impending.[12]

And thus we may Conceive, how Diseases are Convey'd from
distant Countreys or Climates; By the *Animalcula,* or their Eggs, deposited in the Bodies or Cloathes or Goods of Travellers.

Tis generally Supposed, that *Europe* is Endebted unto *America*
for the *Lues Venerea.* If so, *Europe* has paid its Debt unto *America,*
by making unto it a Present of the *Small Pox,* in Lieu of the *Great*
One.[13]

Dr. *Lister*[14] having observed, That the *Plague* is properly a Disease of *Asia,* and Still comes from thence; he adds, That the *Small Pox* is an Exotic Disease of the Oriental People, and was not known to *Europe,* or Even to the Lesser *Asia,* or to *Africa,* till a Spice-trade was opened by the latter Princes of *Egypt,* unto the remoter Parts of the *East Indies;* from whence it originally came, and where at this day it rages more cruelly than with us. Dr. *Oliver*[15] likewise gives it as his Opinion, That we received the *Small Pox* and *Measles* from *Arabia;* and that *Europe* was wholly unacquainted with them, until by the frequent Incursions of the *Arabians* into *Africa,* and afterwards into *Spain,* the Venom came to be Spred as now it is.

The Essential Cause of the *Itch,* appears to be a Vast Number of *Minute Animals,* that make Furrows under the Scarf-skin,[16] and Stimulate the Nervous Fibres; as may be demonstrated by a *Microscope,* Examining the Humour in the little Bladders rising between the Fingers. The Insects contained in a very Small Part of that Humour, fixed upon the Skin of a Sound Person, Either by shaking Hands with the Mangy, or using a Towel or a Glove after him; these do soon insinuate into the Pores, and then quickly multiply Enough to occupy almost all the Surface of the Body. Hence, if the Cure be not so closely followed, as not only to check, but also to kill, all the Animals, they soon increase and become as Troublesome as they were before. In the like Manner is a yett more Filthy Disease communicated. Thus tis that *God Judges you, O ye Whore-mongers and Adulterers!*

M. *Hartsoeker*[17] does not Scruple to say, *I beleive that Insects occasion most of the Diseases which Mankind is attack'd withal.*

Dr. *Marten* suspects, that there is possibly no *Ulcer,* or ulcerated Matter, but what may be stocked with *Animals,* which being of different Species, the Ulcerations may be more or less Violent according to them.

The learned *Borellus*[18] assures us, That Several times he hath seen *Animals* upon *Plaisters* taken from *Fistulous Ulcers;* and he adds, *Thus we are held of many Diseases which come from Invisible Animals, or such as can only be perceived by Microscopes.*

The famous *Mayem*[19] also observed a *Cancerous Breast,* full of these *Animals.*

Dr. *Andry*[20] found, *That* the *Pustles* of the *Small-Pox* are full of them; and so is the Blood and Urine of them that have it: *That in the Venereal Distemper,* there is hardly any Part of the Body that is not gnaw'd by them; *That* in the *Fistula Lacrymalis*[21] the Water that comes from the Eyes is full of them; *That* our *Cancers* are horribly replenished with them, which gnaw upon all the Sieves of the Glands with prodigious Consequences: And, *That* as these *Animals* grow old, they assume *New Forms,* which would be very Terrible unto People, if they could but see the Terrible Spectacles.

Dr. *Marten* is not without Suspicion, That a *Consumption* may often be of this Original; and that these *Animals* or their Seed, may Sometimes be by Parents hæreditarily conveyed unto their Offspring; or Communicated by Sick Persons to Sound Ones, that are too conversant with them. He also supposes, That tho' Great Quantities of these *Animals,* or of their *Eggs,* may be Lodged in our Blood and Juices, yea, and in our Vessels find a Nest which may bring them into Life; yett while our Secretions are duely performed, or usual Evacuations continued, the *Animals* may be Cast out of our Bodies as fast as they are bred there; and their own very Motion may Contribute unto it. But when the Emunctories thro' Cold or any other Cause are obstructed, or any usual Evacuations are Stopped; this prevents their passing off, and many Mischiefs ensue upon it.

While I was thus Entertaining myself with the Speculations of Dr. *Marten,* and his Auxiliaries, upon this *New Theory of Diseases,* I litt on Mr. *Bradly's*[22] New *Improvements of Planting and Gardening;* who maintains, That the *Blights* upon the *Vegetable World* are owing to *Insects;* whereof he discovered Some (a thousand times less than the least Grain of Sand) which found the *Cold* so agreeable an Element unto them, that at a Yard's Distance from a Slow Fire the Heat would burn them to Death. But those Insects he thought overgrown Monsters, to those which have been discovered by M. *Lieuenhoek*[23] (and other Ey-witnesses) whereof above Eight Million may be found in one drop of Water: And Mr. *Hook* proceeded so far as to demonstrate Millions of Millions contained in such a mighty Ocean. A very gentle Air may carry these from one Place to another, and so our Plants become infested with them.

On this Occasion I find his Friend Mr. *Ball,*[24] modestly but very learnedly offering his Apprehensions, That our *Pestilential Diseases* may be of the like Original. In *Europe,* the *Plagues* are brought by Long, Dry, *Easterly Winds,* which Mr. *Ball* thinks, may bring infinite Swarms of these Destroyers; and that most probably they come from *Tartary:* For he has never heard of properly *Pestilential Distempers* any where in the World, but where the *Tartarian Winds* have reached them. When the *Plague* raged in *London,* those places which had

Scents that probably Kill'd or Chas'd away these *Animals,* were kept from the Infection.

This Conjecture about the *Origin of Diseases,* may be as good as many that have been more Confidently Obtruded and more generally Received.

But what *Remarks* are to be made upon it; what *Sentiments of PIETY* to be produced?

"How much does our *Life* ly at the Mercy of our God! How much do we walk thro' *unseen Armies* of Numberless Living Things, ready to Sieze and Prey upon us! A *Walk,* like the *Running* of the Deadly *Garloup,*[25] which was of old called *a passing thro' the Brick-kiln!* What *Unknown Armies* has the Holy One, wherewith to Chastise, and Even destroy, the Rebellious Children of Men? Millions of Billions of Trillions of Invisible *Velites!* Of Sinful Men *they* say, *Our Father, Shall We Smite them?* On *His* order, they do it Immediately; they do it Effectually.

What a poor Thing is *Man;* That a *Worm* inconceivably less than the *Light Dust of the Balance,* is too hard for him!

How much is it our Interest and our Prudence, to *keep resolves in the Love of God!"*

But, O ye Sons of Erudition, and, *ye Wise Men of Enquiry;* Lett this *Enquiry* come into a due Consideration with you; How far a Potent *Worm-killer,* that may be Safely administred, would go further than any Remedy yett found out, for the Cure of many Diseases!

Mercury,[26] We know thee: But we are afraid, Thou wilt kill *us* too, if we Employ thee to kill *them* that kill us.

And yett, for the Cleansing of the small *Blood-Vessels,* and making Way for the free Circulation of the Blood and Lymph, and so to Serve the greatest Purposes of Medicine, there is nothing like *Mercurial Deobstruents,*[27] of which, the *Cinnabar* of *Antimony, Æthiops Mineral,*[28] and the Antihectic of *Poterius,*[29] may be reckoned the principal. But after all, tis time to have done with the *Metaphysical Jargon,* which for a Long Time has passed for the *Rationale* of Medicine. How much would the *Art of Medicine* be improved, if our Physicians more generally had the *Mathematical* Skill of a Dr. *Mead*[30] or a Dr. *Morgan,* and would go his way to Work, *Mathematically,* and by the *Laws of Matter* and *Motion,* to find out the *Cause* and *Cure of Diseases?* The Words of one of them are worth receiving: "Since the Animal Body is a *Machine,* and Diseases are nothing else but its Particular Irregularities, Defects, and Disorders, a *Blind* Man might as well pretend to Regulate a Piece of *Clock-work,* or a *Deaf* Man to tune an *Organ,* as a Person ignorant of *Mathematicks* and *Mechanism,* to cure Diseases, without understanding the Natural Organization, Structure, and Operations of the *Machine,* which he undertakes to regulate.

CAP. VIII. *Raphael.*[1]
Or, Notable Cures, from the INVISIBLE WORLD.

IT is not more *Notorious,* than it is *Astonishing,* that many *Methods* and *Medicines* for the Cure of *Diseases,* have been the Communications of *Dæmons* to our World. That ever Such *Good* should be done by *Evil Spirits* unto the Children of Men! Certainly, not without Some *Evil Designs* of Theirs, at the Bottom of all.

It is well-known, That it was the ancient Custome, for Patients under Various Infirmities, upon the Observation of Certain Cæremonies, to fall asleep in the Temple of *Æsculapius:* and in their Sleep, to Enjoy *Dreams,* which gave them Directions how to obtain the Releef of their Infirmities.[2]

A *Table,* found in the Isle of *Tyber,*[3] where Stood once the Temple of *Æsculapius,* is at this Day to be seen at *Rome;* On which the Greek Inscriptions Record several Strange Cures wrought in such a Way; with the Names of the Patients, who left these grateful Memorials of what they had received.[4]

Very odd is what *Suidas*[5] relates, of a *Jew,* who in the Temple of *Æsculapius* at *Athens* was Ordered in this Way to feed upon *Pork,* that he might be help'd for the *Spitting of Blood.* He found Help; and if he intermitted his *Pork-Diet* but one Day, he would be out of Order upon it. *What Snares were here!*

We are informed by *Diodorus,* The *Egyptians* affirm That *Isis*[6] used Effectually to instruct the Sick, by *Dreams* in their Sleep, how to Cure their Distempers; and the Sick recovered their Health, even after Physicians had quite given them over.

One would wonder, how Several of our Common *Remedies* came to be first of all Thought upon! I hope, I have not Suggested the true *Original* of them. If it be so, God has graciously *Overruled,* and fetch'd a *Treacle*[7] out of a *Serpent!* But if the *Bad Angels* have taught People how to Cure many Diseases, why may not the *Good Angels* be also Considered, and the *Goodness* of the Great God our

SAVIOUR in *their Ministry,* be acknowledged, in the Communication of many Succours to be Miserable World!

Unaccountable and Unintelligible Things, are the *Responsa Raphaelis,* or, Instructions for the Cure of Diseases, which Dr. *Napier,*[8] an old Gentleman of uncommon Devotion and Innocence, had from a Genius of that Name, when his Patients brought their Cases to him; and which are to be seen at this Day in the *Musaeum Ashmolaeanum,* among the Manuscripts lodged there.

Camfield in his *Theological Discourse of ANGELS,*[9] expresses himself willing to refer unto the Head of the *Angelical Ministry,* the Choice Reciets, for which M. *Antoninus*[10] acknowledges himself a Debtor to the Gods; who did use Δι' ὀνειρατων βοηθημὰτὰ δοθηναι.[11]

Of the *Angelical Ministry* conspicuous, or at least probable, in Showing the Sick what to do for a Cure, I will not recite any *Outlandish Instances:* Except *One,* which my Father has transferred out of *Clark's*[12] Collections into his *Remarkable Providences:*[13] And this I will mention for a Reason, anon to be intimated.

One *Samuel Wallas,* of *Stamford* in *Lincolnshire,* had been in a Consumption for Thirteen Years; was worn away to a Sceleton; and for four years had lain bed-rid. Being left Alone on a Lords-day, and reading a Book of Piety, there came to him a person of an aged, but comely and lively Aspect; unto whom he related his poor Condition, adding, That he wholly Resigned himself into the Hands of God, for Him to dispose of him as He pleased. The Stranger said, *Thou sayest very well; Be sure to Fear God, and Serve Him, and Remember to Observe what I now Say unto thee.* "To morrow morning take Two Leaves of *Red Sage,* and one of *Blood-wort:* putt those three Leaves into a Cup of Small Beer; and thereof drink as oft as need requires. On the Fourth Morning take away those Leaves, and putt in Fresh ones. This do for Twelve Days together; And ere these Twelve Days are Expired, thro' the Help of God, thy Disease will be cured, and the Frame of thy Body altered. When thy Strength shall be somewhat recovered, Change the Air; And within a Month shall the Clothes thou hast now on thee, be too strait for thee. He repeted his Charges unto the Sick Man, *To Fear God, and Serve Him.* And the Sick Man asking him, whether he would please to Eat any thing; he answered, *No; The Lord CHRIST is Sufficient for me. And seldome do I drink any-thing, but what cometh from the Rock."* When he came in, tho' it Rain'd, he had not one Speck of Wett or Dirt upon him. When he went out, tho' there were people Standing at their Doors on the other Side of the Street, none saw him. The Directions that had been prescribed were followed; and the Successes that were promised were to Every Ones Admiration accomplished. An Assembly of Ministers meeting on the Occasion, Concluded, That it was One of the *Good Angels,* who had thus appeared.

The Thing advised unto, was an *Agreeable Remedy.* Upon which, I will now relate, That I knew a person, who at about Fourteen Years of Age had great Symptoms of an *Hectic*[14] upon him, and who Said, as he had cause, *I am going apace to the Gates of the Grave, I am deprived of the Residue of my Years.* In this Distress, he betook himself to this *Wallasian Remedy;* And now, *At more than Threescore Years of Age he writes the Story of it!*

But I will proceed now to Two or Three Domestic Examples.

A Woman about Nine Miles off the City where I sojourn, grievously handled with the *Gout,* had a Dream, that her Husband going thither the Gentlewoman of the House he went unto, told him of an *Infallible Cure* for her. She said not a Word unto him of it. But he went the next morning to the place about Other Business. The Gentlewoman being, upon her Enquiry of him, informed about the State of his Wife, She told him, That she had an *Infallible Cure* for her; and sent her by him, a little Bottel of *Aligator-Oyl.* Upon his coming home, she anticipated what he was to have said unto *her,* and Said first unto *him, Come, I know you have brought me home what will Cure me of my Gout.* With Surprize, he told her, *So he had!* She applied it, and was perfectly recovered.

Another shall be this.

A Young Woman [*Lydia Ingram,*] and other Languishing Illnesses fell Ill of a Feavour, which was at Length attended with a very Great Swelling of her Stomach and Sides, and a *Total Suppression of Urine for Ten Days together.* Our Ablest Physicans gave her over for Hopeless: But while she lay so, she dream't that there came into the Room, a Gentleman with the Circumstances of a Venerable Old Age upon his Head and Face; Butt of a Very comely Countenance; of a Middle Stature; and having a Light-Coloured Chamlett-Coat for his Habit. Much such an One as the Learned *Rhodius*[15] reports to have been Seen by the Creeple miraculously cured at *Padua: Vise per quietem Sene, Veste Candida, Salutemque Pollicito, modo Divino fideret Auxilio.*[16] This Gentleman Said, *That Over-hearing the Groans of One in Distress as he pass'd by the House, he could not but come in.* And now, having the Case of the Young Woman more particularly related unto him, he gave her this Advice: *Take a Glass of White Wine, and putt into it a Little Alum; and add the Powder of a burnt Beef-marrow-bone, as much as may ly upon the Lid of the Civet-box now in your hand;* [which was about as broad as a Sixpence:] *Drink this Off; Do it Twice in Three Hours; By the Fourth Hour you shall have Releef.* So he went away. She awoke, and informed the Physicians of what passed; only she forgott the Third Ingredient. They allow'd her to take the *White-Wine* and *Allum,* if she pleased; for they were able to do no more. She took it; but without any Effect. Hereupon she fell asleep again; and the Same Venerable Person came again unto her. He asked, whether she had followed his Advice? She said, She had; but found no Good of it. He asked her, *What have you done?* She told him. He replied; *Don't you Remember the Powder I told you of, to take as much of it as might ly on the Lid of your Civet-box? Alas, you have almost fool'd your Life away. However, go take what I bade you. I beleeve it may do you good yett. There is nothing too hard for God; And so you'l find it!* Which Last Words he also repeted, at his then going out of the Door. She then awaking told her Physicians of the Remedy; whereof she now gave them a more Perfect Account. The Remedy was immediately allowed and præpared; tho' the Physicians derided it as a meer Whimsey, and unlikely to do any Good. She took it; and by the Fourth Hour, she had the Releef proposed; and at one time voided Five Pints of Urine: And from Wednesday at one a clock, to Friday at one a clock, there came no less than Six Gallons by Measure from her. The Suppression returned, and continued Three Days. The Same Venerable Person then came once more unto her, in her Dream; and said, *How dost thou do now, Child?* She Said, *I grow Weaker.* He said, *Have you done as I advised you?* She said, *Yes.* He Said; *Why, did you repeat it?* She said, *No.* He Said, *Why not?* She [afraid] Said, *We can't gett White-Wine.* He look'd very much displeased, and said; *Not White-Wine! There's Enough in the Town; But People that want a Will, Seldome Want an Excuse.* She said, *I am almost gone!* He replied, *You are almost gone indeed! However Take it again; All Things are possible with God.* He then went unto the Door; and now turning about again, he Said with a more Cheerful and Pleased Countenance; *Take it, and give God all the Glory: give God all the Glory! Fare you well.* And so he went out. She accordingly follow'd his Advice; and found present Releef. She went on taking it for twice or thrice a Day, and God bless'd it so, that she Recovered, and quickly came abroad. Yea, She is now above Twenty years after alive; in which time she has had successively Two Husbands; and Seen many other changes.

A Third may be This.

One whose Name is *Thankful Fish,* belonging to *Falmouth,* had except in the *Headache* now and then, Enjoy'd a Good Health till she was Twelve Years of Age. In her Thirteenth Year, she was visited with Sickness and Weakness, for Three Months together, and followed with Fitts that had on them an *Hysterical* Aspect, which so Enfeebled her that she could neither *Step* nor *Stand,* for Ten Years together, but was confined unto a low Chair, in which on a Smooth floor She could sometimes move a little from one place to another. She had a Strong Impression on her Mind, that if she were carried unto *Rhode-Island,* she should *there* find a Cure: But the Physicians there honestly told her *There was nothing to be done for her.* Under this grievous Discouragement, she was told of Several *Miraculous Cures* that occur'd in the latter End of the last Century; and Some that were Cured of Distressing Maladies, While Reading and Thinking on the *Miracles* wrought by our SAVIOUR in the Days of His Humiliation; and Beleeving that He could still do as great Things as ever. She had good Advice given her, to *Pray* much, and ask the prayers of others for her; and hope in the Power and Mercy of her SAVIOUR. By and by, while she yett continued at *Rhode-Island* she heard a mention of a *Malt-Bath;* and tho' her friends were much against her trying of it, but thought her so feeble that it could not be used without unhappy Consequences, yett she was Impetuous and Obstinate for it, and would not be diverted from the perillous Experiment. She had not been Twenty Minutes in the *Malt-Bath,* before she *Died away;* and was taken out, as in a manner *Dead,* and putt into a Bed. Here they kept her warm, from *Tuesday* in the Afternoon to *Friday* in the Evening: All which Time, she lay Senseless, and Eat nothing, but once or twice they poured a few Drops of a Liquid into her Mouth. At length, as one waking out of a Sleep, and greatly Refresh'd and Reviv'd, she found her Strength to admiration Restored. She putt on her Clothes, and got up, and Walk'd about the Room: And on the Day following [which was Nov. 14. 1724] she found herself yett more Able to *Stand* and *Step;* And on the Lords-day, Sennight Ensuing, She, who had formerly been brought unto the Church, on a Chair between two or three Persons, now Walk'd thither on her own Feet, where (not forgetting her *Name*) she signified her Desire to have *Thanks* rendred unto God her SAVIOUR, for the Wonderful Work which He had wrought upon her: And she continues to *Walk* and *not faint,* or complain of Weariness.

[What shall one think of a passage, in the Memoirs of, Mr. *Robert Billig,*[17] One of the shining *Lamps of Heaven,* that were extinguished in 1662. The *Gout* had utterly taken away the Use of his Legs, by a weakness in his Knees and Ancles; and the Use of one of his Arms also; insomuch that he could hardly go a few Steps with Crutches. Having been for Some time in this Condition, and being one Day alone in his Parlour, he felt a Strong IMPULSE upon his Mind, which caused him with much Difficulty to creep up into his Chamber, and there with fervent Prayer pour out his Soul before the Lord. Whilst he was praying, he Strangely found himself Strengthened; and when he Rose from his Knees, not only was his Pain all gone, but he walked as well as ever in his Life. He came with Joy, to his Friends, who were so astonished, they could hardly beleeve their Eyes. This was in, 1658. He continued Serving the Kingdom of God until 1695, when he died about seventy three Years of Age.]

In these Narratives, I am far from the Intention, of Encouraging Unwarrantable *Superstitions,* or *Affectations;* or Countenancing any Dispositions to go out of the *Ordinary Road for Cures.* But thus much I may venture to say: It is possible there may be more of the *Angelical Ministry,* than we are *Ordinarily* aware of, in Leading us to *know* and *use* those Remedies, which our God may bless for our Good under our *Diseases.* The *Good Angels* may by Impressions on the Mind of [shall I say, *His Brother?*] the *Physician,* or, by an *Insensible Manuduction* to the *Friend* or *Book* [suppose an Hint in our, *Angel of Bethesda!*] that may inform us, *How to be cured;* be the *Ministers of God for our Good.* Indeed, they chuse to *be Behind the Curtain,* and Latent and Cover'd under more *Visible Causes,* as may be; and it is for some Reasons best it should be so: But by being in favour with Their Glorious LORD, we may Enjoy Unknown Benefits from the *Angelical Ministry;* and having received them, the Praises of the *Angelical Ministry* are to be rendred unto HIM.

Honest *Manlius*[18] relates notable *Cures* of Persons by Directions in *Dreams* communicated unto them. It looks, as if Good ANGELS directed them. The admirable BOYL,[19] who was no Stranger to *Philosophy,* is yett full in it, that there is a greater Intervention of *Angels,* in our Diseases, and in the Cure of them, than is among *Philosophers* commonly thought for.

The Very Learned *Bartholinus,* in his *Acta Medica,*[20] gives us Relations of *Cures,* which he determines could proceed from none but *Good ANGELS* Immediately operating in them, and for them: *Causa Supernaturalis admittenda, Eaque a DEI ministro ANGELO Procurata.*[21] And he has this Remarkable Passage thereupon: *Certe plures hujusmodi CURATIONES occurrunt QUOTIDIE; cum non raro, Medicis desperantibus, convalescant aegri inter incurabiles numerati:* Not *Rarely,* but Even *Daily,* we see persons that were *given over by the Physicians,* yett most *unaccountably* Recovered: He thinks, the Ministry of Good ANGELS may be concerned in such Recoveries!

A Very Learned *Physician* making these Acknowledgments, methinks, is a Brother to that *Beloved Physician,* who is the only Evangelist that makes the Remark upon the *Hæmorrhoiss* cured by the Immediate Hand of Heaven, *She had in vain Spent her Substance on the Physicians!*

CAP. IX. *Stimulator.*

or, Considerations upon

<u>Pains</u>, Dolours, Aches, in general.

WHAT is *Pain?* Tis a Sensation produced on the *Tension of a Nerve.*

But I address myself to them, who have a more *Exquisite Way* of Knowing *What it is,* than from hearing a Description of it given by a Philosopher. They *Feel* it!

And considering our *Constitution,* of Numberless *Nerves,* with our *Scituation* among objects that may putt our *Nerves* upon the Rack; it is a Wonder, that we feel no more of it. *O Man, Free of Pain,* Wonder at the Mercy of thy God, and Celebrate it with most thankful Praises!

But unto the Man that is *Chastened with Pain,* Lett us now recommend Some agreeable *Sentiments of PIETY.*

Lett not thy *Pain* distract, but lett it quicken, thy *Thoughts;* and *Provoke* thee to Think such Things as these.

Think; "Alas, What have my *Sins procured!* And how much more have my *Sins Deserved!* Under and about my *Pain,* I may now hear the Glorious God Saying to me, *Thy Way and thy Doings have procured these Things unto thee: This is Thy Wickedness! And shall it not be Bitter to thee?*"

Think; "I now taste a very Little of the *Cup* which my dear SAVIOUR, when *God laid on Him the Iniquity of us all,* drank very deeply of! He suffered grievous *Pain* to purchase for me a Deliverance from the eternal Miseries in the Punishment of the Wicked, and the Benefit of my having these my Temporal Miseries made profitable to me."

Think; "How woful, how rueful will my Condition be, and what *Pain* must I undergo, if I dy in ill Terms in Heaven, and must have my Portion in that *Hell,* which is a *Place of Torment,* from whence the Smoke of *the Torment ascends forever and ever!* What shall I do, that being thus *Warned,* I may *flee from the Wrath to Come!"*

Yea, O Christian, Lett all thy *Pains* be so many *Spurs,* to quicken thy Pace in the Race of Christianity: And Lett them hasten thee into those Dispositions of PIETY, which will be rich Compensations for all that thou mayst Suffer from them.

In the Memorials of One under *Pains,* I have mett with a Passage to this Purpose.

"Tho' Violent *Pain* be an Affliction which I have always with a singular Importunity deprecated, yett now being under it, I sett myself to Adore a *Sovereign* and a *Righteous* and a *Faithful* God, as inflicting all my *Pains* upon me. I continually Said, *Lord, If thou wilt bruise and break a Vessel of Clay, which thy own Hands have given a Being to, none may say, What doest thou!* And, *Lord, I am worthy of all the Sad Things that I meet withal, and punished far less than my Demerits.* And, *Lord, I beleeve thou aimest at my Good, and in Faithfulness hast afflicted me.* I consider *His Will* as Ordering my Affliction, and I adored it as a *Sovereign* and a *Righteous* Will, and full of infinite *Wisdome,* Designing Such *Ends* as I ought forever to be Reconciled unto. I considered also my Affliction, as Carrying on my Conformity to my SAVIOUR, who was here a *Man of Sorrows and acquainted with Griefs,* In these Views, I bore my *Pain* with Patience, and had Thoughts full of *Resignation* to the Will of God, and of *Satisfaction* in it, raised in my Mind, Still as it returned in its Rages upon me. I proceeded then to consider, That my *Patience* under my *Pain,* was a *Spectacle* which the Infinite God is gratified in the beholding of, my JESUS having restored my *Person* to His Favour, and making *Intercession* for my Acceptance; My JESUS being also the Author and giver of my *Patience,* And my JESUS being imitated in it; It becomes to the Glorious God a grateful Spectacle. Hereupon, as a Paroxysm of the *Pain* was approaching, I still thought; *Now I am going into an Opportunity of being a grateful Spectacle to my God! And shall not my Love to Him cause me to be gratified with what shall be a Pleasure unto Him? Yea, tho' it be out of my Torture, that there arises a Pleasure unto Him!* Tis inexpressible, What I saw and felt on this Occasion. Surely, My God will not send me to *Hell!* He will send *Heaven* thither with me, if He do!

In what follows wee'l keep as well as we can, to the Maxim of *Bartholinus; In Theatro applausum meretur, qui Idonea non qui multa profert.*[1]

In many *Pains,* we must with a mighty Caution avoid *Repellents.*[2] To *Strike In* that Humor of Vapor which causes the *Pains,* may be attended with Tragical Consequences.

Here is a notable Poultis, to appease *Pains,* and *Aches.*

§ Take *Onions;* Boil them or Stew them in Water, till they be Soft Enough to make a Poultis. Drain away the Water; Beat 'em; and spread 'em to a Good Thickness on a Linen-Cloth. Apply them as hott as the Patient can bear.

§ A Bundle of *TOW* laid and kept hott upon a Pained Place, often quiets and extracts Exquisite *Pains,* and restores Motion to Parts that are benumbed with them.

§ Some that have been Vexed with Obstinate *Pains* here and there (brought by taking *Colds,*) have been Strangely helped, by Wearing a Piece of *Red Bayes*[3] on the Parts affected.

§ In many a *Pain* which vexes us, it would be good Advice, (and not imply a snappish and senseless *Revenge,*) to Say, *Beat it.* A continued *Beating* on the Place, with a *Fist,* or Some other Instrument, has frequently discussed, or perspired *Pain,* to Admiration.

§ Spirit of *Sal-Armoniac*[4] mixt with stale Oil of *Sweet Almonds,*[5] gives a speedy and potent Releef in External Pains.

It is observed, That *spirituous* Ingredients blended with *unctious* ones, are admirable Remedies against *Pains;* and vastly præferable to the *Spirituous* taken apart.

§ It is a Remark of Dr. *Cheyne;* "Providence has been kind and gracious to us beyond all Expression, in furnishing us with a certain *Releef,* if not a Remedy, to the most Intense of our *Pains.* When our Patience can hold out no longer, and our *Pains* are at last come to be Insupportable, we have always ready at hand, a Medicine, which is not only a present Releef, but, I may Say, a Standing and Constant *Miracle.*"

He means, *Opium,* and the Solution of it, *Laudanum.*[6]

It produces its wondrous Effects, by *Unbending,* and *Loosening,* the *Fibres,*[7] which in our *Pains* have a Constriction and Contraction upon them.

The Doctor Says, Whenever *Pain* is become Intolerable, after præmising the proper *Evacuations,* then *Opiates* will certainly re-leeve, and are proper to be administred.

If the Case be attended with *Vomiting,* then Solid *Opium* will do best: If Speedy Releef be required, and there be no Vomiting, then, *Laudanum.* In common Cases, use Vinous Vehicle.[8]

In the *Cholic,* it should be given with Some *Stomach Purge:* as *Elixir Salutis,*[9] or, Syrup of *Buckthorn;*[10] and in those of more Tender Bowels, with Tincture of *Rhubarb.*[11] Especially, if the *Cholic* be in the Lower Bowels, and attended with no Vomiting. In which, an Artificial Vomit may be præmised, if Circumstances do not forbid it.

In the *Stone,* it should be given with Oyl of *Sweet Almonds,* or in Some Soft Emulsion, to lubricate the parts.

In *Hard Labours* of Women, and Sluggish Purifications: In the *Gout* also, and the *Rheumatism,* It ought always to be given with proper *Volantes,*[12] *Anti-hystericks,*[13] and *Attenuants.*[14]

In *Violent Pains,* the First Dose is to be Large; From Thirty to Forty-five Drops of Liquid *Laundanum;* or its Equivalent in *Opium,* from *Two Grains* and an half, to *Three* and an half. And afterwards to be increased, by Fifteen Drops of the Liquid Laundanum, or Half a Grain of the *Opium,* Every Half Hour till the Pain begin to re-mitt: And then an entire Stop is to be putt unto its Adminstration.

The Doctor Says, There is less Hazard of *over-dosing* and *over-doing* in this, than is commonly thought for. I could not well forbear this Communication.

But I desire, it may never be in any other than the hand of a Skilful, Careful, Consciencious *Practitioner.*

Most certainly, *Opium* is either a great *Friend* or a great *Foe,* to Nature, just as it is Wisely or Madly made use of.

CAP. X. *Cephalica.*
or, Cure for the <u>Head-ache</u>
And the <u>Ague</u> *of the Head.*

IT is a Proverbial Expression for a Man of a very Healthy Constitu-tion, *His Head never aked.* But how few are the Men, that can have this affirmed of them? For the *Head* is furnished with a great many *Nervous Parts,* which are of the greatest Sensation; and many *Excre-*

ments are generated in the *Head,* which if they be not in due time discharged, those parts must needs be Vellicated,[1] irritated, and incommoded. Salt, Sharp, Austere Particles, in the Mass of Blood, those which we call the *Animal Spirits,* carried beyond their Sphære, to the *Nervous Parts* of the *Head;* these Cause the *Head-ache,* by vexing the *Fibres* there. A too Quick *Motion,* or a too large *Quantity,* of the *Blood,* or too great a Fermentation or Deflagration[2] in any of the *Bowels,* hurry these Particles to the Membranes of the *Head,* and give *Pains* unto it.

My Friend, Lett not the *Pains* of thy *Head,* chase or keep those *Thoughts* out of thy *Head,* which ought now more than ever, to have a Lodging there.

Think; "What a *Forge of Sins* against the Glorious God, has been this Poor, Vile, Sinful *Head* of mine! How *Empty* has my *Head* been of such *Thoughts,* as a Reasonable and a Religious Mind ought continually to have been replenish'd with! But how *Filled* with Such *Vain Thoughts,* yea, Such *Base Thoughts,* as I can't be *Saved,* if I give a *Lodging* to! What *Wandering,* what *Impure,* what *Covetous,* what *Ambitious,* what *Malicious* and *Envious* Thoughts, has this *Head* of mine, been a Seat unto! *Lord, I am worthy of all the Pains thou dost inflict upon it!"*

Think; "What *Pains* did my dear SAVIOUR suffer in His *Head,* when He felt the *Crown of Thorns* Violently Struck into it! What my SAVIOUR Suffered in His *Head,* has purchased for me, the Pardon of the *Sins,* which has Exposed my *Head* unto all its *Pains:* and my Deliverance from the *Pains* of my *Head,* when it shall be best for me; and the Grace to Employ my *Head,* more as I ought to do, than I have done heretofore."

Think; "I wish that Gracious Hand of my SAVIOUR, may remove the *Pains* which my *Head* is now afflicted withal. But lett it be a much greater Wish with me, That my *Head,* may, like the Forehead of the *High-Priest,* have, Holiness to the Lord, written upon it, and be a very *Holy Head!* That My SAVIOUR, and the *Mysteries* and *Concernments* of His *Kingdome,* and the *Perfections* of God, and the *Works* of His Hands, may be very frequently Entertained in the *Visions of my Head,* with Right *Ideas* of them formed there; *The Right Thoughts of the Righteous!* And my *Head* may say to Him, *Lord, How Precious are thy Thoughts to me; How Great is the Sum of them!* That my *Head* may be full of *Projections* and *Contrivances,* how to serve the Kingdome of my SAVIOUR, and how to do good unto my Neighbour! *O my SAVIOUR, I beg it of thee!"*

Think; "I feel the Truth of that Word, *The Head sick, and the Heart faint.* May the *Rulers* of my People, the *Heads* of our *Tribes,* be such that the whole *Body* may not be putt out of order. May the *Heads* of *Families,* be so well-disposed, that the whole House may be kept from Disorder."

Pained Man; If thou art thyself the *Head* of any Society, pursue this Meditation.

But Now,

Videbis quam levibus, ac tenuis Momenti Medicamentis tuam Valetudinem tueri possis.[3]

Lett those Words of *Manlius* on his *Libellus Medicus,*[4] introduce all the Medicines in Every one of our *Capsula's.*

§ *Hippocrates* for a *Pain of the Head,* fomented it a Considerable time, with *Warm Water,* and then used *Sternutatories.*[5] If this were ineffectual, he opened a Vein in the Nose and the Forhead.

§ In the *Head-ache,* forbear salt, and sharp, and windy, Meats and Drinks.

§ *Baglivi* speaks of a very dangerous *Headache,* after trying all Remedies in Vain, cured by the Juice of *Beet-Roots,* Vigorously snuffed up the Nostrils, divers times in a day.

§ If an *Head-ache* proceed from the suppression of any Excrements, a seasonable Evacuation will soon carry it off.

§ Breathing a *Vein,*[6] and particularly the *Forehead-Vein,* Eases an *Head-ache,* when too much Blood causes it.

§ *Clysters*[7] in hott *Head-akes,* and *Blisters* in cold ones, are oftentimes very significant.

§ The *Paracelsians* cry up *Narcoticks,* to quiet and fetter the Raging Spirits, that make our *Head-ache.* The Oyl of *Guajacum,*[8] has a very strange Vertue to cure a strong *Head-ache.* In stubborn *Head-aches* of a long standing, *Willis*[9] præscribes, the Juice, or Powder, or Distilled Water, of *Millepedes.*[10]

§ Bathing the *Head* in cold Water, has done wonders, in some *Head-akes.*

§ A Dish of *Coffee;*—yea and of *Thea*[11] also;—but especially the former;—is a frequent Releef to Pains of the Head.

§ Anoint the Temples with Oyl of *Nutmegs.*[12] Tis a famous Præscription;—If the Pain be in the Forepart of the Head.

§ I have seen a mighty Efficacy for Pains in the *Head* contracted by Colds, and the ill-digested Humours or Vapours there, in the use of *Spirit of Sal Armoniack;*—the Bottle frequently smelt unto.

§ *Vervain*[13] was cried up for the *Head-ache,* as long ago, as the days of *Terence*[14] and *Tully. Forestus*[15] reports, T'wil cure the Pain, by being putt under ones Pillow. What if it should be kneaded with sharp *Leaven,*[16] and Oyl of *Roses,*[17] and so applied?

§ Take Powder *de Gutteta;*[18] Native *Cinnabar* præpared; half an Ounce, Mix.

A Specific in the *Headache,* and in Convulsive Affections. The most pertinacious Pains in the *Head,* (as we find in Dr. T. *Fuller*)[19] even almost unto Madness, have been happily cured, all other Means failing, with *Pulvis de Gutteta* alone, and an Infusion of *Prim-rose*[20] Flowers, *Betony,*[21] or *Tea.*

§ *Mineral Waters* are the last Refuge of many *Head-akes,* and none of the least.

§ Take fresh *Rosemary*[22] an Handful; Boil for a pretty while, in a Quart of Water. Then with it almost fill a Mug, and lett the Patient cover his Head and Face with a Napkin; So that he may receive the Steam as hott as he can well bear it; and this as long as he finds the Steam strong Enough.

§ One in my Neighbourhood that lay adying of a Cruel *Head-ache,* after the unsuccessful Use of all other means, was cured by nothing but stopping his Nostrils with Wool, and so hindering the Air from that Passage into his Head.

§ Here's an Electuary.[23] Take *Betony,* and *Gentian,*[24] and *Elecampane,*[25] and *Rosemary,* and *Damask-Rose*-Leaves; of Each an Equal Quantity, pound them, and compound them, into an Electuary; Whereof take a Small Quantity Every Night, at going to Bed. Many that have been troubled with an obstinate *Headache,* for many years; This plain Remedy has cured them.

Mantissa.

Gnarus, Amice, Mali, miseris Succurrere deseo.[26]

There is a grievous *Pain,* which we call,

The Ague in the Head.

A *Thorn* is gott into One Side of the *Head,* which (with Intermissions) will shoot forth a *Raging Pain* Every Way, that will reach down into the Jaws; especially if a *Defective Tooth* be there. So great the *Pain,* that the *Patient* loses his *Patience,* and could almost count a *Decollation* worth undergoing for his Deliverance. It will be upon Examination found That on the Outside of the Cranium, and under the Skin, there is often collected an Humour, which distills thro' the *Pericranium* into the adhæring Membrane, and falls down into the Eyes, Ears, Cheeks, Neck, Teeth, and Throat, and sometimes broken Impostumes are thence discharged. Here enters, and fixes the *Thorn,* which causes the *Ague in the Head.* Allow me the Term; since *Tertullian*[27] will have a *Pain in the Head,* the *Thorn*[28] which our Apostle complained of. *Reader,* Look into the *Capsula,* where thou will find our *Thoughts,* on *Pains* are lodged; and find them out, on this Occasion.

§ But what shall be done to pull out the *Thorn?*

The Application of *Hott-Bricks,* has given Ease when the *Pain* has been in its Extremity.

§ An Embrocation[29] with the *Oil of Mint,*[30] has been very useful and helpful.

§ And so has the *Oil of Turpentine.*

§ A Cataplasm[31] of *Beaten Mustard,* with *Rum,* has done some cures.

§ And, so has *Pepper* and *Rum.*

§ And, a Poultis of *Ginger.*[32]

§ Some find a *Mullein-Tea,*[33] to cure, almost miraculously.

§ A Bundle of *Tow* worn on the Part affected, has drawn out the Pain.

§ Beaten *Mustard-Seed,* incorporated with the White of an Egg, Laid on as a Plaister, has been too *Strong* for this Enemy.

§ *Blisters* drawn under the Ears, are one of the most infallible Remedies.

§ Especially, if a *Purge* be added; The *Cephalic Pills*[34] are very agreeable to the Occasion:

Usibus Educto Si quicquam Credis Amicu.[35]

§ But some affirm, That no Remedy is to be compared unto a *Vomit.* It will do, when all other Methods and Medicines fail.

CAP. XI. *Dentifrangibulus.*
or, The Anguish, and Releef, of
The Tooth-ache.

THE TOOTH-ACHE, How frequent a Malady! Two Twigs of the External *Carotid Artery* running under the Ear and entring into the

Inferior *Maxilla,* are disseminated thro' all its Length, into the Roots of every *Tooth,* to carry Blood for their Nourishment. In those Vessels, acrid Humours [together with the Blood] pass to the *Teeth,* and gnaw and vellicate the exquisitely sensible Membrane that coats their interiour *Medulla,* and hence the intolerable Twinges of the *Tooth-ache.* Tis a very surprising Thing, which the learned *Raw*[1] has observed and affirmed; That the Seeds of all the *Teeth* ly hid in the Socketts of the Gums, or Jaws, of a *Foetus;* and that as many Seeds as lay latent there, so many *Teeth* a Man should have in his Life. He was able to demonstrate unto the Eye, the Seeds that were hid in the Gums of a New born Infant. Every *Foetus* contains the Seeds of the compleat Number of Teeth, which are Ever to appear upon Room occasionally made for them, as long as he lives; and they are precisely *Fifty-Two.* Besides the *Thirty-Two* Teeth, which are found in a perfect Man, there are the Trace of *Twenty* more, which are to be found in Every Infant.[2]

So then, there are *Fifty-Two* Tormentors in thy Gums alone, O Man, to which thy Sin has made thee liable, as in the Course of thy Life, they may Arise and Appear and Corrupt; and the Nerve at the Bottom of each becomes uneasy.

If I go to Read unto One under the *Tooth-ache,* a Lecture on our Philosophy of his Distemper, he will give but a Poor Attention to it; He will cry out *Rather tell me What Shall be done to give some Ease unto me.*

But I will first Advise him, how to *gett Good* by his Pain, before I direct him, how to *gett Out* of it.

Under the Torments of this Malady, there are Some Truths to be *chew'd* upon: Some *Thoughts* that if being *Intensely Pursued,* they won't at all Divert or Abate the *Pain,* yett they may cause what is thus *Painful,* to become as *Useful* unto the Sufferer.

Think; "The *Teeth,* wherein I Suffer so much Torture; How much have I *Sinned* with them! The Sin of my *First Parents* was perpetrated by the *Teeth.* An horrid *Sin;* a *Sin* that is *Mine;* and forever to be Bewayled.

I have Employ'd my *Teeth* in *Eating* Irregularly, Inordinately; and Without a due Regard unto the Service and Glory of God, in my *Eating.*

How often have I dug my *Grave* with my *Teeth.* And how justly am I punished with *Pains* in the *Teeth,* which have been so abused!

My *Teeth* are used in my *Speech.* Some of the *Letters* pronounced in *Speaking* are the *Dentals.* In *Speaking* amiss, how many Sins have I been guilty of!"

Think; "Among the *Sufferings* wherein my dear SAVIOUR made *Expiation* for my *Sins,* the Pains which the *Fist of Wickedness* gave to His *Cheek-bone,* were particularly sensible. O my SAV-IOUR, may the *Sins* of my *Teeth,* as well as all my other Sins, thus Expiated, be all forever pardoned. And may I have the Grace for the Time to come, always to *Eat* and *Speak,* in the *Fear of God!"*

Think; "If the *Pains* of the *Teeth,* are so intolerable: If the Continuance of these *Pains* for one Year together upon me, would make me so very miserable; How can I undergo the *Pains* of them who *Dy in their Sins!* the *Pains* in the *Strange Punishment reserved for the Workers of Iniquity!* the *Pains* which will cause *Weeping and Wailing and Gnashing of Teeth,* unto those that are thrown into them! *Pains* which are, no Mortal can say how *Great,* and of how *Long a Continuance.* Oh! Tis a *fearful thing, to fall into the Hands of the Living God!* If His Immediate Hand inflict *Pains* upon me, *how can my Heart Endure* them! O my SAVIOUR, Deliver me from those direful *Pains!* Enable me to Repent of the *Sins* that will Expose me to the *Pains!* How infinitely am I Endebted unto the SAVIOUR, who has delivered me!"

Finally; The *Pains* of the *Teeth,* hasten the Destruction of them. And, *O Man,* when thou dost perceive thy *Teeth* agoing, wilt thou not infer, that thou art thyself agoing after them? Thy *Perishing Teeth* give this Admonition to thee; *O Man, Since the Hardest and Strongest Things thou hast about thee, are so fast Consuming; Do not imagine that the rest of thy Body will remain Long Unconsumed, or that any Bones of thy Body shall not soon Moulder into Dust.*

It is a Passage that *Austin* has in his *Confessions.* L. 9. C. 4. *"Lord,* Thou doest afflict me with *Pain of the Teeth;* and when it was so great that I could not speak, it came into my Mind, to admonish my Friends present, that they should *pray for me,* unto the God of all Health. Writing this on Wax I gave it 'em to read; and as soon as we kneel'd down, the Pain went away. I was amazed, I confess, *My Lord, My GOD;* for I had never found any thing like it, in all my Life."

Tis a Marvellous Indiscretion, in People, to be no more Careful of Præserving a *Good Sett of Teeth;* In the Contrivance whereof the Wise Design of the Glorious Creator has been so Conspicuous! And in the Continuance whereof, the *Speech* is much Concerned; the

Breath kept Sweet; the *Beauty* sett off: and insupportable *Pains* prevented.

If People would betimes use to wash their *Teeth* with *fair Water* every Day; and Wash behind their *Ears,* and about their *Temples,* yea, their whole *Heads,* with *Cold Water;* (and avoid some *Scurvy* Courses and Follies!) they might Enjoy a *Good Sett of Teeth* all their days.

Yea, tho' they have Suffered much in their *Teeth,* by the Neglect of this Præservance; Lett them *Now* take it up; *Now* make use of it. They may find the Benefit of it, the rest of their Days.

> *Tot Remedia ad Sedandos Dentium dolores Prostant,*
> *quot Homines.*[3] Bartholin.

The Number of Remedies for the *Tooth-ache,* is almost as Large as that of St. *Apollonia's*[4] Teeth, which being brought in from the Several Churches in the Kingdom, at the Order of an English King, who was troubled with the *Tooth-ache,* were found Enough to fill Several *Hogsheads.*

§ To prevent the *Tooth-ake* and keep the *Teeth* Sound, frequently rub the *Teeth* with the Ashes which remain in *Tobacco-pipes,* after the rest of the Body has been consumed in Smoke; and then wash the Mouth with fair Water, but lett it not be too cold.

§ It looks like some Disgrace to the *Physicians,* That so many People, even of their own dearest or nearest Relatives, do so commonly ly whole *Days,* perhaps *Weeks* together, under the Torments of the *Tooth-ache* unreleeved. It seems to say, *Syrs, You are Physicians of how Little Value! You can't so much as Cure the Tooth-ache!*

§ Thrust the Eye of a Needle into the Bowels of a *Sow-bug;*[5] and the Matter which it fetches out, putt in the *Hollow Tooth,* if it be such an one that akes: *This* I have heard cried up, as an *Infallible* for the *Tooth-ache,* and I have seen some Success of it.

§ A Thigh-bone of a *Toad,* applied unto an aking Tooth, rarely fails of easing the Pain.

§ *Borellus* tells of a poor Countryman, whose intollerable *Tooth-ache* threw him into Convulsions; That he was cured with *Betony* thrust up his Nose.

§ *Willius*[6] writing *De Morbis Castrensibus,* promises rare Effects from a Decoction of the Shavings of Fir Wood in Beer, held hott in the Mouth.

§ Two or Three drops of the freshly Expressed Juice of *Rue*[7] dropt a little Warm, into the Ear and the Ear Stopt Lightly with Wool upon it. This does Feats in the *Tooth-ache.*

§ Take *Allum,*[8] and melt it; While tis melting mix a little powdered *Ginger* with it. Make it into little Pills, and hold it between the Teeth, so as to bear on the Aking Tooth. It seldom fails of giving Ease.

§ If the *Aking Tooth,* be in any Degree an hollow One, melt a little *Bees Wax,* and mix with it a little *Tobacco Ashes,* And Stop the Tooth with it. It Eases marvellously.

§ If the *Tooth-ache* be from a Defluxion manifestly *Cold,* Boil the Inner Bark of *Elder,*[9] with a strong Vinegar, till all the Liquor be boil'd away. Of this *Bark,* while it is yett hott, putt in the *Tooth* which is afflicted; Monsr. *D'ube*[10] sais, *It will infallibly Ease the Pain.*

§ If it be from a Defluxion[11] Evidently *Hott,* the same Gentleman, directs a Gargarism,[12] with Fair *Water* and Strong *Vinegar* mixed. Or, the use of *Whey.* or Blood-Letting.

§ For this Purpose, *Fuller* has, *An Aluminous Epithem.*[13] Take Burnt *Allum* powdered, Half an Ounce; *Nutmeg* one Dram; *Honey of Roses* Enough to make it an Ointment. Spread it on Paper, and with a Convenient Cloth bind it unto the Side of the Face which is in Pain. *It repels powerfully,* When it is not a Rotten Tooth, but a Sharp Rheum affecting the whole Jaw, and One Side of the Face.

§ Or Apply a Plaster of *Burgundy-Pitch,*[14] mixed with powdered *Nutmeg,* to the Artery in the Temple.

§ To check the Defluxion which causes the *Tooth-ache,* Shavings of *Comfrey*[15]*-root,* made a Paste and applied unto the Temples, may do well. Diverse little Plasters; Especially one of Mastick; have been advised for this Purpose.

§ Or, *Shepherds-pouch,*[16] bruised, and putt into the Ear.

§ A little Bag of *Featherfew,*[17] bedewed with *Rhum,* and made hott between Two Plates over a Chafing-dish; Apply this.

§ *Blisters* drawn behind the Ears, and Repeted, have done Wonders in the *Tooth-ache.*

§ What shall one think of *Hipps*[18] gathered in the Wane of the Moon, in *August,* and worn on the Arm of the same Side with the *aking-Tooth?*

§ They præscribe a Thousand Things, to be held in the Mouth, Especially, to chew *Pellitory* of *Spain.*[19]

And things to be putt into the Hollow Tooth. Especially, a Bit of Lint which is tinged with Oyl of *Cloves,*[20]—or of *Origanum.*[21]

§ Among the Scots, they use a green Turf, heated among Embers as hott as can be Endured, and applied unto the Side of the Head affected.

§ If there's nothing else to be done, *Draw the Tooth!*

§ The *Cerecloth*[22] you'l find in the Chapter of the *Sciatica*, Laid under the *Ear*, does wonders in the *Tooth-ache*.

CAP. XII. *The Prisoners of the Earth*

under,

The GOUT.

With some Notable and Instructive Entertainments

for them.

O Thou Sword Causing Terrour in the Land of the Living; How do the *Sons of the Mighty* tremble before thee! Even, the Swift[1]-footed *Achilles* cannot escape thee! Yea, *All the People, all the Inhabitants of the World, Both Low and High, Rich and Poor together,* feel the Strokes of this *Terrible One.* Tis, *Dominus Morborum;* But Especially, *Morbus Dominorum.*[2]

Tho' *much Study* will be not only a *Weariness,* but also a *Detriment,* unto the *Flesh,* that has the *Gout* Racking of it, yett the *Gouty Patient* has usually more *Strength,* as well as *Time,* to Read; than most People have in many other Diseases; and he may do well to Employ his *Unhappy Liesure,* in the Reading of as many profitable Things as he can. T'wil not only *Divert* him; (which will be one part of the Regimen alwayes to be prescribed under this Malady: but also *Improve* him; and he will be *Doing of Something* to good Purpose, while he is Laid by from his other Business; and he will not *Possess Months of Vanity,* when *Wearisome Nights are appointed* unto him.

We will therefore, for *his* Entertainment make this Article Somewhat Larger than Some of the Rest in this our *Hospital;* It shall be a *Swol'n* Article, that will now Entertain him.

If there be anything in the Remark of *Dolæus,*[3] That *Few fools are troubled with the Gout,* I may expect that my Patient may demand of me, some *Rational Account* of his Distemper; What may be the *Original,* what the *Operation* of it. He may Look to be (*Cured,* I will not say; perhaps he knows his Distemper too well, to Look for *That,* but I will say,) *Treated,* not as a *Carter* or a *Porter,* but as a *Philosopher.*

Now, if this may satisfy him, we will *Talk* a little, of what is now Commonly *Talk'd* about the Matter.

The *Bones,* particularly at the *Joints,* are covered with certain *Membranes,* which abound with a Vast Number of *Glandules,* (a sort of Small, Soft, Spungy, Porous Bags.) the Office whereof is, (like a Sieve) to separate from the Mass of Blood which circulates thro' them, a certain Mucillaginous Liquor or Jelly, which is by the Anatomists called, The *Synovia,* and which is to the Joints very like the Smooth Slippery Mixture of Grease and Tar, with which we anoint the Naves of the Wheels in Jacks and Clocks and Carts and Coaches, to give them an Easy Motion. In a Sheep or a Calf newly killed, if you cutt at the Joint a little above the Hoof, while it is yett warm, this Liquor will be visible to the Eye of any Enquirer after it. Upon which Liquor, if you drop a little Vinegar, it will make a Considerable Coagulation, which you may be a little instructed from. Now, foul, sharp, Scorbutic Humours, bred in the Stomach, associate themselves with the Circulating Blood. Wonder not, that you find me upon the *Stomach* here; For, whatever *Fernelius* and Company may Suggest, *Helmont* and *Etmuller,* and *Boerhave,* and *Sydenham,* as well as *Sennertus*[4] and *Riverus*[5] and *Bonetus,*[6] and a whole Army of Oracles, determine the Rise of the *Gout* ordinarily to be in the *Stomach.* We may suppose the Humours of an *Ill-Digestion* there, to be of what we call *Military Shapes,* and not fitt for an Association with the more *Peaceable* particles of the Blood. Nature has a Conflict with them: and laies hold on the first Opportunity for a Depuration; which it finds when it comes to pass thro' the *Mucilaginous Glands,* which doing the Office of Strainers to the Blood, retain those ill-figured Humours like a Sieve (as we said,) stopping the muddy Settlings: And there they prove to the Mucilage, like *Rennet* unto Milk: which at last grows into a *Tophy,*[7] like a Chalk-stone or a Lime-stone; and in the mean time causes most grevious Inflammations. The *Drelincourts,*[8] and other Gentlemen, that have opened the *Gouty Joints,* have sufficiently detected the *Stagnated Jelly* there. To illustrate this a little more, it has found, that the *Sweat* of a *Gouty Part* (which is always more offensive than any other) mixed with the Slimy Liquor in a Calfs or a Neats Foot, just warm after the Creature is killed, will Strangely Thicken it. These Humours thus as it were

Dropping on the Joint, the *Name* of, The <u>Gout</u>,[9] has been produced, (as well as the *Pain* of it) ; The French, *La Goute,* coming from the Latin, *Gutta,* which signifies a *Drop;* and hence flowes through an Irritation of the Nerves, a Misery *almost* æqual unto *That* which has been compared unto, *A Continual Dropping in a very Rainy Day.*

Before we go any further, there is this Remark very Obvious unto us. The Patient may have more Cause to Entertain his *Gout* very *Thankfully* as well as *Patiently,* than he may be well aware of. His *Gout* may be a *Real* (however a *Severe*) *Favour* to him. A *Fever* might probably Enough have Siez'd him, and kill'd him, if his *Blood,* in the Effervescence of the Battel, had not chas'd the Enemy into the Quarters it is now Retreated to. The *Groans* of the *Gout* may have such *Songs* as these intermixed with them ; *The Lord hath Chastened me Sore, but He hath not given me over to Death.* And, *Why should a Living Man Complain? A Man for the Punishment of his Sin?* My Friend, Instead of Lying on thy Couch, thou mightest have been lying in thy *Grave,* if a God who *in wrath Remembers Mercy,* had not sent this Rough Messenger, to rescue thee.

A noted Physician who (they say) died of the *Gout,* writes, *The Gout is so far from being a Distemper, which we should be solicitous to Cure, that in most Circumstances, it is the only Releef the Constitution can have against much greater Evils.*[10]

Thus we are approaching to the *Sentiments of PIETY* to which the *Gout* should Stimulate the Afflicted Patient.

They tell us a Story, that One *Limenius,* an old Musician of *Thebes,* mentioned by *Cardan,*[11] did use to cure *Gouty People* by the sweet *Music* with which he entertained them. If the *Sentiments of* PIETY which *Gouty People* are to be now Entertained withal, have not the Same Effect which the Notes of the *Theban* had, they may however have a Better and a Greater. The Blessings of an *Healed Soul,* are the Best of Blessings.

O Thou Afflicted; the *Bastinado*[12] upon the *Feet* is a very common, tho' no very Easy, Punishment in many Parts of the World ; Every body knows the Manner of inflicting it. *Hill,*[13] in his History of the *Ottoman Empire,* mentions an English Gentleman Cured of the *Gout,* by a *Turkish Mob,* in an Abusive and Revengeful Way, employing this *Bastinado* upon him. Heaven is now laying thee under a *Bastinado.* Acknowledge the *Justice* of Heaven in it ; and lett *Repentance* have its *Perfect Work.* Make this Acknowledgment: *Lord, in the Worst of my Pains, thou dost punish me less than what I have deserved by my Sins. To Suffer intolerable Pains that should give me gnashing of Teeth without any Intermission, and make the Cries of my Torment ascend forever and ever; is what my Iniquities have deserved.* But then, Examine, Syr, Whether your *Gout* be not the Natural and probable Effect, of some Intemperance, wherein you have indulged yourself; and *Consider your Wayes.* It may be that you have not been so careful about your *Diet* as you should have been. It may be you have the *Tartar* of the *Wine* you have drunk, Sticking to your Joints; Or, it may be, as *Hippocrates* observed so long ago, *Men have not the Gout before the Use of* Venus, You may charge yourself with some *Veneral* Irregularities. If you find any of this *Guilt* upon you, it becomes you to *Humble* yourself before the Glorious God: Humbly *Confess* and *Bewayl* your Sinful Follies; Humbly *accept the Punishment* of your *Iniquity;* and Repair to the Great *Sacrifice* of your SAVIOUR for the *Pardon* of it.

Languishing Man, If thy *Gout* will not bring thee down upon thy *Knees,* thou hast a Distemper worse than the *Gonagra,* (or, *Gout in the Knees*) upon thee. If an *Asa,*[14] troubled with the Gout, and Exceedingly *Diseased in His Feet,* think Skill in *Physic,* (wherof his Name would intimate his being of a Race pretending to it,) may Excuse him from *Seeking to the Lord,* and he will *not seek unto the Lord, but unto the Physicians;* his Fault can have nothing said for the Excusing of it. But every thing that *Setts a Man a Praying,* is to be esteemed so far a Kindness to him. A *Gouty* Man made a *Praying* One, will be an *Happy* One. There will be little Need of suggesting to him, what is now to be *Pray'd for.* Begin, My Friend, and the *Spirit of Grace and of Supplications* will be *nigh* to thee; will *help thy Infirmities.*

How Reasonably would the *Pains* of the *Gout* lead the Sufferer to think on the *Pains* of that HELL, which the Book of Truth calls, *A Place of Torment;* and where a Glorious LORD whose *Resurrection* from the Dead has *victoriously* declared His *Revelation* forever to be relied upon, has *given Assurance to all Men,* that God can and will bring dreadful Circumstances on the *Bodies* as well as the *Souls* of the Wicked! While the *Soul* remains yett united unto the *Body,* the Sentiments of *Delight* or of *Trouble* raised in the *Soul* from Things occurring in the *Body,* have no more than what we may call *Occasional Causes* in those Things, but Really proceed from the Glorious GOD, with His *Immediate Providence* and Concurrence as the *Universal Cause,* perpetually Executing His own Established *Law of Nature,* That there shall be Such and Such *Sentiments* produced on such and such *Occasions*. On the Stretching or the Piercing of a *Nerve*, thence come the Sentiments of *Torment* in the Mind: It is a God always and every where at Work, for the Execution of His own Law, that raises them. When the Union between the *Soul* and the *Body* is dissolved, and the *Spirit returns to God that gave it*, the same God can yett more Immediately, even without the mediation of any *Nerve*, raise the like Sentiments of *Torment* in a guilty Mind: and, that he will do so, may be strongly argued from the Anguish felt by Some under the Terrors of a *Conscience* under a Load of *Guilt*, who have said concerning the *Torment* of being *Burnt Alive, This is but a Metaphor to what I am suffering!* But the *Soul* of the Wicked Man shall be anon reunited unto his *Body* that there may be yett further Sentiments of *Torment* given him; and a *Strange Punishment* inflicted on *The Workers of Iniquity*. Who can Doubt of this, that Beleeves our JESUS to be a *Teacher Come from God;* or that Beholds how Unpunished in this World a *Just God* leaves the Horrid Things done by the worst of Men unto those who are *more righteous than they?* Now lett the *Gouty* People, that are *Chastened with Pain on their Bed, and the Multitude of their Bones with Strong Pain*, fall into serious and awful *Meditations*, on the *Pain*, which will be the Portion of them, on whom an Allpowerful God will make known the *Power of His Anger*. Lord, *Who knows the Power of thine Anger?* Tis Good Advice; *Descendamur Viventes, ne descendamur morientes*.[15] The *Gout* is by *Paracelsus* called, *Morbus Tartareus*. What Stimulations may it give unto *Meditations* on the Dreadful Things undergone in the *Tartareous*[16] *Regions!* Man, What if every *Joint* of thee, as well as one or two, had the *Gout* of it, and thy *Head* and *Stomach* at the same Time tortured with it, and this *Pain* vexing of thee for seven years together? Truly, This were but a very little Emblem of the Miseries, to which thou art obnoxious, until thou escape the tremendous Danger by a Flight unto thy only SAVIOUR, and a Life of PIETY resolv'd upon.

In the Sacred Scriptures, When *Hardness of Heart* is mentioned, the Word, πωρο is made use of. The Word is used among *Physicians*, for that *Knottiness* which an Inveterate *Gout* brings upon the *Joints* of them that are tortured with it. With *Budaeus*,[17] tis *Durities in Artubus;*[18] which has been pronounced *Incurable*. My Friend, If thy *Gout* bring thee not unto such *Sentiments of PIETY*, or, if thy *Heart* be not sensibly moved and mended with them, thou hast something worse than a *Gouty Knottiness* upon it.

I have seen a Servant of God, under sore *Pains* of the *Gout,* making his Pious Reflections, on the Sufferings of our SAVIOUR, when he could complain, *They pierced my Hands and my Feet.* Under the *Gout,* the *Patient* (and one who would be indeed a *Patient*) will do well to take into his Contemplation, the *Pains* Endured by our SAVIOUR, when He made His Complaint, *My Hands they and my Feet have dug / / ev'n as a Lion would; / / my Bones, I may tell all of them; / / they Look and Stare on me. / / Like Water am I pour'd, and all / / my Bônes are out of Joint; / / my Hearts like Wax; in the midst of / / my Bowels tis dissolv'd. / / My Strength is like a Potsherd dried, / / and my Tongue joins my Jaws: / / And thou hast brought me down into / / the Dust where ly the Dead. / /* Sing it, if thou canst! But consider these *Pains* of thy SAVIOUR, as Declaring the *Demerits* of our Sins; as proclaiming the *Love* of our SAVIOUR unto unworthy Sinners; as purchasing our Deliverance from *Eternal Pains,* and Spiritual Advantages to arise unto us from the *Sufferings of this present time.*

And why should not much *Prayer* to Heaven be Employ'd now, as well as on other Occasions? The Apocryphal Epistle of King *Abgarus*[19] unto our SAVIOUR, praying Him to come and heal him, and help him, Supposes the *Gout* then upon him.

This is very Sure; The *Gout* is a Misery, under which a Marvellous *Patience* is called for, under Such a Misery, a Consummate *Patience* (more *Precious* than *Gold* under the *Trial* of the *Fire*) will be *found unto Praise and Honour and Glory.* With what Concern have I read of Several Poor Gentlemen, in whom the Torments of the *Gout,* have produced Such a Disorder of Mind, that they have laid Violent Hands on themselves, and *chose a Strangling* or Stabbing, *rather than Life!* No, Syr; Say rather, *I will bear the Indignation of the Lord, because I have Sinned against Him!*

§ But now, what shall be done for the Releef of the *Grievous Malady?* It has hitherto been the Queen among the *Medicorum Opprobria.*[20] However, without minding an *Italian Physician,* Lett us not altogether *Despair:* Something may be done. The *Tree,* whereof the *Leaves are for the Healing of the Nations,* may afford a *Leaf* that will do Wonders for us. The præscription of that Great Emperour *Charles* V. who, after many Victories was Conquered by the *Gout,* and said, *The best Remedies for the Gout are to Weep and to Bear;* this anon will not be the only one that we may have recourse unto.

The Cure of the *Gout* will not alwayes be a Jest; nor that Versicle always an Oracle; *Tollere nodosam nescit Medicina Podagram.*[21]

I am sorry for the Satyr of *Dolaeus* upon us; who sais, *Few Patients are to be mett withal, that will observe any Rules.*

Tis true, A Great Prince afflicted with the *Gout* might very well Say to the Physicians, *They were at best, but good Guessers.* However, lett us then *Guess* a little.

Tis beyond *Guess*, what I shall first of all quote from the Incomparable *Sydenham*, who had been above Thirty years troubled with the *Gout*, and may be a little harkened to.

One thing he sais, is this; *I Confidently affirm that the greatest Part of those who have Perished in the Gout, have not been so properly killed by the Disease, as by Improper Applications of External Remedies.*

Another thing he sais, is, *We must not attempt the Remedying of the Joints alone, Without a Care of the Whole.* Adding, *Whatever does assist the Blood in discharging the Vicious Humours that are mixed with it, cannot but answer the Intention of Cure, be the Method and Medicine what it will.*

It is possible, there may one day be found out Some *External Application,* so Emollient, and Relaxative and Attractive, that it may first of all Dilate the Pores of the Scarf-Skin, and then with a penetrating Volatility so Rarify the Coagulated Humour as to bring it into a Condition for Transpiration, and then Cause an Easy and Copious Exsudation of it; and the weakened Joint shall be therewithal Corroborated. It is possible at the same time there may be found out, some *Internal Anti-arthritic,* which may at the same time Inwardly Concur to Sweeten the Mass of Blood, and otherwise dispose of the ill-figured Particles floating in it, and at once dissolve the Thickened Moisture in the Joint, and Carry off the Humour from the Blood by some other Channels. *Who can tell?* Gentlemen Physicians, Employ yett more of your *Studies* and your *Prayers* on this Occasion! We hope, Tis not come to a *Ne Plus Ultra,* with you.

It is reported of *Budaeus,* That he Proposing to teach a Method for the utter Extermination of the *Gout,* the Lady became so angry, that she Siezed upon Every Part of him, and made sad Work with him. *Ipsum Auctorem ita Concussit, ut nil Integrum ei reliquerit.*[22] The Fate of *Budaeus* will not Intimidate me. I will go on with my communications.

§ In the mean time, the *Gouty* Patient cannot be too much afraid of Repellents. They are fatal and cruel *Murderers!*

§ *Blisters* made with *Cantharides,*[23] have done Wonders for the Easing and Helping of the *Gout.*

§ By Washing of the Feet Every day in *Urine,*[24] and applying of *Blisters,* the Malady has been to admiration totally cured.

§ Dr. *Brester,*[25] a famous Physician of *Hamburgh,* returning out of *England,* carried this, as one of the Notable Things he had there mett withal. A Celebrated Cure for the *Gout,* by a Bath for the Feet with the Urine of a *Cow;* Especially, if that Liquor were also Drank in the Spring-Season, by which the whole Mass of Blood is diluted and purified.

Borellus tells of an Abbot who was Cured of a Sad *Gout,* by abstaining from all manner of drink. Such was his Abstinence, that he drank not a Drop for Six years together. My *Podagricks* won't make this Experiment. But I wish they would see to it, that their *Drink* both for *Quality* and *Quantity,* may be such as *Wisdome* would oblige them to!

§ Some will mightily cry up an Ointment of *Comfrey*-Leaves.

§ *Burning* of the Place affected, with *Touchwood,* or with *Moxa,*[26] has had a Strange Effect; for the Releef of the *Gout.*

Hippocrates burnt with Raw-Flax.

Ten Rhyne,[27] a Dutch Physician writes a Treatise to prove, That the *Gout* is from a *Venemous* and *Malignant Flatuosity;* a pernicious Vapour which is gott in between the Bone, and the Membrane that immediately covers it, and so inflames it with Tumor and insupportable Torment. And he mightily Commends *Burning* for it. As the grand Remedy used in the *Oriental* Parts of the World.

§ *Purgatives* are more proper to *Prevent* than to *Remove* the *Gout;* Yett *Purging* in Conjunction with *Bleeding,* used before the Access of the Fitt, Monsr. *D'ube* sais. *It Sometimes produces stupendous Effects.*

§ A *Milk-Diet* for Some time entirely kept to, has done Wonders for the Releef of *Gouty* People. Hear the Words of a Learned Gentleman in the *Acta Medica* of *Bartholinus: Nonne Unico Solius Lactis Usu Medico vel nuper Sanatos Legimus Arthreticis Podagricisque cruciatibus Correptos?*[28]

Both *Celsus* and *Pliny* assure us, that the Vertues of Milk for the *Gout,* were Celebrated many Ages ago.

The Learned observe that a *Milk-diet* is exceeding friendly to the *Nerves.*

§ *Antiscorbuticks*[29] are commonly *Antiarthriticks* too.

§ Some that have been dismally handled with the *Gout,* have by the Use of *Bears-Grease* internally taken, obtained a Strange Deliverance.

Quæry: Whether the *Oil of Sweet Almonds,* or *Sperma Ceti,*[30] or some other such Unctious Liquors, inwardly used, in a Sort of *Diet* of them, would not so sheathe the Tormentors, as to Ease the Patients wonderfully?—But then, Cautions must be used, that an *Ill-Habit* of Body be not introduced:

§ In the *Miscellanea Berolinensia,*[31] there is a *New Specific for the Cure of the Gout.* It is, Drink for Three Days after the First Fitt, Twelve Pints of *Diet-Drink* made of *Guajacum, Sarsaparilla,*[32] *Squchanthus,*[33] *Polypodium,*[34] and *Hermodactylus.*[35] The Drinking of This, Three Days, rarely misses of Curing the Patient.

§ *Quincy*[36] sais, There may be almost Wonders done with *Camphire* in the *Gout:*

§ *Vander Heyden*[37] Commends, a *Poultis,* made of Crums of *White-bread,* (or, he sais, rather the powdered Root of *Marsh-Mallows*)[38] boil'd up to a Consistence in New Milk; and pounded with Oil of Lillies, or Fresh *Butter;* mixed with a small Quantity of *Saffron.*[39]

§ Some have been much Eased, by putting their Feet or Hands, into a Bath, made of *Castile-Soap,* as hott as they can Endure it.

§ Here's our famous *Fuller's*[40] Balsame; For *New England* has had its *Fullers,* as well as *Old.*

§ Take two Ounces of *Saffron.* Two Ounces of *Castor;*[41] Half a Pint of *Brandy;* Half a Pint of *Sallet-Oyl.*[42] Beat the *Saffron* and *Castor* to Powder. Putt all into a glass Bottel, Stop'd and Bound very close. Boil it for seven Hours. With this *Balsam* Chafe the grieved Part. But always mix with it a small Quantity of *Oil Peter.*[43]

This Balsame, is the Older, the Better. The Part in Pain must be rub'd with an hott Clothe, and bathed against the Fire. It will drive the Pain before it, if it be *not* settled. If it *be,* it will kill it in Thrice doing.

§ Some Gentlemen have been sensibly Releeved, by a *Water* distilled from the Contents of a *Bullock's Pannels,*[44] newly killed: Fomenting the Part affected.

§ Old *Lucian*[45] brings in the Priests of that—*Goddess, That*

Uncontroul'd makes all Physicians noddies;[46] as having *Temples round begirt with Elder-branches.* There's a Key to it in *Marcellus de Medicina,*[47] who sais, that *Elder* with *Grease,* is of great Use in the *Gout.* And *Scribonius Largus*[48] writing, *De Podagra Frigida,* confirms it.

§ In the *Boylaean*[49] Receits, there is;

A Speedy Remedy for Arthritic Pains

Dip a Feather in good Spirit of *Sal Armoniac;* and gently moisten the Parts affected, or, Take one Part of *Sal-Armoniac,* and three Parts of *Spirit of Wine.* Shake them together; and then dip old, but clean, Linnen Rags in this Mixture; and apply them to the Parts affected. Shift them.

There is added.

A Medicine that almost presently appeases the Pains of the Gout.

Take of *Black Soap* four Ounces; Choice *Wood-Soot* finely sifted, about a Dram. Add unto these about half the Yolk of an Egg. Incorporate 'em diligently; Spread the Mixture Thin, and apply it warm.

§ To appease *Gouty Pains;* take *Linseed,*[50] and with a Little Water, beat it in a Mortar. Lett it be well-rub'd, that the Medullary Part may be Separated a little from the Husk, and make the Water White. In this Liquor dip Clean Rags, till thoroughly wett, and apply them warm to the Parts affected. Shift them every Hour or two.

§ When the *Gout,* Leaving the Extream Parts, flies dangerously to the *Head* or *Stomach,* a *Sinapism*[51] applied unto the Feet, will be as likely as any Thing to bring it back again.

§ A Gentleman in *Germany* releeved his *Gout,* in this Manner. He gathered *Mullein,* when it was in the Flowre, and cutt a good Quantity of it Small, Stalk, Flowre, Leaf, and all; and boil'd it in a pail-full of the *Forge-Water* taken from a Smith's Trough: and then putt into it a Large Piece of *Chalk* in Powder. In this Water he bathed his Feet, Legs, and Knees, as hott as he could Endure it in a Tub till the Water grew cold; He then buried this Water, with the Ingredients, in his Garden.[52]

Using This upon the first Symptom of a Fitt approaching, it always prevented the Fitt, So that he never had any Pain, Swelling or Lameness. If he omitted the Use of this Remedy, he Suffered Racking Fitts of the Gout, which confined him to his Bed, a Month or Six Weeks together; twice in a year at least; chiefly Spring and Fall.

§ Some Gentlemen, who have been sorely handled with the *Gout,* have upon Experience reported and asserted; That filling a minute Leathern Bag of about the Dimensions of one's middle Finger, with powdered Brimstone,[53] and so wearing it any where about their Bodies as to have their Flesh warming of it, they have never had any *Grievous Fitt,* or any more than a *Gentle Touch,* of the *Gout,* after it. But this wants more Confirmation.

§ Some eminent Physicians, besides *Borellus,* have told us Remarkable Things of Gentlemen cured of the *Gout,* by having their *Dogs* to sleep with Them. But, *Wo to the poor Dogs,* who have undergone the *Transplantation!*

§ *Valleriola*[54] and *Heyden*[55] give Instances of Gouty Persons releeved by Transporting Fitts of *Anger,* or of *Terror;* I am far from Recommending the Experiment. But if any of you *Arthriticks* can gett such a Cure as *Antonius Fayus*[56] tells of, by a Transport of *Joy,* I shall be heartily glad of it.

When the Fitt is past, it is the Advice of Dr. *Strother,* To bury the Gouty Part under *Hott Sand* about a Quarter of an Hour together, Twice or Thrice a Day. This will presently supple the Joint, and give new Life and Strength and Vigour to it.

§ It is of Good Consequence, that the *Mind* should be kept *Easy* and *Cheerful,* when the *Gout* is torturing of the *Body.*

Agreeable *Company* may afford its Lenitives.[57]

Reading may afford many Serviceable and Comfortable Entertainments. The Influence which the Reading of *Curtius*[58] and of *Livy*[59] has had, for the Recovery of *Health* to some Eminent Persons, has been celebrated. The *Gouty* may find Histories, that shall not be stuffed with the *Romances* in the former, or the *Prodigies* in the Latter of these.

They forbid *Study,* to men under the *Gout.* But if the Great *Erasmus*[60] had kept unto that Rule, how many Lucubrations of inæstimable Value, had we been deprived of.

Cardan observes, *Habet Podagrosus maximam temporis Partem in sua Protestate. Gouty* People have more Time to Command than other People. They should mightily study *How to improve their unhappy Liesure unto the best of Purposes:* and yett, not in such Severe Studies, as to inflame and enrage the Malady.

A Waggish Fellow Sings,

> The *Gout's* Enrag'd by Care and Sadness:
> The best *Oyl* for't, is that of *Gladness.*

Among the Scribbles of the Bantering *Lucian,* the Learned know, there is a Farce, wherein he represents the *Gout* as a Goddess, whose Priests are the *Gouty People.* While she is boasting of her Invincible Power, she is informed that certain Quacks from *Syria* had Threatened and Undertaken to dispossess her. Offended at their Præsumption, she sent her trusty Executioners to torment them wonderfully. When the Wretches had in Vain applied all their most Potent Remedies, they betake themselves to most humble Supplications, wherein they confess that she had conquered them. On this Confession, she recalls the Tormentors and is contented with her Acknowledged Victory.

I will not commend the *Tragopodagra* of *Lucian* to the Reading of my *Gouty* Patients: Because I do not think that any can be much Edified by reading so lewd a Writer.

And it may be some will think, that in Reading the *Gout-Raptures* of Dr. *Willit,*[61] they do not find that any uncommon Charms of Witt are to be mett withal. But A little to suit the Intention of *Reading,* We will here insert some Heads of the fine Oration with which *Pircheimer*[62] brings in the Lady *Gout,* as making her *Apology,* against the Complaints of them who say, they suffer by her.

The Lady, first hopes that her Judges will not be prejudiced by the Clamorous Accusations of them that cried out upon her; inasmuch as tis well-known, the Best in the World, underwent the Clamours of a calumnious Multitude.

She sais, They could not with any face complain of her Visits to them; for she never Visited them until they not only Invited her, but Even Compelled her unto it. *Ita Vivunt, ineo ita bibunt, ut Etiam me invitam, Saepiusque Reluctantem in suum Contubernium Pertrahant, ac festinate Compellant.*

She sais, That her Accusors Laying upon her, the blame of the Pains they undergo, have indeed none to thank but themselves; *Penitus immemores, Vitam suam Corrupissimam, ac pessimis Vitiis Contaminatam, tot Malorum Causam esse.* Very commonly, she sais, they are People of such Luxurious Manners, that they are altogether unworthy to have Health continue with them.

She observes, If she were so bad a Companion as People would make for, how comes it then to pass, that when Persons are siezed with other Distempers, their Friends come to them with a Sorrowful and Condoling Aspect; but whenever *she* first gives her Company any where, presently the Friends of the Patient all come about him to make merry with him. Every one, *In Risum Solvitur, accurit, jocatur, et ferme Congratulari*[63] *Videtur.*

She then putts her Clients, in Mind, of the *Honours* that she helps 'em to; Every one gives *Place* to them; Every one allows them to *Call* for what they will; Every one allows them to *Sitt* or to *Ride,* as if they were Persons of the best Quality; and Persons of the best Quality complement them. Nay, their Friends take Pleasure in bringing to them all the *Talk of the Town;* and they have more Intelligence, than if they were walking on the *Exchange* every day.

She affirms, that she often obliges them, to prosecute their *Business* in the most Thoughtful and Gainful Manner, while she rescues them from thousands of Dangers, which in going Abroad, they would be exposed Unto. Yea, How many might have been *Hanged* for an Hand in a Plott, if She had not *Imprisoned* them? Their Heads have been saved through her Laying them by the *Heels!* Yea, She declares, That for the Cultivation of their *Minds,* they are more than a little Endebted unto her. Be sure, She gives them Opportunity for it. Particularly, she makes them notable *Rhetoricians;* Enabling them to *Disguise the Matter,* they talk about, as *Rhetoricians* do, For scarce one of them will ever confess the *True Cause* of her coming to him. And for *Astrology* and *Philosophy,* She appeals to them, whether their very Bodies do not now furnish them with more Knowledge and Presage, than any *Almanacks* could ever pretend unto. She makes them also *Physicians* to an high Degree: and putts 'em on Reading indeed Every thing that may accomplish them. All this too, she does for nothing! Yea, she Removes and Even Destroys, that Contagion of the *Body,* which would obstruct the *Soul* in conversing with its most proper Objects. *Dum Corpus debilito, Animum Sano; Dum Carnem affligo, Spiritum Corroboro; Dum Terrenum Expurgo, quod Caeleste est introduco:*[64] *Dum Temporarium adimo, quod Immortale est Confero.*

She asserts, That she prolongs the *Lives* of Men, by driving to the Joints, that furious Matter, which would else fall on the nobler Parts, *Et perquam facile Spiritum extingueret Vitalem.*[65] Yea, she cures their *Vices,* at a Rate beyond all the *Divines* in the World. She knocks down, and keeps low, the *Pride* of Men; and mortifies their Ambition, making *Men Remember that they are but Men.* She prevents their Meddling with the Affairs of other Men. She Scourges them for their Criminal Excesses, and brings them to *Repentance;*

and putts a Stop to their *Debaucheries.* Nor Can *Angry People* under her Charms, vent their Anger as they would, if she did not restrain them. She goes on with a Relation, [*Which t'were to be wished, might be always True!*] That by Weaning Men from this World, and showing them the Vanity of all things here below, she awakens them to Serious PIETY, and brings them to the Sincere and Fervent *Worship* of God; and helps them to Glorify Him in a particular manner with a Religious *Patience* under His afflictive Dispensations. How *Humble* also doth she render those that are under her Institution! *How Modest!* How *Courteous!* How free from a *Revengeful* Temper! And how full of *Compassion* to others that may be under the same, or any Calamity! With what *Assurance of Success* do you usually address one of these Patients, when *Alms* for the Releef of the Miserable are to be asked for! So that the Lady upon the whole Concludes, *Accustatores meos Communi vestro Calculo unanimiter Condemnabitis.*[66]

Lest *Pirckheimer* should not have said Enough, *Cardan* will come with an Oration, and it is no Longer, *Apologia,* but, *Encomium Podagrae,* that must be the Title of it. It were well, if what he sais, were more universally verified. *Qualem hominem facit Podagra! Pium, Castum, Continentem, Prudentem, Vigilem. Nemo tam Dei Memor, quam qui a Podagrae Doloribus detenetur. Qui Podagram Paritur, oblivisci non Potest, quod Caeteris omnibus sui Contingit, se esse Mortalem.*[67] In short, The *Gout* makes People Wise and Good; Mindful of their God and of their *End;* and Every thing that they should be.

Reader, If thou dost not in thy own Experience find it so, thy *Gout* has not had its due Effect upon thee.

A Gentleman has Lately Published a Treatise Entituled, *The Honour of the Gout.*[68] which I have not yett had the Opportunity to meet withal.

Cap. XIII. The *Gout's* Younger Brother,
or, The <u>Rheumatism</u>, and <u>Sciataca</u>, *quieted.*

HERE comes a *Gout,* wherein Help is more commonly hoped for.

A *Rheumatism,* called, A *Bastard-Gout,* Lies in Wandring Pains of the Joints, which proceed (as we must say, till we can talk to better purpose,) from a Volatil Acid falling on the Membranes of them.

The Lower Part of the Back Sometimes is more particularly

Siezed with such Pains. And then, the, *Sciataca,* or, *Hip-Gout,* becomes the Name of the Malady.

There is more of *Pain* than of *Peril* in the Distemper. But it calls for much *Pitty* in the Spectators, as well as *Patience,* in the Sufferers.

O Thou Child of Sorrow, Under all thy Dolours, with an Exquisite and Excellent *Patience,* glorify the Righteous God who inflicts them upon thee. Confess, *Lord, Thou dost not punish me as my Sins deserve. These are not the Great Pains and of Long Continuance which my Sins against an Infinite God have made me worthy of.*

Wait Patiently till Gods Time arrives for the Removal of thy Calamity. It won't be *at once;* it must be *waited for.* Be *Patient,* and beleeve, *God has meant all this unto Good.*

So improve this *Time of thy Visitation* (in a Troublesome Sense it may be called *so,*) that *Repentance* may have its perfect Work, and that upon a *Faith* in the *Sacrifice* of a SAVIOUR (who for it became a *Man of Sorrows and acquainted with Griefs,*) thou mayst have some Assurance that thy *Repented,* Bewayled, abhorred Sins are *Pardoned.* Butt lett thy present Condition, wherein thou hast the *Use of thy Limbs* taken from thee, Stirr thee up very particularly, to Lament thy former *Inactivity* in the Service of God; Thy being so Listless and Lifeless in all Motions for the Serving of God, and the Saving of thy Soul; And Resolve, with the Help of God, that if He Restore thee, thou wilt be more *Active* in Doing of Good, yea, *Doing with thy might, What thy Hand finds to do.*

Water-Gruel and *Patience,* are sometimes pleasantly præscribed by them who See, [I say, *See,* for you may be sure, they don't *Feel!*] the *Rheumatism.* The Meaning however is Good. Beware of all preposterous Managements; And Submitt unto a *Liesurely Cure.* Be sure, *Water-Gruel* is as one may say, even a *Specific Diet* for it.

§ Strange Cures of a *Rheumatism* have been wrought among us, by nothing but keeping to a Diet of Whey. I knew a Gentleman, Who, whenever a Fit of the *Rheumatism* took him, always found a Cure by following this *Whey Diet.*[1]

§ For a *Scorbutic Rheumatism,* tis directed by *Willis;* Take the Infusion of *Stone-Horse*[2] *Dung,* made in Wine or Ale; in any proper Stilled Water twice or thrice a day; to four or six Ounces.

§ In People of a Robust Constitution, *Blood-Letting* is not only Seasonable, but also will *do Wonders.* In Persons of a Feeble Constitution, it must be more Cautiously ventured on.

§ An usual Method in the *Rheumatism,* has been; To correct the

Sharpness of the Humours, with the Testaceous Powders;[3] *Crabs Eyes and Claws, Oister-shels, Eggshels,* and the like; A Dram four times a day in some warm Vehicle, for Six or seven Days.

Then, To Sweat with Decoctions of *Quajacum,* and *Sassafras,*[4] and the like. The Sweating to be Repeted Every Three or Four Days; and between Each time, the Alkalious Powders to be taken.

Then a gentle Purge.

Briefly, *Corrigents* and *Catharticks,* are the general Method for the Cure of a *Rheumatism.*

§ Honest *Woodman*[5] præscribes a Cure for a *Rheumatism,* without Bleeding, Sweating, or Vomiting. "Take *Sweet Mercury*[6] finely Levigated, one Dram; *Scammony,*[7] Two Drams; *Electuarium Lenitivum,*[8] One Dram and an half; Oil of *Juniper,*[9] four Drops; with Syrup of *Saffron,* make a Maws for Pills; which divide into Twelve Doses."

Give one of these every other Night, at going to Bed; which will seldome fail to give Three or Four Stools, the Day following. Do this, till about Six, Eight, or Ten be taken. Woodman sais, *It never yett fail'd me in curing the Rheumatism.* Yea, he adds, *when they have been Continued until Twelve or Fourteen were taken, I have known them give great Releef in the Gout itself.*

I doubt, Master *Woodman's* Patients might have many of them, too much of a *Venereal* Addition to the Rheumatism, else his Pills would not have been altogether so potent with 'em. Our People are generally Strangers to that Circumstance.

§ In *Rheumatic* Pains of the Loins, (known from those of a *Nephritic* Sort by the Patient rising with Difficulty, and as if cutt through the Middle, after bowing down to the Ground) *Baglivi* says, There has been great Success of taking a Pint of Milk-Tea Every Morning.

§ For the *Sciatica,* our People find great Releef, by *Rum,* which has had *Castoreum* steeped in it.

§ Here is a *Cerecloth.* Take one Pint of *Linseed* Oil; Eight ounces of *Red Lead;* Four ounces of *White-Lead;* Three ounces of *Castile-Soap;* the *Leads* must be Powdered fine, and Sifted thro' a fine Lawn Sieve. These must be Incorporated, in a well-glazed Pipkin, over a gentle Fire; and you must keep Stirring of it until it be brought into a Consistency for a Plaister.

This Plaister has had incredible Success in the Curing of the *Sciatica.*

Yea, and the proper *Gout* itself has been strangely releeved by it, Especially, if used at the *Beginning*.

Applied unto the Joints of the Jaw, and under the Ear, it also helps the *Tooth-ache,* to admiration.

CAP. XIV. *Flagellum.*

The <u>Stone</u>
[And other Diseases of the *Kidneys* and *Bladder*]

THE STONE!—

Animus meminisse horret, Luctuque refugit.[1] No; I will rather thus utter my Outcry: Great God, *Thorough a Fear of Thee my Flesh is with a Trembling Siezed; and of thy* awful *Judgments I am very much afraid.* Among the *Scourges,* which the Wrath of the Glorious God employs on a Sinful and Woful World, the *Stone* is most certainly One of the most Horrible to be thought upon. There are Some, which are by Way of Eminency called, *Grievous Diseases,* Most certainly the Stone is to be numbred among them: Tis one of the *First* Magnitude among them. If the *Gritty Bread* of the Captives, obliged them to those *Lamentations, He hath broken my Teeth with Gravel-Stones,* how Lamentable is the Case of them, who are *broken with Bladder-Stones!* In this direful Malady, that Word is accomplished in the Extremity of it, *The Wheel is broken at the Cistern.* But the Torments of being *Broken on the Wheel* are, at least, in regard of their Duration, to be accounted not so Formidable. We seem to countenance the poetic Fiction of our Original, and proclaim ourselves, *Durum Genus,* if the *Stone* be not unto us, a very *Affecting Spectacle.*

They that have hitherto been *Præserved* from the tremendous Distemper, are to be first of all call'd upon. Syrs, Be Thankful, Be Thankful, to the Glorious God, who has hitherto preserved you, and think, *O Thou Præserver of Men, what shall I do for Thee? How shall I speak and live the Praises of my gracious Praeserver?*

What are *You* Better than the Sufferers? They that are groaning under the Hideous Tortures of the *Stone, think you that these are Sinners above all Men,* who are not with such *Groans* piercing the Ears of their Neighbours? *I tell you, Nay;* But Except you be humbly sensible of the *Free-Grace,* which has thus distinguished you, you may likewise all justly become the Sufferers.

Consider the *Sins*, for which the Glorious God might justly break you between the *Milstones* of His Wrath: And be Swallowed up with Admiration at His *Forbearance!*

The Times whereat you often in a day have the *Urinary Excretion* performed with *Ease*, are Times which invite you very frequently to lift up your Hearts unto God with such an Acknowledgment as This; *O, My most merciful God, I bless thee, that the grinding Torments of the Stone, are not now grinding of me.*

Every Day, when you make your *Prayer to the God of your Life*, Will you not particularly pray for this, *Lord, Lett not grievous Diseases be inflicted on me?* And shall not your Preservation from such *Grievous Diseases*, be a particul[ar] Article of your *Thanksgiving* to God?

One arriving to near *Threescore*, proposed it, That he would keep a *Day of Thanksgiving* unto the Glorious God, in a Singular Manner to give Thanks for this; *That he had gott on so far towards the Close of his Pilgrimage*, Helped Hitherto, *and kept free from the Grievous Diseases*: And Especially, *That his Way thro' the Wilderness had hitherto been Encumbred with none of the Stones, which make to be Evil, all the Days of those that are afflicted.*

Your *Gratitude* unto the God who has *Redeemed* you *from this Adversity;* should be particularly Expressed, in your Contributing all you can, to the Releef and Comfort of the Miserable.

But now, O you that are the *Miserables* [*Emphatically* so, *Eminently* so!] Now you are thus *overthrown in Stony Places*, may the *Words* of your SAVIOUR be *Sweet* unto you: such *Words* as are now to Entertain you.

What an *Horror of Sin*, should be produced in you, by the *Dismal Effects* of it, whereof you are so sensible? In every Pang of the Pain given by the *Stone*, lo, *the Stone cries out of the Wall*, and from the tortured Membranes of the Part where it lies, its Voice is this, *Thy Way and thy Doings have procured these things unto thee; This is thy Wickedness; Because it is Bitter, and reaches down unto thy Remotest Bowels.* Truly, *Si non essent peccata, non forent Flagella.*[2] Sin which brought all *Death* into the World, has brought this *Horrible Way of Dying* among the Rest. Oh! Lett none Entertain Light Thoughts, of an *Evil* so mightily offensive to God, so dreadfully punished in His Creatures! None but *Fools* will *make a Mock of Sin*. Wherefore, Lett the *Stone*, which thus falls upon you, cause you to fall down on your Knees before the Glorious God, with all the Contrition and Confession of the most serious *Repentance*. With a

Repenting Soul, Cry out, *Lord, I have Sinned, and I have done very foolishly.* And make your Flight unto the *Sacrifice* of your SAVIOUR.

But then the *Lusts,* which are the Dispositions to Sin, in your Souls; may you be so happy as to slay them upon this Mortal *Stone!* Lett such an *Aversion for Sin* be raised in you, by the Apprehensions which the *Stone* shall give you, that your Sinful Dispositions may perish as by a Messenger coming from the *Quarries of Gilgal.*[3] Yea, Lett this *Stone* that is now within you, be That, at which you will dash the *Bratts,*[4] when you feel the *First Motions* of any Sin stirring in you.

But you, my Friends, if any in the World, are they to whom it may be said, *Ye have need of Patience.* In you, as much as in any, there is an Opportunity for *Patience to have its perfect Work.* Tis by a Consummate *Patience,* that you are to *Glorify* God.

You are a *Spectacle to Angels,* as well as to *Neighbours,* in all your Sufferings. And when you are Suffering of *Terrible Things, Now* for you to whisper not One Word, that shall have in it, the least murmur against the *Justice* and *Goodness* of the Glorious God, but on the Contrary, to keep Admiring and Adoring of Him, as a God infinitely worthy to be Loved and Served and Praised forever; To Express nothing but such a *Faith* as this; *Tho' my God slay me, yett will I trust in Him;* And, *I will beleeve Him a GOD of unfailing Mercies and Compassions, Even tho' I am Consumed:* Verily, This will be to the *Angels,* as well as to the *Neighbours,* a most Lovely *Spectacle. God will be glorified* in you. Yea, the Infinite God Himself, who is infinitely more than all the Spectators in the World, will with Delight behold the *Spectacle.* And you are all this while but under a Præparation for *Astonishing Foelicities* which are prepared for you in a *Future State;* where your *Stone* shall be turned into a *Radiant Jewel* of the *Crown* which is laid up for you; and the *Trial of your Faith, shall be found unto Praise and Honour and Glory at the Appearing of JESUS CHRIST.*

To Engage your *Patience,* Consider what an *Holy* and *Righteous* GOD, He is, who is now smiting of you. Tis true, You are now *Stoning to Death.* But humbly say, *Lord, Thou hast been so Blasphemed by my Sins, that I deserve thus to dy for my Blasphemies!*

I have known an Excellent Person, marvellously *Patient,* when dying of the *Stone;* who, being asked, How he could bear so much *Dolour* with so much *Patience,* replied, *The Thought of my Sins, I find Enough to work Patience in me!* [It was my Grandfather.][5]

Think, "Any thing out of *Hell,* short of *Hell,* is less than what my Sins have deserved. But if the *Torment* of the *Stone* be so bad, what is *Hell,* that *Place of Torment,* which my Sins have deserved! But oh! what Regards do I owe to the Glorious Redeemer who saves me from that *Indignation and Wrath, Tribulation and Anguish."*

But *Patience* must proceed further than so, and Acquiesce in the Divine *Sovereignity,* and acknowledge: *O Thou Sovereign Lord of all: What am I before GOD my Maker, but as the Clay before the Potter! My God, If Thou wilt please to take this poor, mean, vile Peece of Clay, and to dash it in Peeces against a Stone; I may not, I will not say unto thee, what doest thou!*

Man, Hast thou not another Disease to be complained of! Even that which the Word of God calls, An *Heart of Stone?* An *Heart* which will not receive Impressions from that Word! Lay to Heart, the *Stone* in the *Heart,* and lett *That* become uneasy to thee!

A Servant of God under Strong *Temptation* to Sin, cries out as being *Pricked in his Reins,*[6] or, as if he had a *Stone* in his *Kidneys* tearing of him.

Syrs, You have Enough to wean you from *this World,* and make you *Willing to Dy.* Yea, you may stumble upon this insupportable *Stone,* into those Terms, *My Soul chuseth Strangling, even Death rather than Life: I Lothe it, I would not Live always.* But oh! Resolve, *I will wait all the days of my Appointed Time.* Methinks, Honest Groenvelt[7] gives good Advice, Where the Case of the *Stone* is never so desperate; "Lett the Patient be advised, not to abbreviate his Life, thro' Impatience, but with Fortitude and Constancy becoming his Christianity, Expect Deliverance from the *Supreme Physician,* who only by His Almighty Power, can sett Limitts, and a Period unto all Misery."

I have known some Aged Servants of God, much afflicted with the *Stone,* find their Affliction wondrously Abate and Asswage, as *Age* has advanced on them. *Lord, I know Thou canst do Every thing!* I know One, praying with a Society of Christians, had this Petition: *Lord, Lett us not go Roaring to Heaven!* He had *Roar'd* under the *Stone.* But soon after this, applying himself to the *Urinary Excretion,* he fell at once into a Swoon, and Suddenly and Silently went away to a *Better World.*

In the Memoirs of Mr. *James Creswick,*[8] an Excellent Minister, I find: He was one of a very Exemplary Patience under Tormenting Pains of the *Stone.* His Executor had a Box containing above Six hundred *Stones,* that came from him, or were found in him, some of which were above an Inch and half long. But he would frequently Say, *Lord, I am Thine; and Thou canst do me no Wrong. I had rather have Health of Soul, in a Body full of Pain, than Health and Ease of Body, with a distempered Soul.*

The *Stone,* in *Galens* time, was pronounced Curable by Nothing but a *Manual Operation.* And indeed, Since a Cure by all other Medicines, even by *Millepedes* themselves, (Cried up for such a powerful Dissolvent in the Case, by others as well as *Hartman,*)[9] is rarely hoped for, the *Manual Operation* is now with much Success very commonly practised. The *Ish Calaphot* (which a Learned Man takes to be the Original and Etymology of the Name *Æsculapius,*) that is to say, *The Master of the Knife;* He tis that must go about the Cure. What shall be done, when the *Stone* is of (or anything near) such a Magnitude, as that mentioned by *Hildanus,*[10] which weighed no less than Two and Twenty Ounces, I know not. I know, what a *Celsus* would have done upon it. However, The Practice of *Lithotomy,* Especially since the *Franconine* has been so improved by the *Collotian,*[11] comes now to be reckoned among the Favours of Heaven to a Wretched World.

Christian, Intending with Courage to undergo the *Manual Operation,* Thou wilt first Thoroughly *make Ready for Death.* Mourn for, Turn from, Every Sin; Say, *What have I any more to do with Idols?* Look to the *Blood* of thy SAVIOUR, that thou mayst be *Cleansed from all Sin.* Give thyself up to God, with a Soul sincerely sett upon a *Return* unto Him. Embrace thy REDEEMER in all His *Offices,* that thou mayst be brought back unto God. *Leave nothing undone,* which God would have thee to *Do* before thou *dy.* Then call together a Number of thy *Christian Friends,* and in a convenient Portion of Time sett apart for that Purpose, Lett them with *United Supplications,* Cry unto God, that He would graciously Appear, and give a Good Issue to the Distress now upon thee.

And now, with a Soul full of affectuous Thoughts, on the *Anguish* which thy SAVIOUR underwent for thee, when the *Iron entered into His Soul,* Submit Courageously to what thou shalt find ordered for thee.

What *Bartholomew Dias*[12] called by the Name of *Tormentoso,* King *John* afterwards called, *The Cape of Good Hope.* This *Tormentous Malady* may be rendered such, by a right Behaviour under it.

§ *Ligon*[13] relates, astonishing Effects of this Remedy for even breaking, and bringing away, *Stones* and *Gravel.*

Take the Pizzle[14] of a *Green Turtle;* dry it with a Moderate Heat; and pulverise it. Of this take as much as may ly upon a Shilling, in Beer, Ale, or White-Wine. It works a speedy Cure! Yea, the *Turtle-Diet* will do Wonders for the *Stone.*

§ *Borellus* affirms, a *Ptisan*[15] made of what grows on the *Wild-rose*[16] dried in the Oven; has delivered many that were afflicted with the *Stone.* But he sais, it must be used a pretty while together.

§ The great *Boyl* mightily commends a Distilled Water of *Arsmart,*[17] in the *Stone.* And many others have sett the Value of a Secret upon it, for its Efficacy in such Cases.

§ In Fitt of the *Stone,* tis one of the *Boylaean* Receits. Take *Sack,* or in the Want thereof, *Claret,*[18] and by Shaking or otherwise, mix with it as well as you can, an Equal Quantity of *Oyl of Walnuts;*[19] of this Mixture give from four or six to eight or ten Ounces at a Time, as a *Clyster.*

§ And so is This; Take Powdered *Crabs Eyes;* Dissolve them in White-Wine Vinegar. Drink from two Spoonfuls to six.

§ There is a Strange Passage related by honest *Philip Woodman.* A Gentleman, who had been many Years troubled with the *Stone* in his Bladder, and found no Help from the most able Physicians, filled *Three Stone-Bottles* with his *Urine,* as he successively voided it. These *Bottles* he covered with a Tile, or Slate, and buried them something deep under Ground, where they could not be disturbed. For the Present he felt no Releef; but after about Six Months, his Disease began to decrease; and in a few Months more he grew perfectly well, and so continued. He was told, before the Experiment was made, that he would find no Ease, till the *Urine* began to Vanish, and that as *that* Vanish'd, the Disease would go off. I know not what well to make of it. Be sure, All *Sacraments,* which call in Help from *Dæmons,* (whereof I see not, that *this* must be one,) are dangerous Things; the *Remedies* worse than the *Diseases* they are used for. Be warned, Reader, Be warned against going to the *God of Ekron.*[20] Do not *Acheronta Movere.*

§ An old Man incureably tormented with the *Stone,* forever found a Strange Releef of his Torments, by a warm Draught of *Mutton-broth and Beer* mixed.

§ The Duke of *Wittemberg*[21] taught *Luther* to releeve himself under Pains of the *Stone,* with a Strong Decoction of *Juniper-Berries* in Wine and Water.

§ For the Prevention of the *Stone;* Much Use of *Ground Ivy,*[22] in all the ways imaginable, is never Enough to be Commended. It will also answer a Thousand other good Intentions.

or, use much of our *Samp-Diet.*[23]

§ An Eminent Person who had been tormented with the *Stone*, found this Releef. "I took twelve Grains of the *Salt* made of the *Stones* which were taken out of Men; I dissolved the said Salt in a Little Water; and then I putt all into a Glass of White Wine, and drank it off, and walked about my Chamber near two Hours: At the End whereof I had great Need to make Water, and I Voided (with Violence) a Large Glass full of Gravel, which was so gross and so rugged, that it caused me to void near a Pint of Blood. The same thing happened to me three times; and Every time I voided Blood: Which made me Judge, that I should have taken Less of the Said Salt. The Said Stones were Calcined in a Potter's Oven, and after they were Calcined, I Extracted the Salt out of them with distilled Rain Water. The faeces I Calcined again and Extracted the Salt as before; which I repeated so often, till the Said Stones yielded no more Salt. *Note,* That to make this Salt for a *Man,* you must take the Stones taken out of *Men;* and for a *Woman,* those that are taken out of *Women.*"[24]

Ⅱ Tis no rare thing for People to be afflicted with <u>Gravel</u>.

§ Take an Ounce of Syrup of *Marsh-mallows,* mix with Two or Three Spoonfuls of *White Wine.* Warm it on the Fire; And add an Ounce of Oyl of Sweet Almonds; and slice into it a Quarter of an Ounce of Nutmeg. It has been a very Successful Remedy.

§ Here's a *Wonder-Worker!* Take of *Nettle-Seed,*[25] of *Parsley-Seed,*[26] of *Burdock-Seed,*[27] about half an Ounce (*ana*) more or less. Make a gentle Decoction of these, in a Quart of *White Wine.* Sweeten a little Glassful, (or four or five Spoonfuls) of this, with some Syrup of *Marsh-mallows;* and give it unto the *Patient.* I wish he be a *Patient!*

§ A Tea of (unbruised) *Linseed* is a marvellous Thing.

§ So is, the *Red Blisters* found on *Oister-shells,* pulverised.

§ In very Tedious, Dolorous, Desperate Fitts of the *Gravel,* there has been an Immediate and an Astonishing Success of this plain Remedy; Take half a Gill of *Molasses,* and the Same Quantity of *Hogs-Fatt,* united.

§ Take the thick Skin that is found in the *Gizzard* of a *Cock* or *Hen;* Dry it until it be pulverable. Give it in any convenient Vehicle, from a Scruple to two Scruples.

§ Take the Juice of *Onions,* two Spoonfuls; *White Wine* half a Pint, or more. Mix them for a Draught. This gives present Ease; and if repeted for some time, they tell me it quickly cures.

Ⅱ An Appendix, relating to
Urinary Diseases

In all *Urinary Diseases,* (which are commonly very *Uneasy* Ones,) the most proper *Sentiments of PIETY,* will be;

That we have been too Insensible of our Dependence on the Glorious God, for keeping all the Various and Numerous *Wheels of Nature* in a *Regular Motion* for so many years: The least of which being disturbed, what a troublesome *Confusion* follows!

That the *Pains* which we *Suffer,* are much less than what we Deserve.

That the *Sin* which has brought these *Pains* into the World, (and what our great SAVIOUR could not Expiate, without being *Acquainted with Griefs,*) must be an *Evil,* to be inexpressibly Bewayled and Abhorred.

Repentance must be carried on to its *perfect Work,* by these Calls from the *Lower Parts of the Earth.*

If any thing *Disorderly* or *Incautelous* in our *Drinks* has brought any of these Diseases upon us, the Fault is to be repented of.

And if the Patient hath been at any time guilty of any *Venereal Miscarriages,* CONSCIENCE, Do thine Office upon him.

Ⅱ The Anatomy has not hitherto discovered any other Way for the *Urine,* than thro' the *Blood,* [As it neither has the Passages that carry *Milk* to the *Dugs!*] yett there is most certainly a Nearer Cutt from the *Stomach* and *Intestines,* by the Convenience whereof Remedies may come Entire and little altered, unto the *Reins* and *Ureters.* We need not quote an *Hochstetter,*[28] or a *Diemorbroeck,*[29] or a *Fuller,* or the *Philosophical Transactions,* for this. The Quick Descent of Things from the *Stomach* into the *Bladder,* which we see Every day, renders it unquæstionable. There are some *Direct Passages* from the *Stomach* to the *Bladder;* ordered by a Gracious Providence, to prevent an immoderate Distension of the *Blood-Vessels* upon Drinking, which would follow, if all were to pass through the Lacteals into the Blood.[30]

§ The Strangury is a Disease too well known, wherein the Urine is Evacuated by Drops, with a continual Desire of the Evacuation; and great Heat and Pain in the Neck of the Bladder.

Sometimes there is only a *Dysury;* wherein the *Urine* is voided with a due Quantity, but with great Heat and Pain in the Parts, giving a *Difficulty* to it. But sometimes it proceeds to an *Ischury,* which brings a *Total Suppression* of the *Urine* with it.

It is usually Caused, by an Acidity in the Urine, which is produced from a Vicious Digestion in the *Stomach:* which therefore is in the first Place usually to be looked unto.

§ In a *Strangury,* the *Stomach* should first be Cleansed from its Acrimonies; It may partly be done by gentle *Vomits,* which are of wondrous Use, not only in This, but also in all Urinary Diseases. After which, there may be some Use also of gentle *Purges.*

Turpentine taken from half an Ounce to six Drams, Opening its Body with the Yolk of an Egg, and made into a Potion, with Two or Three Ounces of *Parsly Water,* has been highly commended, for both of these Purposes.

§ One was delivered from an Obstinate *Strangury,* by nothing but using to drink Water tinged with a little *Rum.*

§ All the *Alcalious Powders,* are of use to correct the Sharp *Serum,* and unlock the Passages of the Bladder; *Crabs* Eyes and Claws; *Oyster* Shells; and *Egg* shells. And so is, the Juice of *Stonehorse Dung,* half an Ounce, or more, given in a glass of White Wine.

§ Spirit of *Nitre,*[31] dulcified, given from Twenty to Thirty Drops, is admirable.

§ *Wood-lice* are a Specific.

§ Oil of *Sweet-Almonds,* and Syrup of *Marshmallows,* with a little *Balsam of Sulphur* terebinthinated.[32] What think you, of such a *Linctus,* to be now and then a little taken of it?

§ Six or Seven Cloves of *Garlick,* bruised with Two or Three Ounces of *Rhenish* Wine. Strain it, and so Drink it, every Morning and Evening for Three or Four Days. This gives great Releef in any *Strangury.*

§ A *Strangury* caused by drinking of New Ale or Wine, is presently removed by Drinking about half a Dram of Powder of Nutmegs, and about the same Quantity of Chalk, in Powder.

§ A Plaister to the Navel, made of *Block Soap* one Ounce; and *Saffron in Powder,* half an Ounce; Tis a powerful Thing, to force Urine, in *a Strangury;* Seldom failing to do it, in two or three Hours time.

§ An <u>Ischury</u>, or Stoppage of the *Urine,* is help'd like a *Strangury.* To which may be added, Clysters of Urine, Turpentine, and the Diuretic Herbs.

If there be an Inflammation of the Parts, *Bleeding* may be proper.

A Cold, Thin, Spare Diet may be proper.

§ Pills of powdered *Nutmeg,* and *Saffron,* and Woodlice, with *Turpentine,* may be of good Significancy.

§ Take Venice-*Turpentine*[33] dried a little at the Fire, Two Drams; Juice of *Liquorice,*[34] and Powder of the same, one Scruple. Mix them; and make Pills as big as Pease; and roll them in Powder of *Millepedes. Dolaeus* cries up these as Excellent Pills.

§ For *Suppression of Urine* give about a Spoonful of bruised *Mustard-seed* in any convenient Vehicle.

§ Some have had a *Suppression of Urine* releeved by powdered *Mouse-dung,* when other Means failed.

§ Or, Lixiviate[35] Water with *Ashes;* Drink freely of it.

§ If the Use of *Cantharides* has caused, any Trouble to the Urine, and the Vessels of it; Large Draughts of *Milk* soon remove it. Especially if *Marsh-mallows* be boiled in it.

Syrup of *Marsh-mallows* gives a Strange Releef in these Cases.

§ A Decoction of Common *Mallows* and *Garlick,* in White-Wine, drank morning, noon and night, is a great Secret for the forcing of *Urine. A Secret* which *Every body knows of.*

§ A <u>Dysury</u>, or Sharpness of the *Urine,* Every body knows that half a Dram of *Sal-Prunellae,*[36] or of the best *Salt-Petre,*[37] dissolv'd in a little Water, or small Beer, drunk Every three or four hours, will cure it.

§ An Acrimony of the *Urine,* Decoctions of *Mallows* presently help it. Or, a Scruple of *Gum Arabick,*[38] dissolv'd in a Glass of White-Wine, drank Every six or seven hours. Or, Whites of *Two Eggs,* beaten to a Water, adding an Ounce of *Parsley-Water,* and of Syrup of *Violets.*[39]

§ If the *Heat* of *Urine* be caused by *drinking* too *hard,* Large Draughts of *Common Water,* duely repeated, soon releeve the Criminal.

§ For *Sharpness of Urine,* give about half an Ounce at a Time, of *Ground Ivy* in any Convenient Vehicle.

§ *Etmuller* mentions One who on drinking Wine always fell into a *Dysury,* and made Bloody Urine; but was always Cured by taking *Oil of Sweet Almonds.*

§ A *Stoppage* and *Sharpness* of Urine may proceed from indurated *Faeces* in the Strait Gutt, which may compress the Neck of the Bladder. An Agreeable Purge releeves immediately.

§ In all Diseases of Urine, the Body must be kept open by *Clysters,* or *Laxatives.*

§ Among the *Urinary Diseases* is to be reckoned a <u>Diabetes</u>; wherein the Body is destroy'd, by voiding Large Quantities of *Urine:* Sharp Humours bred in the *Stomach,* which mixing with the Blood melt it into a *Serum.* And an *Incontinency of Urine,* when it is not retained in the Bladder, as it should be; which may proceed from a Weakness of the Sphincter-Muscle there.

§ In a *Diabetes,* the Acrimony of the Blood must be corrected. A few Ounces of *Lime-Water,* drunk three or four times a day, is of good use in this Case. And so is *Milk,* or *Whey,* drunk plentifully, especially if *Red hot Iron* have been often quenched in it.[40]

§ The, *Decoctum Incrassans.* Take of *Gum Arabic* powdered grossly, Three Ounces. Boil it in Water (carefully stirring it, that it may not burn to the Bottom) from *Two Pounds,* to *Twenty Eight Ounces;* and Sweeten it with Four Ounces of Syrup of *Marshmallows.*

This mightily thickens acrid Humours that are too thin, and Sheathes up the Sharp Salts that are in them. It is a good Remedy against *Scalding Urine,* and it helps in a *Diabetes,* as well as in tickling Coughs.

§ *Hartman* speaks of *Steel,*[41] as the Grand Releef under a *Diabetes.*

§ *Snails* burnt, and the Ashes taken, seldome fail of curing this Distemper.

§ For *Incontinency of Urine,* and the Beginning of a *Diabetes:* Cutt off the Necks of well-blown *Sheeps Bladders.* Of the remaining Membranes, putt a good Number one over another into a Covered Pott; Where being gently, but fully, dried in the Oven, pulverize them. The Dose, as much as may ly upon a Sixpence.

§ Or, Powder of a Burnt *Toad,* hung in a Bag, about the Neck.

§ For *Incontinency of Urine,* a *Mouse* flay'd and dried in a warm Oven, and powdered, and so drank at Night in a Glass of Red Wine, or any proper Vehicle; (repeated Eight or Ten times,) tis an Incomparable Remedy.

Take of the *White Substance* (Looking like Chalk) which is found in *Flint-Stones;* Dry it, and make it unto a Powder. Of this Powder give as much as may ly upon a Shilling, to a Child that cannot hold its Water. Lett it be done for eight or ten days. T'was hardly ever known to fail of curing the poor little Pissabeds. The Dose increased and continued, may do for Elder People.

Cap. XX. *Variolae trimphatae*
The
Small-Pox Encountred.

IT is an *Hard Chapter* that we have now before us. There is a *Great Plague* which we call, The SMALL POX, wherein *the Misery of Man is great upon him:* A Distemper so well *known,* and so much *Felt,* that there needs no Description to be given of it.

So Few among the miserable Children of Men do now Escape it, that the *Enquirers after Causes* have Suspected the *Original* of this Malady, to be some *Venom Connate* with every Man, (Derived, they'l tell you, from the *Maternal Blood* unto him) which lies Dormient and Buried, until it be fired by *Contagion,* and then furiously breaking out from its unknown Lurking-Place, it mixes with the whole Mass of Blood, and makes the Terrible *Disturbance,* and Even *Destruction,* the *Fear* whereof holds Mankind in a very uneasy *Bondage.*

But this *Old Notion* loses much of its Authority, by our Considering that it is a *New Distemper.* Tho' the Learned *Bartholinus* to that Quæstion *an deformis hic Morbus Antiquis fuerit notus?* answers, *Non ausim dubitare,*[1] yett, all that is quoted from *Hippocrates* and from *Aetius*[2] and *Galen,* will not remove the *Doubt* of other Learned Men upon it. Nor will they see, that *Celsus* (the *Tully* of the Physicians) has described so livelily our *Small-Pox,* That one may say, *Ovum Ovo Similius non sit.*[3] Tis Evident unto us, that the *Ancients* were unacquainted with it: It is one of those *New Scourges* whereof there are Several, which the Holy and Righteous God has inflicted on a Sinful World. It is not many Ages ago, that it was brought into *Europe* thro' *Africa;* on the Wings of those *Arabian Locusts,* which in the *Saracen* Conquests did *spread over the Face of the Earth.* It seems, as if the Constitution of the *Earth,* and of the Air, and of *Humane Bodies,* has altered in Successive Ages; From whence *New Maladies* have arisen, which the præceding Ages were Strangers to; (and the *Symptoms* and *Effects* of *Old* ones have mightily altered;) And probably more will yett arise. Hence (as the *Leprosy* grows less common, so) *New Fevers* appear. But the proper *Plague* has never yett visited the vast Regions of *America:* Howbeit *Pestilential Fevers* little better than *That,* have *there* made most fearful Ravages.[4]

It begins now to be Vehemently Suspected That the *Small-Pox* may be more of an *Animalculated Business,* than we have been generally aware of. The *Millions* of — — — —[5] which the *Microscopes* discover in the Pustules, have Confirmed the Suspicion. [What would a *Nieuentyt*[6] now say, Reading Job. VII.5.[7] upon it?) And so, we are insensibly drawn into *New Sentiments,* about the *Way* of its *Conveyance,* and the *Cause* why tis convey'd but once; All which,— *Non Sunt hujus Loci.*[8]

The *Sentiments of PIETY* to be raised in and from this *Grievous Disease,* are what I am first and most of all to be now concerned for.

And now, O *Mankind* in general; Wilt thou not from the View and Sense of this *New Evil Devised* against thee, Humble thyself *under the mighty Hand of God?*

Glorious God, Such a Sharp, and indeed such a New Rebuke of thine upon us, Correcting us for our Iniquity, and Consuming our Beauty as a Moth, (yea, as a Lion,) Why, Why must it come upon us? Righteous art thou, O Lord: yett lett us Reason with thee of thy Judgments!

The Answer which Heaven thunders down upon us, is; *Ah, Sinful Generation, a People Laden with Iniquity, a Seed of Evil-doers, Children that are Corrupters; They have forsaken the Lord! And Why are ye Stricken more, Even with Strokes that were unknown to the more Early Ages? Tis because ye Revolt more and more!*

The Distressed *Children of Terror* having such a *Fearful Expectation* of this *Fiery Indignation* to *devour* them, and Seeing that, *Sceptra Ligonibus aequat*[9]—Even *Stars,* yea, *Crowns,* are struck down by it; They are Certainly Stupid out of Measure, and more Foolish, than the *Wild Asses Colts,* if they do not Immediately Turn and Live unto God, and gett into such a *State of Safety for Eternity,* that they may be *Ready* for whatever *Event* this *Distemper* may have upon them, and not be *Afraid with any Amazement.*

The Advice, is; And, Oh! *Behold an Angel with a flaming Sword* over thee giving of it; *Præpare to meet thy God,* O thou Traveller thro' an *Hatzar-Maveth,* a Land where *Fiery Flying Serpents* are hovering Every where about thee!

Be Restless, until the *Things that accompany Salvation,* and the *Evident Tokens* of it, be plainly to be found upon thee: Until thou art able to say, *My Mind by a New and a strong Biass given from Heaven unto it, is come to make the Serving and Pleasing of the*

Glorious God, the Chief End of my Life: And I now go to God, for that which I have heretofore gone to Creatures for. The Blessed God is now more to me than this World; The Enjoyment of Him is a Blessedness præferrible with me, to all the Pleasures and Riches and Honours of This World. Able to say; *Every Thing of a Glorious CHRIST is precious to my Soul, I prize Him in all His Offices; I prize Him with all His Benefits; I would fain have Him to fulfil in me all the Good Pleasure of His Goodness.* Able to say; *There is no known Course of Sin, Condemned by the Continual Reproaches of my Conscience, wherein I indulge myself; if I am Surprised into any gross Act of Sin, I feel my Bones broken, till a Repenting Faith has restored me to the Peace of GOD. The Lusts of indwelling Sin, I seek, I Sigh, I Long for a Deliverance from them.* Able to say; *I Love my Neighbour; I am glad, when it goes well with him; I am grieved when it goes Ill with him. If he do Evil to me, I durst not so much as wish Evil to him.* And able to say, *it is my Delight and Study to do Good; And I Labour to be a Faithful Steward, of the Talents wherewith my SAVIOUR has betrusted me.* If thou canst not yett say such Things, *Give no Sleep to thine Eyes, nor Slumber to thine Eylids, until thou canst.*

And then, What wouldst thou do, if the *Summons* were certainly brought unto thee, hearing thyself Summoned within *one month* to *appear before God the Judge of all?* Surely Thou wouldest without any Delay, Sett apart Some Time to go through a *Process of Repentance* and *Lay hold on Eternal Life.* Instructed from the Gospel, In these Moments of *Agony for Eternity,* thou wouldest cry to God, That with Displays of *Sovereign Grace* He would Quicken thee to *do what thy Hand finds to do,* that thou mayest be Saved. Thou wouldest Poenitently confess the Things, in which canst upon *Examination* find, that thou hast offended Him. Thou wouldest *Carefully with Tears* beg it of the Compassionate God, that He would *Pardon* all thy Offences, for the sake of the *Sacrifice* which His Beloved JESUS has offered up to the Divine Justice for thee. Thou wouldest Plead that *Sacrifice* for thy *Atonement,* with Cries that would pierce the Heavens. And then thou wouldest give thyself up unto God, with *Dispositions* and *Resolutions* of all possible *Obedience* unto Him; With a *Respect unto All His Commandments. All this* wouldest thou do. Then do it; Even *all this.* Do it *Just Now.* Lett it be done without *any more adoe.*

Finally; Be Inquisitive, What hast thou *left undone,* that if the

Pulls of thy *Last Hour* were now upon thee, thou wouldest wish *that it had been done?* My Friend, suppose thyself within a Few Minutes of thy *Expiration;* Suppose thyself in all the awful Solemnities of a Death-bed; Suppose thy *Life* just agoing, and thy *Soul* presently to appear before the tremendous Tribunal of God. Now under the Illuminations of such a Supposal, ask thyself, *what should I wish to have done before I come to this?* Go do it out of hand. Lett it be done with all the *Dispatch,* with all the *Concern* imaginable.

There is an *Epitaph* upon one laid in *West-Minster-Abby,* which has in it such Terms as these; *One who thro' the Spotted Vail of the Small-Pox; rendered a pure and unspotted Soul to God.* Shouldest thou *Dy* of the *Small-Pox,* after such a Conversion to God, *This* may be thy Happy *Epitaph.* And as it is Expressed on the *Grave-Stone* of another there, who dy'd of the like Distemper, thy Happiness will be, *Ex Igne ac Tunica Molesta Evolasse ad Coelos:* To fly away for Heaven, out of as Burning a *Coat,* as what *Nero* putt upon the ancient *Martyrs.*

But I may now suppose the Person thus *Præpar'd,* become a *Patient.*

Being Visited with the *Small-Pox,* there are many Exercises of PIETY, which there will be a Call unto; Among which there will be none more Pertinent than that of the deepest *Self-Abhorrence,* and *Self-Abasement,* from a Sense of the *Original Sin,* which will oblige us to cry out, *Unclean! Unclean!* and Confess, *Lord, I am a Filthy Creature!*

My Friend, What a *Loathsome Creature* art thou! *Loathsome* even to Thyself as well as to all that are about thee. Thy *Sin* has rendred thee so unto the Glorious God, who is *of Purer Eyes than to behold Evil, and Cannot Look upon Iniquity.* It should render thee so unto Thyself; *Loathing thyself in thy own Sight, for thy Iniquities, and for thy Abominations.*

There is a *Poison Within* thee, the *Poison* of an *Evil Heart which departs from the Living God.* By *Temptation* as by a *Contagion,* the *Poison* makes horrible *Eruptions.* All the nasty *Pustules* which now fill thy *Skin,* are but Little Emblems of the *Errors* which thy *Life* has been filled Withal. Make thy Lamentation, *Lord, From the Sole of the Foot, even to the Head, there is no Soundness in me; nothing but putrifying Sores.*

In the *Wearisome Nights* that are *Appointed* for thee, thy Complaint is, *My Skin is broken and become Lothesome.* Thy *Bed*

Comforts thee not; thy *Couch* does not *Ease thy Complaint;* perhaps thou art *Scared with Visions,* and things of a *Frightful Aspect* appear before thy closed Eyes. Now lett *Repentance* have its *perfect work.* And lett thy Condition lead thee to a *Repenting Sense* of the *Sin* which has provoked and procured this Calamity for thee, and is Livelily Resembled in it. Poenitently say, *Lord, My Wounds do Stink and are Corrupt, because of my Foolishness!*

Lett this Apprehension of thy *Loathsome Sin,* drive thee to the *Blood* of thy SAVIOUR, for the *Pardon* of it; That thou mayst be *Cleansed from all Sin.* At the same time, Importunately Sollicit for the SPIRIT of thy SAVIOUR, to Expell the Malignity of *Sin* that is Lodged in thee, and send up thy *Groans* unto Him, for His *Purifying Influences.*

While some are very *sorely* handled by this Noisome and Painful Distemper, others are favoured with a more *Gentle Visitation.* If this be thy Case, Be very Thankful to a Compassionate God; Thankfully own, *it is of the Lords Mercies that I am not consumed, because His Compassions fall not.*

There is One Circumstance of this Disease (which an acute and famous Anatomist, methinks, yett gives but a very weak Reason for;) It has hardly ever been seen, that any after having Suffered it *Once,* comes to Suffer it a *Second time.* There are Several other *Fevers,* it may be *Six* or *Seven* sorts of them, that may have the Same Observation made upon them; *No Man undergoes them Twice.*[10] It is to be hoped, *O Man,* That this observation will be verified in thy *Moral Experience;* and that the *Grosser Sins,* which thou hast once *Repented of,* thou wilt *Never again* fall into them.

But thus having *Sought First,* what is *most* of all to be Sought for, and Serv'd the *Kingdome of God and His Righteousness,* from the *Calamity* that is come upon us, we may the more hopefully proceed unto the Work of Encountring and Conquering the *Adversary.*

An *Adversary,* which *wilt thou play with him as with a Bird?* No, He will *fill* thy *skin* as with *barbed Irons.* And *shall not one be cast down at the Sight of him? Who can come to him with his double Bridle? Sparks of Fire Leap out of his Mouth: His Breath kindles Coals. When he raises up himself the mighty are afraid, He Spreadeth Sharp pointed Things, upon* our Clay. He makes our Blood to *boil as a Pott:* He makes our Humours *Like a Pott of Ointment.*

Yett lett us be of *Good Courage;* yea, be *Very courageous.* There is a way to Manage him!

⫾ Unknown is the Number of *Lives,* which the Glorious God has made our *Sydenham,* the Instrument of Saving, by teaching us a New and a Right Method of treating the *Small-Pox,* and reclaiming People from the Madness of *Killing one another with Kindness,* and praeposterous Proceedings.

I am willing to treat my Friends, with what I know of the *Sydenhamian* Method. But at the same time I must advise them, That from a Difference of *Seasons* and of *Climates,* there may happen some Circumstances, that may require Proceedings, wherein this *Incomparable Method* must not be Strictly in all Points adher'd unto. The Malady call'd, *Variolae,* is not without its *Varieties:* yea, I have myself[11] seen *Anomalies* in the *Small-Pox* wherein a *Sydenham* himself might not be entirely relied upon. There is now then an *Irregular Small-Pox,* in which it may not be Easy to fix Rules for an *Unchangeable Regimen. A Skilful* and *Thoughtful* PHYSICIAN must be always near the *Patient,* [*My Friend,* Make *Sure,* and then make *Much,* of such an One!] And this *Physician* will take his Measures from the *Indications* as he finds them. Nevertheless, *For the Most Part,* they will *Both* of them find their Account, in Receiving and Remembring Such Things, as I will deliver in the Ensuing *Aphorisms.*

I. The Distemper we call, *The Small-Pox,* is usually distributed into Two Sorts; The *Distinct* Sort; and the *Confluent* Sort; The *Symptoms* whereof have some Difference; and the *Way of Managing* must be also a Little Different.

By not being aware of *This,* what *Mortal Errors* have been often run into!

II. By how much sooner the *Pocks* come out before the Fourth Day of the Illness, Ordinarily so much the more they will prove of the *Confluent Sort:* However Sometimes there are Accidents that may keep a Restraint upon them.

III. If the *Face* be very full, tho' the *Body* should not be so, yett the Sick is in as much danger, as if Every Member of the Body were crouded with them. And tho' the *Body* be full, yett if there be Few in the *Face,* the Danger is not so great.

IV. Very *Violent Symptoms* at the *first Arrest* of the Disease, and particularly, *Convulsions* in Children, you must not be always frighted at them: They very commonly introduce very *Moderate Effects,* and the most *Comfortable Issue* that can be look'd for.

V. I am going to mention the Enemy, of which I may say, *Thou shalt Fight neither against Small nor Great, so much as this!* All possible Care, must be used that the *Ebullition*[12] *of the Blood* may not *Rise too high;*

Either by *Hastening* the Patients too *Soon* unto their Beds, or by *Confining* them too *much* there:

Or, By heaping on too many *Cloathes,* (which ought not to be more, than what they are in their Health us'd unto:)

Or, By keeping the *Air* of the Chamber too Close and too Hott: (which in Summer may allow of a little Ventilation:)

Or, By giving of pretended *Cordials,* and *Expellers:*[13] (Vile *Expellers,* which have Millions of times *driven* the poor *Souls* out of their *Fired Mansions!*)

Too hasty an Assimulation of the *Variolous Matter* has most certainly *Slain its Ten Thousands,* yea, the most of the *multitudes, multitudes,* that ly *Slain* by the Hand of this *Destroyer* in the *Valley of Death.*

VI.   On the other side, unseasonable *Vomits,* and *Purges,* and *Blood-Letting,* may happen too much to diminish the Necessary *Ebullition.* However, if there be a Just Suspicion, that the *Small Pox* coming out will prove of the *Confluent Sort,* an *Emetic* may be useful; yea, a *Phlebotomy* may be Needful.

O *Wisdome,* How *Profitable* art thou to *direct!* And how Requisite art thou to the *Physician!* How often to be Exercised!

VII.   Yett the Patients must not be Exposed unto Injuries from the *Cold.* And if the Pustules happen to strike in, or the Swelling of the Hands and Face to fall, from *Such* an Accident, (and a Return to the *Warmth* of the Bed be not Enough to do it) there may be some Recourse to the otherwise Exploded *Cordials* and *Expellers.* However still have a Care of being too lavish in them; *Repeted Ebullitions* of the Blood are very Dangerous Things!

VIII.   When the Distemper appears, Lett the Patients forbear the Use of *Wine* and *Flesh:* And I again say, of *Cordials* and *Expellers,* and all *Inflamers.* Don't lett 'em Swallow *Fire-brands!* Leave *Nature* undisturbed. It is hardly known, that *Nature* fails of doing its Part for Thrusting out the *Small-Pox. Forcing* it, is the most likely way of *Hindring* it.

Lett their Ordinary *Drink,* be *Small Beer,* gently warm'd with a Toast. And lett 'em drink their Bellyful!

Their *Diet,* Lett it be Oat-meal gruel, or Barley-gruel, or Milk-porridge; (One Third, Milk, Two Thirds, Water.)

Roasted Apples are no Forbidden Fruit.

Nay, *Roasted Apples* with *Milk,* may now and then be allow'd of.

But nothing too *Hott;* nothing too *Cold;* nothing too hard of Digestion.

IX.   Tho' I said, what I Said; Yett, at the time of Maturation, When the Purulent Particles flowing back on the Blood threaten to poison it, three or four Spoonfuls of *Generous Wine,* Morning and Evening, may, (if your Physician see no Fevourish Prohibitions,) be allowed of.

X.   Lett not the Patients be (as I have said once already) too *Soon,* or too *Much,* Confined unto their Beds.

Lett them keep up as Long as ever they can.

If the *Small-Pox* be of the *Distinct Sort* (in which Case there usually needs little to be done,) I know not why they should ly *Stiffling* and *Baking* and *Roasting* in their Beds; for whole Days together, if there be so much of *Summer* as will permit them to rise with *Safety.*

Be it how it will, If they should be *taken out* of their *Beds,* once or twice Every Day, all the time of their Illness, they might on many Accounts fare the Better for it. [Only, Be Sure, The Inconveniencies of taking any *Cold,* must be carefully *Watch'd against!*]

And when they are Abed, Lett them *Change their Place* ever now and then, to curb any *Sweat* they may fall into. The less they *Sweat,* the better.

Some at the very Point of *Death,* yea, Thought actually Dead, have been saved by nothing, but being *taken out of Bed.*

Young Persons are sometimes afflicted with a Total Suppression of Urine. Lett them only be *taken out of Bed,* and Led once or twice cross the Room; they are help'd immediately!

XI.   Anon, If the *Small-Pox* don't come out well, the Medicines called *Paregoricks,* have a Success to be wondred at: Your *Liquid Laudanum* (Fourteen Drops, for a Grown Person; Children will not want it:) or, *Diascordium,*[14] and the like, mixed in a Small Quantity, with some agreeable Distilled Water, will check the *Boiling Blood,* and Nature will freely then cast out the Morbific Matter.

XII.   Strong *Young Men,* and such as have inflamed their Blood by Free Drinking, may have Occasion to Bleed in the Arm, when things are hereabouts. Lett the *Doctor* See how it is!

XIII.   In the *Confluent Sort* of the *Small-Pox,* there comes on a

Salivation, just upon or soon after their First coming out. This having preserved the Lives of the Patients, uses to cease about the Eleventh Day. But a *Swelling* of the *Face* and *Hands* must then Supply the Place of it; without which, they must *go to their Long Home.* Tho' the Swelling of the *Face* also should a little abate, yett if the Swelling of the *Hands* continues and increases, there can be no Surer Sign of Recovery. The Way to keep this *Discharge of Nature,* in an Orderly Condition, is, To *Drink Freely* what was formerly allow'd; and be sure, such Drink as will provoke no Sweat upon them: And therewithal to Take what shall presently be mentioned. I will only first observe, what has been in Part already observed, and what cannot be too often inculcated; That as a *Temperate Regimen* is generally the *All in All,* for the management of the *Small Pox* in all the Kinds of it; [Certainly, The Way to bring a great Company of People handsomely and quietly out of a Room, will not be to throw in *Fire-Works* among them!] So, to prevent the too Exorbitant *Ebullition of the Blood,* there can be nothing more adviseable, than the free use of Some Innocent Liquor, which will allay the Heat that Scorches and Wearies the Patients. Besides the *Small Beer* aforesaid; a Decoction of *Bread,* and a Small Quantity of Calcined *Hartshorn,*[15] in a Large Quantity of *Water,* Sweetened with Sugar, may be Very Soberly advised unto. And so may a Convenient Mixture of *Milk* and *Water,* if the Stomach be not overcooled with it.

XIV.   What was just now promised shall now be Mentioned. The Benefit of *Narcoticks* in this Case, is inconceiveable. Tho' my *Sydenham* a long while commended *Liquid Laudanum,* yett anon he came to Praefer *Diacodium:*[16] (only, where this might happen to be nauseated; and then to the *Liquid Laudanum:*] I say, *Diacodium:* An Ounce of This, in *Cowslip Water,*[17] or some other such Distill'd Water. It should be given about five or six in the Evening, before the *Restless Fitt* usually comes upon the Patients. Give this, Every Day after there appears Occasion for it; yea, it may be done from the very Sixth Day after the first Invasion. To some young Men, of what we call a very *Sangiune Complexion,* an Ounce and Half will be requisite for a Dose. Yea, when the *Small-Pox* do flux very much, this Anodyne may be given Every Eighth Hour. The Efficacy of this Remedy, Surpasses Imagination! We now *come to this Leviathan, with a Double Bridle!*

XV.   Besides the Intention of Bridling the *Ebullition of the Blood,* there may be something also necessary, to conquer the *Putrifaction.*[18] And for this Purpose, we scarce know of any thing better than that on the Fifth or Sixth Day, the Patients come to have the *Spirit of Vit-riol*[19] dropt into their *Small Beer,* so as to make it a *Little Acid.* Lett this be the *Ordinary Drink;* and Lett them *Drink freely,* I say, *Drink Largely* of it. If they Drink not Enough of it, (which it would be Strange if they should not!) then mix that *Spirit of Vitriol* with a proper Syrup, or some Distilled Water and Syrup; and give them now and then of That! It has done Wonderful Things! When the Blood of Young People, and Such as have been too much acquainted with the Bottel, has raged with Such Violence that it has broke out of the Arteries into the Bladder, and they have made *Bloody Urine,* which is as desperate a Symptom as the *Small Pox* can be attended with; yett even *Then,* this Course has brought all to rights. My *Sydenham* seems almost in the Transport of an *Archimedes*[20] at this Discovery.

XVI.   When *Children* have the *Small-Pox* of the *Confluent Sort,* a *Looseness* usually follows them, as a Salivation does People of Riper Years. But it must not be Stopt. Thousands have been kill'd, by stopping this Provision of Nature, for the Evacuation of the Morbific Matter.

XVII.   If in the *Confluent Sort* of the *Small Pox,* the *Spittle* be baked so tough by the preceding Heat, that the Patients are nigh Strangled; use a Gargarism, [*Small Beer,* or *Barly-Water,* with *Honey of Roses,*] and Syringe the Throat often with it.

If they are at the Last Gasp of *Choaking,* a *Vomit* may be given very seasonably.

XVIII.   I have known an Instance, That one taken with the *Small-Pox* was thought siezed with only a *Fever.* They plied the *Soles of his Feet* with *Pigeons:* and the Consequence of it was, that he had no *Small Pox* above his Waste, but enough below it: His *Head* and his *Breast,* was kept also very Easy, all the time of his Illness. Whether Such Doings are Adviseable, or may be ordinarily practised without Hazard,—*melius inquirendum.*[21] However my *Sydenham,* allows Epithems to the *Soles of the Feet,* in the *Small-Pox* of the *Confluent Sort.* From the Eighth Day, he allows to grown People, *Garlick* Sliced and Wrapped in a Cloath; to be repeted Every day.

XIX.   *Experto Credo:* after all the Methods and Medicines, that our *Sydenham* and others rely upon, I can assure you There is nothing found so sure and safe as *this,* procure for the Patient, as Early as may be, by *Epispasticks,*[22] a plentiful Discharge at the Hand-Wrists; or Anckles, or Both; and keep them running till all the Danger be over.

When the Venom of the *Small-Pox* makes an Evident and Violent Invasion on the Nobler Parts, this Discharge *does Wonderfully*. If there be no such Danger, there is less Occasion for this or any other *Anxious Administration*.

XX. When the Patients are on Recovery, and the Pustules are falling off, and they have begun to feed upon Flesh, (especially, if they have been violently handled) *Bleeding* in the Arm, will be seasonable, and may prevent very Ill Effects of a Depraved Blood. And a Little *Purging* will now also come in Season: So all is concluded,—*Si quid novisti rectius istis.*[23]

⫿ But we will not content ourselves with *One Doctors Opinion*. Wherefore, tho' I will not oppress my Friends, with an Ostentatious Heap of *Collections,* which it were Easy to introduce on a Subject handled by so many Writers, I will call in Two more, who may be Enough with our *Sydenham* to constitute, a *Council of Doctors,* on the present Occasion.

The Ingenious *Woodman,* observes, That in the Assaults of the *Small Pox,* the *Constitution* of the Patients, is very much to be considered, whether it be what we call, *Flegmatick,* or *Cholerick. Blood-letting* is fatal in the *former;* but in the *latter* it may be very Expedient, yea, Necessary, at the Beginning of the Distemper. Yett, if great *Malignity* attends it, *Bloodletting* must be omitted, whatever Symptoms may seem to demand it.

If the *Stomach* be clogg'd with Gross Humours, a *Vomit* may be given at the Beginning, which may prevent a Future *Looseness*.

A *Costive* Belly, is much præferrible to a *Loose* One. Yett there may be Occasion for a *Clyster*.

If a *Looseness* happens before the Eruption, it must be Suppressed. But, if it happen after the Suppuration of the Pustules, and be not very Violent, there needs little notice to be taken of it. While it continues, or if it be fear'd approaching, lett the Drink be a Decoction of *Hartshorn*.

No Drinks whatsover must be given actually *Cold.* The *Small Beer* may have a little *Saffron* infused in it.

Opiates are very Good; not only to check a *Looseness,* but also to promote all Intentions.

If the *Pocks* retreat, because of a *Looseness,* Take *Venice-treacle* one dram; Oyl of *Cinamon*[24] Six Drops, *Laudanum* one Grain: Mix. give it Every Two or Three Hours.

If *Choaking* be fear'd, give a Vomit out of hand.[25]

If the *Eyes* do suffer very much, often drop into them *White Rose-Water,* wherein *Saffron* has been infused.

If a *Cough* be very troublesome, lett the Drink be a Pectoral Decoction of *Hysop,*[26] *Colts-foot,*[27] *Liquorice,* and the like, Sweetened with Syrup of *Poppy-heads.*[28]

If a *Cold* be taken after the Eruption, so that the Pustules retire, and Languors follow, the Party must be covered very warm, and *Cordials* be given, and *Blisters* be applied unto the Legs and the Feet; From whence if an *Heat of Urine* arises, it may be cured with Draughts of *Whey,* which has a few Grains of *Gum Arabic* dissolved in it.

He breaks off so. "More People are lost, thro' a præposterous use of Needless Remedies, which destroy the Regular Ferment, and check the Expulsive Efforts of Nature, than thro' the Vehemence of the Disease."

The celebrated *Pitcairn,*[29] would have the Patient *Lett Blood,* while the *Fever* does Last; yea, tho' the *Small-Pox* do begin to come out. But I doubt, he is *Too Universal* in this Direction. Do Thou, *O Discreet Physician,* determine when to *Bleed.* However, I must say, I have seen an astonishing Success of *Bleeding,* when the *Second Fever* has greatly threatened the Patient. And I have seen many a Life Lost, in a Complement unto the *Physicians* who have earnestly forbidden it. If on the Fifth, Sixth, Seventh or Eighth Day after the *Small-Pox* be come out, it goes in again; This Gentleman sais, A *Vein* is to be again opened, and *Cantharides* in Powder must be Laid unto the Neck.[30]

When the *First Fever* is over, and the *Small-Pox* is come out, he would have the Patient often drink any of the Simple, Distilled, Insipid Waters usually sold at the Apothecaries; in which lett *Sheeps-Dung*[31] be infused for some Hours, and then add Syrup of *White Poppy.*

Besides *Water-Gruel,* he commends a Drink of *Barly-Water,* with Syrup of White-Poppy, which will mightily assist the important *Salivation.*

Ⅱ But have we no *Præservatives,* to defend us from the *Invasion* of this dreadful Distemper, or from the *Violence* of it when it has invaded us?

Our *Sydenham* thinks, That *Purges* duely used before the *Infection* be taken, do hopefully præpare the Body, to feel *Fewer* of the *Small-Pox* and of the *Better Sort.*

In a Time and Place of much Infection, perhaps there is, [Give me Leave to say, *After a due Improvement of the NINETY-FIRST PSALM!*][32] no Præservative Comparable to that of a Bit of *Myrrh,* carried in the Mouth of Persons who have already had the *Small-Pox,* and fear not the Return of it, yett if they Visit Many and Nasty Sick Chambers, may have their Spirits horribly poisoned with it. It may do well for *Them* therefore to Employ this Præservative.

It has been thought that *Infection* commonly Siezes first on the *Salival Juices.* If *so,* the less we *Swallow our Spittle,* the better, where we are in danger of being infected.

Mantissa.

To the foregoing Entertainments, that there may be nothing Wanting, it is fitt that I should add at least a few Delibations[33] from what the valuable Dr. *John Woodward*[34] has written, in his Treatise about, *The State of Physic.*

He observes, Dr. *Sydenham* went a little too fast and too far, into the *Cooling Method,* under the *Small-Pox,* and in his Later Time a little quitted it.

The Physicians Chief Care in this Distemper, must be to steer and rule the *Passions,* and keep up the *Hopes* of the Patient. The *Stomach* is very much, the Seat of the *Passions;* in which Bowel also is found the *Source of the Matter;* that being sent from thence into the *Blood-Vessels* with which it has a very notable Communication, is the Cause of the *Small-Pox:* And a Disturbance here, is quickly felt in the Blood, with pernicious Consequences.

If the Physician be consulted in the Beginning of the Distemper, he has an Opportunity of Superseding the use of almost all other Medicines, by casting out much of the Morbid Matter with a *Vomit.* This Operation being dexterously managed and effectually pursued, the Patient is marvellously Releeved: All the symptoms, not only of the Stomach, which indicate for this Operation, but of the whole Body, Remitt unto Admiration. Yea, There have been Instances, wherein the Vitious Matter in the Stomach happening to be little, and not over-boisterous, a *Vomit* seasonably interposed, has discharged almost all the Matter, and the Pustules that began to show themselves, have disappeared. And in other Instances, where such an Evacuation has been made in Season, the Pustules have not only proved very Few, but also begun to turn a Day or two sooner than even the most Favourable Sort use to do.

A *Putrid Phlegm,* in Conjunction with a *Biliose Matter,* seems to be the Cause of the *Small-Pox;* which by the Luxury of the Later Times, is now more generated in us, than it was in our Ancestors.

In this Distemper, the *Diet* must be Plain, Thin, Light, Exactly Temperate. *Liquids* must not be too plentifully taken. High *Cordials,* must not be given in great Quantity, and without great Caution. If the Fever lower too much, then some Small Drops of such things may be given.

The *Acids* commonly præscribed, are too much of the same Nature with the *Salt,* that constitutes the chief Peccant Principle in this Disease. And *Absorbents*[35] don't answer Expectation.

In Case of a *Diarrhaea,* the main Care of the Physician, must be, to support the Patient and Remove Obstacles, that the Passage of the Peccant Matter downwards, may not be hindred, and so Stopped in the Intestines as to be turned back into the Blood; and appease the Tumults of the Stomach, so that it may cease any longer to send the Matter down.

To the Gentlemen who are for *Purging* in the *Small-Pox,* we may address the Words of *Horace;*

> *Periculosae Plenum Opus Aleae*
> *Tractas, et incedis per Ignes*
> *Suppositos Cineri doloso.*[36]

My Doctor finds, that of all the Remedies to Encounter the *Small-Pox,* there are none Comparable to the Sweet *Vegetable Oyls,* Especially the *Oyl of Sweet Almonds,* and such Unctuous Medicines, which may be mixed with Pulps, or Conserves, or Mucilages, for such as can't well take them alone. These wonderfully contribute unto the Frustrating and Subduing of that sharp and hott Matter which all the Mischiefs of the *Small-Pox* may be ascribed unto.

But all along, in the several *Stadia* of the Distemper, incredible would be the Benefit of Seasonable *Vomits.* Only, they must be Sufficient Ones, and well-adapted. And among these, the *Ipecacuanha* appears one of the most manageable, and of the most Easy Discipline.

In the End of the Disease, these will be of great Consequence, to prevent very grievous Consequences.

But I have now a further Story to tell you. What if we should find out a Way, that the Contagion of the *Small-Pox,* may not (by the *Salival Juices,* as tis commonly thought,) enter the *Stomach,* and make a furious and fatal *Combustion* in the Phlegmatic and Biliose Matter there, nor enter the *Lungs* more immediately, as with many perhaps it may; but enter by the *Outworks* of the Citadel, and carry off what it has to sieze with very gentle Symptoms, and when it reaches the Stomach in that Way yett be presently conquered with an easy *Emetic* there? This is the Story, which I have now to tell you. And hundreds of Thousands of Lives will be soon Saved if my Story may be harken'd to.

Appendix.

There has been a *Wonderful Practice* lately used in several Parts of the World, which indeed is not yett become common in our Nation.

I was first instructed in it, by a *Guramantee*[37]-Servant of my own, long before I knew that any *Europeans* or *Asiaticks* had the least Acquaintance with it; and some years before I was Enriched with the Communications of the Learned Foreigners, whose Accounts I found agreeing with what I received of my Servant, when he showed me the Scar of the Wound made for the Operation; and said, That no Person Ever died of the *Small-Pox*, in their Countrey that had the Courage to use it.

I have since mett with a Considerable Number of these *Africans*, who all agree in one Story; That in their Countrey *grandy-many*[38] dy of the *Small-Pox:* But now they Learn This Way: People take Juice of *Small-Pox;* and cutty-skin, and putt in a Drop; then by'nd by a little *sicky, sicky:* then very few little things like *Small-Pox;* and no body dy of it; and no body have *Small-Pox* any more. Thus in *Africa,* where the poor Creatures dy of the *Small-Pox* like Rotten Sheep, a Merciful God has taught them an *Infallible Præservative.* Tis a *Common Practice,* and is attended with a *Constant Success.*

But our Advice of this Matter, as it comes from Superiour Persons in the *Levant,* is what may have most Attention given to it.

Our first Communication comes from Dr. *Emanuel Timonius*[39] R.S.S. who writes from *Constantinople,* in *December,* 1713. To this Effect.

The Practice of Procuring the *Small-Pox,* by a Sort of *Inoculation,* has been introduced among the *Constantinopolitans,* by the *Circassians* and *Georgians,* and other *Asiaticks;* for about Fourty Years.

At the first, People were Cautious and Afraid. But the *Happy Success* on Thousands of Persons for Eight years now past, has putt it out of all Suspicion. The Operation has been performed on Persons of all *Ages,* both *Sexes,* differing *Temperaments,* and Even in the Worst Constitution of the *Air;* And none that have used it ever died of the *Small-Pox;* tho' at the same time, it were so malignant, that at least *Half* the People died, that were affected with it in the 'Common *Way*.

They that have this *Inoculation* practised on them (*he sais*) are subject unto very *Sleight Symptoms,* and hardly sensible of any Sickness; nor do what *Small-Pox* they have, ever leave any *Scars* or *Pitts* behind them.

They make Choice of as Healthy a Young Person as they can find, that has the *Small-Pox* of the best Sort upon him; On the Twelfth or Thirteenth Day of his Decumbiture. With a *Needle* they prick some of the Larger Pustules and press out the Matter coming from them into some Convenient Vessell of *glass* (or the like) to receive it; which ought first of all to be washed very clean with Warm Water. A Convenient Quantity of this Matter being thus collected, is to be Stop'd *Close,* and kept *Warm,* in the Bosom of the Person that carries it (who ought rather to be some *other person* than what Visited the Sick Chamber for it, lest the Infection of the *Small Pox* be convey'd in the *Garment* as well as in the *Bottel,* and the intended Operation be hurt by the Infection being first convey'd *Another Way.*) and so it should be convey'd as soon as may be, to the Person that is waiting to be the *Patient.*

The *Patient* being in a *Warm Chamber,* is to have several *Small Wounds* made with a Surgeons Three-edged *Needle,* or with a *Lancett,* in Two or more Places of the Skin; (the best Places are in the *Muscles* of the *Arm:*) till some Drops of Blood follow: And immediately lett there be dropt out a *Drop* of the Matter in the glass, on Each of the Places; and mixed well with the *Blood* that is issuing out. The *Wound* should be covered with half a *Walnutt-shell,* or any such *Concave Vessel,* and bound over, that the Matter may not be rubbed off by the garments, for a Few Hours. And now, lett the Patient (having *Fillets*[40] on the Wounds) keep *House,* and keep *Warm,* and be careful of his *Diet;* The Custome at *Constantinople* is, to Abstain from *Flesh* and *Broth,* for Twenty Days, or more.

They chuse to perform the Operation, Either in the Beginning of the *Winter,* or the *Spring.*

The *Small-Pox* begins to appear sooner in some than in others, and with lesser Symptoms in some than in Others: But, *With Happy Success in all.* Commonly *Ten* or *Twenty* Pustules break out: Here and there One has no more than *Two* or *Three:* Few have an *Hundred.* There are some, in whom no *Pustule* rises, but in the Places where the *Insition* was made; And here the *Tubercles* will be puru-

lent. Yett Even These, have never had the *Small-Pox* afterwards, tho'
they have Cohabited with Persons having of it. No Small Quantity
of Matter will run for Several Days, from the Places of the *Incision.*
The *Pocks* arising from this Operation, are dried up in a short time,
and fall off; partly in thin skins; and partly vanishing by an Insensible
Wasting.

The Matter is hardly so thick a *Pus,* as in the common *Small-
Pox;* but a thinner kind of *Sanies.*[41] Whence it rarely Pitts; Except at
the Place of the *Incision,* where the *Cicatrices*[42] are never worn out,
and where the matter is more of the Common Sort.

If an *Apostem*[43] should break out in any, (which is more frequent
in *Infants,*) yett there is no fear, for tis heal'd safely by Suppuration.
They scarce ever use the Matter of the *Insitious Small-Pox* to serve
the Designs of a *New Insition.*[44]

The *Inoculation* being tried on such as have had the *Small-Pox*
before, it had no Effect upon them.

Dr. *Timonius* affirms, That he never yett observed any *Bad
Consequence* of the Practice which now so many do come into.

But it is in *the Mouth of Two or Three Witnesses,* that the Thing
must *be Established.*

We shall again see, this *Leviathan* is not so *Fierce,* but that there
are some who *dare to stir him up.*

Since this Communication from Dr. *Timonius,* we have another
from an Eminent Person, whose Name is *Jacobus Pylarinus,*[45] the
Venetian Consul at *Smyrna.* Tis entituled, *Nova et Tuta Variolas
Excitandi per Transplantationem Methodus.*

This Gentleman observes, That this *Wonderful Invention* was,
first, *à plebeia rudique gente in Humani generis adjumentum, in
saevissimi morbi Solamen detecta,* found out, not by the *Learned*
Sons of Erudition, but by a Mean, Course, Rude Sort of People, for
the *Succour of Mankind* under and against One of the most Cruel
Diseases in the World. He seems to look on it, as a marvellous Gift of
a Good God, unto a miserable World. It was rarely, if ever, used
among *People of Quality,* until after the Beginning of the present
Century. A Noble *Graecian* then in distress for his Four Little Sons,
lest the *Small Pox* might bereave him of them, Consulted with *him,*
about using the *Inoculation* upon them. At first, his *Ignorance* of the
Matter, made him decline giving him any Advice upon it. But a
Graecian Woman who was a notable *Inoculatrix* happening to come
in while they were discoursing of the Matter, told them so much

about it, that the *Experiment* was Resolved upon. The Woman managed, in her Way, upon all the *Four Sons.* The Three *younger,* all of
which were under Seven years of Age, felt a very gentle Illness, had
a very *few pustules,* and in about a Week all *Fever* and *Hazard* was
over with them. The *Eldest,* about Eight years old, was taken with a
Malignant Fever: and (tho' he had not many *Pustules*) narrowly
Escaped with his Life. *Pylarinus* imputes this, to an Atrabiliarious[46]
and otherwise Humourous and Unhealthy Constitution of the Lad,
and a *Neglect* of using such *Preparatory Expiation* of his Body,
as they had been advised unto. But upon this *Happy Success, Mirum
quam multas Nobiliorum Familias, ad Imitationem troxit!*—It was
wonderful to see; what a Multitude of *People of Fashion* presently
followed the Exemple. So that at this day every one does without any
Hæsitation, and with all the Security imaginable, practise the *Transplantation;* Except here and there a few *Cowards* that are afraid of
their *Shadows.* Indeed, the *Turks,* whose Faith in Fate, is as we know,
and who are a more Indocible Sort of Animals, do not yett much
come into it.

    Pylarinus, instructed by his Greek Operatrix, directs; To take
a *Proper Season* for the Insition. She would use it only in the *Winter;*
but he thinks the *Spring* may do as well.

    The Fermenting *Pus,* must be taken from the Mature *Pustules*
of a *Good Sort,* in a Young Person; of a Good Constitution, kept warm
in a close Viol, and hastened unto the Application.

    The *Air* of the Chamber must be kept very Temperate.

    The Greek *Operatrix,* prick'd more Places, and less Fleshy
Ones, than *Pylarinus* approved of: With an oblique Stroke pricking
the Places with an Iron or Golden *Needle;* and with the same Needle
dropping and thrusting the *Pus* into the Wound; and so binding all
with *Fillets.* Her Way was thus to prick, the Forehead, the Chin, both
Cheeks, both Wrists, and both Insteps. This was doubtless over-doing.
Pylarinus affirms, that Some have done the Business, *Unico duntaxat
Vulnusculo ad Brachium inflicto;* with no more than *One Little Insi-
tion* in the Arm, and it has done very well. [*So it has been with such*
Africans, *as have shown me the Marks of their Inoculation.*]

    They must not keep their *Beds* more than is necessary.

    Wine, Flesh, Broth must be laid aside.

    The Ferment comes into Action, Sooner in some than in others.
Usually the *Small Pox* appears on the *Seventh* day; Sometimes on the
very *First.*

The *Symptoms* prove Remiss or Intense, according to the Various Constitution of the Bodies.

The *Small Pox* proves, of the Distinct Sort; And there will be but *few* of them; it may be *Ten* or *Twenty;* rarely an *Hundred*.

In some few, the *Insition* has produced no *Small Pox* at all; but the Persons have afterwards been, in the *Common Way,* taken and handled with it, like other People.

The *Wounds* made for the *Insition* prove often Very Sore. And with some they degenerate into *Apostems;* yea, These do swell sometimes, and rise, and fall, and rise again. There has also happened on this Occasion, an *Abscess* with Suppuration, in some Emunctory[47] of the Body: But this is a very Rare Occurrence.

In fine: *Pylarinus* affirms, It was hardly ever known, that there was any *Ill Consequence* of this Transplantation: *Quinimo rite recteque tractata, et in Corporibus per Peritum Medicum apte praeparatis, certissimam promittit Salutem.* The Business being well and wisely managed, and the Body being by a *Skilful Physician* well-prepared; you may depend upon it (*he sais*) in an ordinary Way, there can be *nothing but a good Isssue of it*.

But, I remember, I spoke of *Three Witnesses*. I will therefore add: *Kennedy*[48] says, That in the Little Time that He was at *Constantinople,* he was assured of *Two Thousand* that had lately undergone the Method of the *Small-Pox Inoculated;* and there were no more than two who died under it, and the *Death* of these was entirely owing to their own Ill Conduct in Exposing themselves.

Hitherto you have nothing but *History*. But a little *Philosophy* and *Speculation* may be now asked for; and an *Enquiry into Causes* a Little Endeavoured. No doubt, among the *Wise Men of Enquiry,* there may be found, *So many Men so many Minds*. Every Gentleman may form his own *Hypothesis;* and some of the Later and more Modern Curiosity, will try how far the *Vermicular Scheme* will carry them thro' a Solution of these and all *Appearances* in this Distemper.

I have seen the Point after this *Pothecary* manner talk'd about. The venomous *Miasms*[49] (Lett *That* Word serve at the present) of the *Small Pox,* entering into the Body, in the Way of *Inspiration,* are immediately taken into the *Blood* of the *Lungs:* And, I pray, how many *Pulses* pass before the very *Heart* is pierced with them? And within how many more they are convey'd into all the *Bowels,* is easily apprehended by all that know any thing, how the *Circulation of the Blood* is carried on. At the same time, the *Bowels* themselves are En-

feebled, and their Tone impaired, by the *Venom* that is thus in-
sinuated. Behold, the Enemy at once gott into the very *Center* of the
Citadel: And the Invaded Party must be very Strong indeed, if it
can struggle with him, and after all Entirely Expel and Conquer him.
Whereas, the *Miasms* of the *Small-Pox* being admitted in the Way of
Inoculation, their Approaches are made only by the *Outworks* of the
Citadel, and at a Considerable *Distance* from the Center of it. The
Enemy, tis true, getts in so far as to make Some *Spoil,* yea, so much
as to satisfy him, and leave no *Prey* in the Body of the Patient, for him
ever afterwards to sieze upon. But the *Vital Powers* are kept so clear
from his Assaults, that they can manage the *Combats* bravely and,
tho' not without a *Surrender* of those Humours in the Blood, which
the Invader makes a Siezure on, they oblige him to *march out the
same way he came in,* and are sure of never being troubled with him
any more. But perhaps the Few Words, that I wrote, in my Introducing of the Story, may be as much to the Purpose, as all of this *Jargon.*
I'l have done with it.

I durst not Engage that the Success of the Trial *here,* will be
the same, that has been in all the *other Countreys* where it has been
tried hitherto: tho' we have seen it succeed well in very *different
climates.* Nor am I sure that if it should be made upon a Body, where
the *Blood* is already nigh upon the Point of some unhappy *Fever,* this
may not help to set *Fire* to such a Thing. But I am very confident no
Person would miscarry in it, but what *would most certainly* have miscarried upon taking the Contagion in the *Common Way.* Wherefore,
if it be made at all, (and all the *Scruples* that some have about the
Tempting of Providence be also gott over,) I advise, that it be never
made but under the Management of a *Physician,* whose Conduct
may be much relied upon, and who will wisely *Præpare* the Body for
it before he *Perform* the Operation. *I have done.*

I am now able, as an *Eywitness,* (and more than so) to give a
more full Account of the *Practice,* which until *Now* I could only propose as a Matter at a greater Distance.

About the Month of *May,* 1721, the *Small-Pox* being admitted
into the City of *Boston,* I proposed unto the Physicians of the Town,
the unfailing Method of preventing Death, and many other grievous
miseries, from a tremendous Distemper, by Receiving and Managing
the *Small-Pox,* in the Way of *Inoculation.* One of the Physicians had
the Courage to begin the Practice upon his own Children and Servants;[50] And another Expressed his Good Will unto it. But the rest

of the Practitioners treated the Proposal with an Incivility and an Inhumanity not well to be accounted for.[51] Fresh Occasion I saw, for the Complaint of a Great Physician; *"Heus, quanto Dolore auger, dum video Naturae ministrum Medicum, Hostem ejus devenisse!"*[52] The Vilest Arts were used, and with such an Efficacy, that not only the Physician, but also the Patients under the *Small-Pox Inoculated* were in hazard of their very Lives from an Infuriated People. But I myself had thrown into my House in the Dead of the Night, a fired *Granado,* charged with Combustible Matter, and in such a Manner, that upon its going off, it must probably have killed them that were near it, and would have certainly fired the Chamber and speedily have laid the House in Ashes. But the merciful Providence of God our SAVIOUR so ordered it, that the *Granado* passing thro' the Window, had by the Iron in the Middle of the Casement such a Turn given to it, that in falling on the Floor, the fired Wild-fire in the Fuse, was Violently shaken out some Distance from the Shell, and burnt out upon the Floor, without firing off the *Granado.*[53]

The Opposition was carried on with a *Folly,* and *Falsehood,* and *Malice,* hardly ever known to be paralled'd on any Occasion; And in the Progress of the Distemper many Hundreds of Lives were Lost, which might have been Saved, if the People had not been Satanically filled with Prejudices against this *Method of Safety.*[54] However, the Practice went on, and tho' the Physician was under Extreme Disadvantage on more Accounts than one, yett he was attended with Vast[55] *Success.* The Experiment has now been made on *Several Hundreds* of Persons; and upon both *Male* and *Female,* both *old* and *young,* both *Strong* and *Weak,* both *White* and *Black,* at all Seasons, of *Summer* and *Autumn* and *Winter:* And they have generally professed, *they had rather undergo the Small-Pox Inoculated once every year, than undergo the Small-Pox once in their Lives after the Common Way, tho' sure to Live.*

I shall now communicate our *Way of Proceeding,* in the Practice.

I. We make usually a Couple of *Incisions* in the *Arms,* where we usually make our *Issues;* But Somewhat Larger than for *Them,* (Sometimes in an *Arm* and in a *Leg.*)

II. Into these we putt Bitts of *Lint,* (the Patient at the same time turning his Face another Way and guarding his Nostrils,) which have been dipt in some of the *Variolous Matter,* taken in a Vial, from the Pustules of one (if we can find such an one) that has the *Small Pox* of the more Laudable sort now turning upon him; And so we cover them with a Plaister of *Diachylon.*[56]

III.   Yett we find the *Variolous Matter* fetched from those that have the *Inoculated Small Pox,* as Agreeable and Effectual as any other. Yea, and so we do, What is taken from them that have the *Confluent Sort.*

IV.   In four and twenty Hours, we throw away the *Lint;* and the Sores are dressed once or twice, Every four and twenty Hours, with Warmed *Cabbage-Leaves.*

V.   The Patient continues to do things, as at other Times; Only he does not Expose himself to the Injuries of the *Weather,* if *That* be at all Tempestuous. But we find, the *Warmer* he keeps himself, he afterwards finds himself no Loser by it.

VI.   About the *Seventh Day,* the Patient feels the *Usual Symptoms* of the *Small-Pox* coming upon him; and he is now managed as in an Ordinary *Putrid Feaver.* If he can't *hold up,* he goes to *Bed.* If his *Head* ake too much, we putt a Common *Poultis* to his *Feet.*[57] If he be very Qualmish at the *Stomach,* we give him a gentle *Vomit,* yea, We commonly do these things *almost of Course,* (Especially give the *Vomit*) whether we find the Patient want them or no. If the *Fever* be too high, in some Constitutions, we Bleed a Little. And, finally, to hasten the *Eruption,* if it come on too slowly, we putt on an *Epispastic.*

VII.   Upon or About the *Third Day* from the Decumbiture, the *Eruption* begins. The Number of *Pustules* is not alike in all. In some, they are very Few. In others, they amount unto an *Hundred.* Yea, In many they amount unto *Several Hundreds.* Frequently, unto more than what the Accounts from the *Levant* say is usual there. But in some, there is not what may be fairly called, *A Decumbiture:* the *Eruption* is made without their suffering one Minute of any Sensible *Sickness* for it. *Young Children,* even such as are dandled on the knee, and hanging on the Breast, Seem to fare the best of any under this Operation.

VIII.   The *Eruption* being made, all *Illness* Vanishes; There's an End on't; Except there should be something of the *Vapours* in those that are troubled with them. There is nothing more to do, but keep Warm; Drink proper *Tea's;* Eat *Gruel,* and *Milk-Porridge,* and *Panada,*[58] and Bread and Butter, and almost any thing equally Simple and Innocent.

IX.   Ordinarily the Patient Sitts up Every day, and Entertains his Friends; yea, Ventures upon a *glass of Wine* with them. If he be too Intense upon Hard *Reading* and *Study,* we take him off.

X. Sometimes, tho' the Patient be on other accounts Easy Enough, yett he *Can't Sleep* for diverse Nights together. In this Case, we don't give them *Opiates* or *Anodynes;* because we find that they who have taken these in the *Small-Pox* are generally pestered with miserable *Boyls* after their being Recovered. So, we lett 'em alone; Their *Sleep* will come of itself, as their *Strength* is coming on.

XI. On the *Seventh* Day, the *Pustules* are all usually come to their Maturity; (some, on the *Fifth:*) And soon after this, they go away, as those of the *Small-Pox* in the *Distinct Sort* use to do.

XII. The Patient getts abroad quickly; and is most sensibly *Stronger,* and in better Health, than he was before. The *Transplantation* has been given to a *Woman* in Childbed,[59] Eight or Nine days after their Delivery and they have gott rather Earlier out of their Childbed, and in better Circumstances than ever in their Lives. Those that have had ugly *Ulcers* long running upon them, have had them healed on and by the *Transplantation.*[60] Some very Feeble, Crazy, Consumptive People, have upon the *Transplantation* grown Hearty, and gott rid of their former Maladies.

XIII. The *Sores* of the *Incisions* do seem to Dry a Little in the Three or Four Days of the Feavourish Præparation for the Eruption. After this, there is a *Plentiful Discharge* at them. The Discharge continues for some Days after the Patient is quite well on other accounts. But the Sores dry up soon Enough of themselves; we count the *Later* the *Better.* If they happen to be Inflamed, or otherwise Troublesome, we presently help them in the way we do any ordinary Sores.

XIV. The *Transplantation* has been tried on such as have gone through the *Small-Pox* formerly in the Common Way; and it has had no Effect upon them; Except perhaps an Hour or Two of harmless Indisposition, about the Time when the *Irruption* should otherwise have been made upon them.

It has been unhappily given to some few, that have already newly received the Infection in the Common Way. The Eruption has then been presently made in Two or Three days after the *Incision,* and they have undergone the *Small-Pox* in the Common Way; hardly Escaping with their Lives: Tho' Some have thought, the Running of the Sores in these, has been Some Advantage to them.

Two or three have died under or soon after the *Inoculation,* from a Complication of *other mortal Distempers.* An Indian Servant getting a Violent Cold, fell into a *Pleuretic Fever,* that killed her. Another Person that had long been under a Crazy *Melancholy* and *Consumption,* utterly refused all Sustenance and *starved herself to Death.*[61]—But of all the Hundreds that have been under a *Regular Management,* we know not of one but what Rejoices in their having undergone the Operation.

Cap. XXI. *Kibroth Hattaavah.*
or, Some Clean Thoughts, on,
The <u>Foul Disease</u>.

THE Sins of *Unchastity* are Such Violations of the *Good Order,* which the GOD of Nature has præscribed unto the Children of Men, wisely to govern the *Appetites of Generation;* Such Trespasses on the Rules, to be observed for the Comfort and Beauty of *Humane Society;* such Pollutions of a *Body,* the Maker whereof has *Desired* it for an *Holy Temple* to Himself; that we have no Cause to wonder at what the Divine Oracles have told us: *The unjust Shall be Punished; but CHIEFLY they that walk after the Flesh in the Lust of UNCLEANNESS.*—

A Great King Once had a *New Testament* presented unto him, fairly Bound and Guilt, with that Sentence of it, inscribed in Golden Letters on the Cover; <u>Whoremongers and Adulterers God shall judge</u>.

The Threatenings and Fulminations against these Crimes, uttered by the Voice of the Glorious God, in the Book which He spreads as a *Firmament* over His Church, are very Terrible.

And how terribly do we see them Executed!

Among other *Judgments* which even in This World overtake the Vicious, who *being past all Feeling, have given themselves over unto Lasciviousness, to Work all Uncleanness with Greediness;* there is of Later time, inflicted a *Foul Disease;* the Description whereof, and of the Symptoms that attend it, would be such a *Nasty Discourse,* that Civility to the Readers will Supersede it; and the Sheets of the Treatise now before him, Shall not be stained with so much Conspurcation.[1]

The Common Tradition, is; That *America* first convey'd this Great Pox to *Europe*, in requital whereof, *Europe* has transmitted the *Small Pox* to *America*.

Doubtless a Mistake! Dr. *Patin*[2] has written a Curious Dissertation, to prove that this *Foul Disease* is of greater Antiquity. And Mr. *Becket*[3] having with much Curiosity Enquired after it, finds, That in the English Nation more than Six Hundred years ago, it went under the Name of *Brenning,* or *Burning,* which Signified what is now called, *A Clap,*[4] and was not left off till this Appellation came in the room of it. There were then in the Stews,[5] *Muliores habentes Nephandam Infirmitatem.*[6] And the Stews, whereof the most famous, was under the government of the Bishop of *Winchester,* (a Bishop of a Church, you may well say that is the *Mother of Harlotts!)*[7] were forbidden on certain Penalties to keep any such Dangerous Creatures. However, the Plague, is not of such an Early Date, as they imagine, who fancy, that they find something like it in *Hippocrates;* or they who fancy, that it is mentioned even in the Sacred Scriptures; and who therefore have provided even from the Old Testament *A Saint,* unto whose Protection, or Compassion the *Brent Bruits*[8] may betake themselves. The nearest Resemblance of it in Antiquity, seems to be in the Condition of the Adulteress, in the Holy Land; who, upon drinking the *Water of Jealousy,* had the Parts of Generation (called, *The Thigh*) Siezed with a *Rottenness;* and she became *a Curse among the People.* But This was an Infliction Extraordinary and Miraculous, What we now call, *The French Pox.*[9] Tis a *New Scourge,* which the Vengeance of a Righteous God, has not until the *Later Ages* inflicted on the growing Wickedness of the World: and was no more Known in the *Former Ages,* before the *Sixth Chiliad,*[10] than the *Leprosy of the House* is in ours. But a *Sore Scourge* it is, unto the unhappy Criminals, who bring it on themselves, and list themselves among *The Fools in Israel:* Yea, and unto those more *Innocent Ones,* who have the Unhappiness to be *yoked* in the Married State with the *Beasts* which bring it unto them; and never can make you a Reparation. *Lett us adore the Justice of the Glorious God in the Matter!*

An eminent Italian published an *Advertisement,* That he could furnish People with an *Infallible Præservative,* the use of which would keep them, from ever being infected, with the *Foul Disease.* People applying to him for his *Infallible Præservative,* he furnished them with a Picture of a Miserable Transgressor Languishing under the Effects of the Detestable Distemper, his Flesh wasted, his Visage

Wan and Lean, his Eyes hollow, the Bridge of his Nose Eaten away, ugly Ulcers running upon him; *All horrible!* And he said with it, *When you are under Temptation to go into a Baudy House, take out this Picture, and look attentively with some Deliberation upon it; And if after this, you can go in!—who shall I say, has the Driving of you?*

But, alas, this *Infallible Præservative,* has not proved so. The Rueful Spectacles of People, not in *Picture,* but in *Person,* perishing under the *Foul Disease,* have not Effectually restrained Multitudes from venturing upon the *Fireships,* and going on *as An Oxe unto the Slaughter.* Tis astonishing, to read what vast Multitudes one single Practitioner in the most *Public Manner* pretends to have had under his Cure, for this *Secret Disease,* as they call it: Besides the huge Numbers, that Stand in the *Bills of Mortality*[11] for it, either more *Openly* in Express Terms, or more, *Covertly* under the Term of a *Consumption.*[12] How justly may our SAVIOUR calls *ours* also, *An Evil and an Adulterous Generation!* A famous Preacher in *Switzerland* said, *If the Old Punishment of Stoning Adulterers to Death were now in fashion, it may be Suspected the Stones of the Neighbouring Mountain, would not be Enough to serve the Execution.* One would fear, whether he who spoke at that rate in *his* Days, would change his Note, if he were to rise from the Dead, and preach in *ours.* How numerous are the Morsels of *Kibroth Hattaavah!* What Numbers are the insatiable *Graves of Lust,* filled withal.

And now, what shall be Said, unto the Unhappy Creatures, upon whom the *Lues Venerea* is fulfilling the Divine Menace to the *Whoremonger, A Wound and a Dishonour shall he gett,* when he so destroys his own Soul!

Wretches, Because you would not *remove your Way far from the Strange Woman,* you are now *Mourning at the Last, when your Flesh and your Body are Consuming.*

Your *Foul Disease* is too filthy and odious to have the nasty Symptoms of it mentioned. But a good Man, Who had never been under your *Defilement,* and so was not under your *Distemper,* and who could Appeal to Heaven for it, *My Heart has never been deceived by a Woman, and I have not laid Wait by my Neighbours Door;* yett he had an Illness (*Bartholinus* thinks, the *Ulcus Syriacum;* somewhat like what we call, the *Yawes!*)[13] which produced Complaints, that your Case is more uncomfortable filled withal. *My Flesh is clothed with Worms,* [*Worms* without a Metaphor; your

Abominable *Ulcers* are by glasses found Swarming with 'em!] *My skin is broken and become lothsome, yea, my Leanness rising up in me bears Witness to my Face; My Bones are pierced in the Night Season, and my Sinews take no Rest.*

Having thus been in the *Ditch,* which none but the *Abhorred of the Lord* fall into, and feeling the *Nasty Pickle* in which you are come from thence, With what Inexpressible Regret and Remorse, must you *Abhor* yourselves, and Cry out, *I have sinned, and I have done very foolishly.*

Shut up with the *Leper,* Cry out, *Unclean! Unclean!*

Every *Pain* and *Smart* that you feel, in the Progress of the Cursed Contagion that you have taken, Speaks to you, with so many *Lashes,* in such Words as those;—and, methinks, they should sting like *Scorpions!—Thy Way and thy Doings have procured these things unto thee. This is thy Wickedness, Lett it reach to thy Heart, and break thy Impure Heart within thee.*

Thou Fool, call thyself by thy proper Name, and Humble thyself Exceedingly; Lett no *Humiliation* appear too *Low* for thee.

It may look almost like a Prostitution and Profanation, to cloathe such an *Impure Case* as thine, in the *Holy Style* used by and for the Servants of God. Yett, for once, I will say; when *thy Sore is running in the Night, and Ceases not;* now *Remember* God. *Remember* how Wickedly thou hast rebelled against the Commandments of God; *Remember* how Agreeably and Reasonably and Righteously God is now chastening of thee; *Remember* what Warnings God has given thee, that these are but the *Beginning of Sorrows,—Except thou Repent!* And so, *Be Troubled.*

Think: *What have I brought myself unto!—But, my SOUL, my SOUL, my Impure Soul, is in much more woful Circumstances than my Body. Oh! The Turpitude of what I have been guilty of!*

Lett thy Sin, be now *Repented* of; and not only with the *Attrition,* of a Sorrow for thy having Injured *Thyself,* but with the *Contrition* of a Sorrow for thy having displeased the Great God,— *Thoroughly Repented of.*

But, what a wonderful Display of *Sovereign Grace* will there be in it, if thy *Repenting* of this Iniquity, may prove an Occasion of thy Coming to a *Perfect Work* of *Repentance* for *All* thy Evil-doings!—

Wherefore, as the *Motto* on the Hospital, for the forlorn Invalids under this Vengeance, is, *Post Voluptatem Misericordia,*[14]—

we will say, However *Despair* not; There is yett *Mercy* for thee. Become a true Poenitent and there is a Reserve of *Mercy* for thee. *Tho' thou hast gone a whoring, Yett Return to me, Saith the Lord; For I am merciful, Saith the Lord, Only Acknowledge thine Iniquity,* and Earnestly plead the Sacrifice of thy SAVIOUR for a *Pardon;* and lett the *Stolen Waters* of *Sin,* be no longer *Sweet,* but *more Bitter than Death* unto thee!.

As for any Remedies under this *Foul Disease,*—You are so Offensive to me, I'l do nothing for you. You shall pay for your Cure. Lett *Poscinummius*[15] practice upon you for all me. And I shall not care, if he take the Italian *Cortegiana's* Way for your Cure, [a Quarter of an Ounce of *Coloquinesda*[16] infused in a Quart of Proper Wine] which will keep you in Torment for three Days together.—Gett ye gone to the *Cheirurgeon.*—And when he has made a *Thorough Cure,* —Then, *Sin no more.* Don't *Return to Folly any more.* If you do,— *Fools bray'd in a Mortar,* I have no more to say to ye.

CAP. XXII. Malum ab Aquilone.[1]

or

The <u>Scurvy</u>, discoursed on.

THE *Northern* Parts of *Europe,* and the Parts of *America* derived from them, have been of late Years, grievously infested with a Disease called, *The Scurvy:* Wherein the Blood and other Juices, have a fix'd and sharp *Salt* grievously depraving of them; and the Effects thereof are very Deplorable.

I will not enter into the Dispute, whether this Disease were known unto the Ancients. While some imagine that *Hippocrates* means it, when he speaks of the *Swell'd Spleen,* and of the, Ειλεος πματπτς, or, *Volvulus Sanguineus;*[2] and that *Galen* means it when he speaks of the *Vitiligo nigra;*[3] yett others will by no means allow, that those two Gentlemen have given us any tolerable Account of the proper *Scurvy.* *Pliny* may seem to have had more Knowledge of this Disease, when he mentions the *Stomacace,*[4] and *Scalotyrhae,*[5] found in the Army of *Germanicus*[6] near the Sea. And he that gave the Name of *Gingipedium* to the *Scurvy,* did well enough consider the Condition of the *Teeth* and of the *Feet* in this Distemper. But so far as we are informed, The *Scurvy* had its Origin in the *Northern* Parts of

Europe, and was for a long while peculiar to the People near the *Baltic* sea, who gave unto it, the Name of *Schoerbuck,* or *Scorbute,* by which it is now distinguished. The Glorious LORD who has all Diseases at his Command, saying to one, *Go,* and it *goes;* to another, *Come,* and it *comes;* has ordered this Executioner of His Wrath upon the Sinful Nations, to pass the Ancient Limits; and particularly to Visit the *English* Nation at such a rate, that it is thought there are few *English* People, especially of them who *fare well,* but what are *Ill* of it, and more or less tainted with it.

Among all our Maladies, there cannot be found such another *Proteus.*[7] It appears in a Vast Variety of Shapes; and sometimes the Symptoms are very distressing and calamitous. A Gentleman who wears the Name of *Eugalens,*[8] pretends to enumerate, the Maladies which may go under the Denomination of the *Scurvy,* or are Attendents and Consequents upon it; and the Number arises to *Seven times Seven* with him.

The Infected Person has many Humbling Things to think upon.

One of the first Circumstances, wherein the Distemper appears, is, *A Spontaneous Lassitude.* The Invaded Mortal grows *Weary, Heavy, Listless;* tho' he does nothing to tire himself, nor is he willing to do any thing, if he could help it. But lett the *Weary* Patient think; *Lord, How Naturally, how Criminally, am I weary of Well-doing! How little Heart have I to the Work which thou hast given me! How little do I stir myself up to do the Work, which a dying Man ought to do with all his Might!*

My Friend, Lett thy *Head-ache* bring into thy *Head* such Thoughts as these: *Lord, My Head has been too destitute of those Thoughts, which are proper to be lodged in a Temple of God! But, oh, what Vain Thoughts have been lodged there!*

Lett thy Perishing *Teeth,* cause thee to think, *How much have I Err'd in my Feeding!*

Lett thy Odious *Breath,* cause thee to think, *in Speaking, how much has my Throat been like an Open Sepulchre!*

Lett thy Pained and Cramped *Limbs,* cause thee to think, *how Irregular have I been in my Motions! How Indisposed for moving as and where I should have done!*

Lett thy broken *Sleep* cause thee to think; *what a drowsy Creature have I been in the Service of my God, and of my SOUL!*

Lett thy bad *Stomach* putt thee in Mind of thy Neglecting to *Digest* that *Word,* that should be *more to thee, than thy Necessary Food.*

Lett thy hideous *Ulcers,* Cause thee to Reflect on the Ebullitions and Prosecutions of thy *Lusts,* which have rendred thee full of *Putrifying Sores.*

Idleness is often the Cause of the *Scurvy.* Repent of it, O Man, if thine have been so to thee.

Be sure, the *Scurvy* is a lively *Emblem* and *Image* of that Vice. *Idleness* is a *Scorbutic* Affect of the Mind. It will be attended with as pernicious Consequences as any *Scurvy.* Tis as much to be dreaded, as much to be deprecated. *Awake, O Sluggard, and Sett about thy Business!* The Learned *Wedelius*[9] has written a Dissertation, to show, That the Malady wherein *Lazarus* lies an Invalid at the Rich Mans Gate in the Gospel, must be the *Scurvy.* O *Invalid,* lett thy *Scurvy* provoke thee in the Methods of *Piety* to prepare for *Paradise;* and it will not be long before thou shalt be *Comforted.*

Monsr. *D'Ube,* in his, *Poor Mans Physician,* writing about the *Scurvy,* has these religious Passages, which are not unworthy to be transcribed.

"There are *Divine Causes* (of Diseases) by which we understand God Himself, as the Absolute and Principal Cause; Or the Angels and the Dæmons, as Instrumental Causes; being made use of by Almighty God, to afflict us Mortals with Diseases. These *Divine Causes* have so ample a share in this *New Distemper,* that we may justly, with *Hippocrates,* admonish our Physicians, That after they have Enquired into the Nature of Distempers, they ought to have a special Regard unto the *Divinum,* or *Supernatural,* in them; the Interpretation of which, has not a little puzzled some of our Physicians.—The *Scurvy,* some time a Foreigner to our Climate, has been since introduced by God Himself, altering the Constitution of our Air, to chastise us.

—The Nature of this Monstrous Distemper, together with its Various Symptoms, are Evident Signs, that the Same is sent among us by God, as a *Scourge for our Sins;* there being scarce any Part of our Body on which this Disease does not leave very Evident Marks, and Convincing Proofs, of our Iniquities. Thus, our *Ey-sight* is corrupted, and our *Eyes* are inflamed; which have so often been the Idols of our Love and Flatteries. Our *Gums* are full of Ulcers, and the *Teeth* ready to fall out of the Head; which have so frequently Served as Instruments to Revile God and our Neighbours. Our *Mouth* and *Breath,* even from the bottom of our *Lungs,* emits such a nauseous Stench, as is scarce Supportable. The *Legs* are full of Ulcers, and scarce able to support the Weight of the Body; to putt us in Mind, how often they have been accessary in promoting our Luxurious Debaucheries. The same Application may be made, of the Ulcers and Gangrenes (attending this Distemper) in the Inferiour Region of our Bodies; as well as the Palseys, Pains, Fainting Fitts, and other Symptoms, which are the common Attendents of the *Scurvy*.

If then, this Chastisement is owing to our Sins, What have we to do else, than to have recourse unto the Mercy of God; which we are most likely to obtain, by Acknowledging the Heinousness of our Trespasses, and Endeavouring to Correct them by following as well the Doctrine as the Footsteps of our SAVIOUR."

Dr. *Cheyne* observes, There is no *Chronical* Distemper more *Universal,* or more *Obstinate,* or more *Destructive* to our Nation, than the SCURVY. Scarce any one *Chronical* Distemper, but owes its Origin to it; or has a Degree of this *Evil* in it. Yea, scarce any Single Individual of the *Better Sort* is altogether free from it. The same Gentleman observes, That he scarce ever saw it wholly extirpated, in such as have had it in any Degree. Because it requires a Conduct so intirely contrary to the *Habits* and *Customs,* and *Appetites* of our People, who will Surfeit on an *Animal Diet,* and on *Strong fermented Liquors,* tho' they Dy for it. The Bare Laying of Those aside, has even *fastened the Teeth when dropping out,* and marvellously Recovered the Languishing.

§ The *Scurvy* is a *Chronical* Disease. The Patient must have *Patience.* The Enemy is not *presently* to be Conquered. It requires *Time* and *Patience.*

§ One Sais, That *Sobriety is the Bane of the Scurvy; and Intemperance is the Mother that brings it into the World.*

§ The *Scurvy* is by the *Italians* and the *Venetians* called, *Mal de Terra,* or, the *Earth-Disease;* Because, tis their common Practice, to cure it, by Digging an Hole in the *Earth,* into which the Patient is putt, and all but his Head Covered over with *Earth.*[10]

§ *Salt-Meats* must not be liv'd upon.

§ The *Belly* must be always kept open. *Laxative* Things must be given; but not *Violent* ones. *Bleeding* is generally hurtful, except a Strong Pain of the Side, or an *Asthma,* do call for it. *Vomiting* must not be much used; but it may be needful, if the *Stomach* much heave that Way; however the Strength must be considered.

§ Spirit of *Sal Armoniac,* now and then taken in a glass of Wine, is an Excellent Thing for the *Scurvy.*

§ And so is *Whey,* with the Juice of Orange or Lemon in it.

§ *Limons* do Wonders, for the Releef of the *Scurvy.*

§ In the *Scurvy, Mustard* is reckoned a Specific.

§ Every Body knows many Specificks for the *Scurvy,* found in the *Vegetable Kingdome.*

It may be, none superiour to *Sorrel.*[11] The French do wisely to Cultivate it very much. Tea's and other Drinks made of it, are noble *Anti-scorbuticks.*

But *Scurvy-grass*[12] does not well in some hott Sorts of *Scurvies.* The Spirit of *Scurvy-grass,* cried up so much, has not answered Expectation.

§ *Garden-Cresses*[13] are of such Vast Use in this Distemper, that the *Parisian* Physicians have ordered a great Quantity, to grow near their General Hospital.

§ Take two handfuls of *Water-Trefoyl,*[14] and Lett it work instead of *Hops,* in about Eight Gallons of Wort.[15] Lett the Patient use it for his Ordinary Drink.

Among the *Boylaean* Receits, this is called, *An Excellent drink for the Scurvy.*

§ Take the dried Leaves of *Garden-Cresses* and *Juniper-Berries;* Equal Parts, each. After they are Well-Powdered, incorporate them with a Sufficient Quantity of despumated[16] Honey. Take the Quantity of the Bigness of a Walnut in a Little Wine. *D'Ube* cries up this as a pretty Opiate.

§ As a *Præservative,* (and so likewise a *Restorative,*) hear Master *D'Ube.* "I must Recommend to you one Remedy more, which is Easy to be had, costs little; and yett is of great Consequence against this Disease. Gather of *Juniper-berries,* when they are quite black, in the Beginning of *September.* These keep for your Use; and take five or six of them Every Morning, fasting. This removes the Scorbutical Obstructions; Consumes the Superfluous Humidity; and fortifies the Parts that are debilitated."

§ *Woodman* in his *Medicus Novissimus* tells you; "I recommend *Cream of Tartar*[17] as the greatest *Anti-scorbutick,* I ever mett with, in the whole Republic of Physick. By the Use of it, I have both seen and done Wonders; insomuch, that in a Manner I have thrown by all other *Anti-scorbuticks,* Except a very few, which are interlaced with the Use of the *Cream of Tartar.* Tis such a Safe and Cheap Remedy, that the meanest Persons may use it; For which Reason I make it here public; tho' I know, t'wil gett me Envy from those, who would not, if they could, do Good in their Generation. If you find no Alteration for the better in three or four days time, Lett it not discourage you from a further Use of the *Cream of Tartar,* but persist with Patience for some time in the use of it; and you will find (with Gods Blessing desired) Success, as I have often done. Lett me give you this only Caution in using it; That if by taking it four times a Day (*from half a Dram to a Dram!*) it should occasion above Three Stools in Twenty four Hours, Either that the Dose may be lessened, or you may omitt taking it Once or Twice a day, as there is Occasion. It may be taken in any thing, as, Wine, Beer, Ale, Whey, Posset-drink. But the best way of taking it, in the Morning and at Night, is in a Porringer of Water-gruel, Sweetned with Sugar: which at once will be very pleasant, and serve for a Breakfast and Supper, as well as a Medicine for the *Scurvy.*"

§ *Willius* writing, *De Morbis Castrensibus,* prescribes, as an Excellent Remedy for the *Scurvy;* A Decoction of *Trefolium Fibrinum*[18] in Beer, to be drunk Largely and Continually.

Scorbutic Ulcers, often washed with Lime-water, till the Ill Habit of the Body be mended, have had some Releef.

CAP. XXIII. *Moses.*
or, one *Drawn out* of,
The Dropsy.

AMONG the *Thousand Figures of Dying,* one is, The *Lamp of Life* drowning in a *Dropsy.*

When the *Water* of this *Dead Sea,* is contained only in the Cavity of the Belly, tis Called an *Ascites.* But if it be in the Legs and other particular Fleshy Parts, tis called an *Anasarca.* If it occupy the Fleshy Substance of the Whole Body, tis called a *Leucophlegmatia.* If the Belly be distended with much *Wind* as well as Water, tis called a *Tympany.* But if the *Head* be the Seat of it, and the Flood reach the Top of the Mountains, then it is called an *Hydrocephalus.* There are other Parts of the Body, which have their *Special Dropsies.*

Doubtless, the Original of this Malady, is much owing to a *Depauperated Blood,* which having lost its due Texture, breeds a *Lympha* that by Stagnation or Acrimony swells or breaks the Vessels. And a Weak Influx of the Animal Spirits on the Cutaneous Fibres no doubt may contribute also unto it.

Whether the Patient Labour under an *Hydrocephalus* or no, he has as Bad a Malady, and one too much akin to it, if under a *Dropsy* of any sort, he be destitute of the *Godly Sentiments,* which it would naturally call him to.

When the *Hydropical* Person feels the Waters from the *River of Death* flowing in upon him, What Cause has he to make that Cry, *Save me, O God; For the Waters are come in unto my Soul. I am Come into deep Waters, where the Floods overflow me.* My Friend, This was the Cry of thy *Dying* SAVIOUR. Make it; and plead the *Death* of thy SAVIOUR, that thou mayst be Saved from Sinking in those deeper and blacker *Waters,* the Troubles of a Guilty SOUL: and in the *burning Lake,* whereof the *Torment* is forever and ever.

The *Tumid State* of the Patient under a *Dropsy,* may justly putt him in mind of the *Pride,* for which all Men living (tho' some above others) have cause to Humble and Abase themselves, before the Glorious God, who *knows the Proud afar off.* Think, "Lord, What a *Tumified Wretch* have I been, in my high *Thoughts* of My *Self, Oftime* at my *self,* and *Claims* for *my* self: What an *Abomination to the Lord:* Pardon me, O my GOD! give me to shrink into *Nothing* before thee!"

Pride is the *Dropsy* of the Soul. And considering the *Vanity* of it, it may more particularly be called, *A Tympany.*

The Patient beholding the *Inæquality* in the Parts of his Body: Some Enormously *Tumified,* while others are as much *Emaciated;* May do well to Reflect upon that *Unæqual Christianity,* wherein he has too frequently (and most People have too commonly) Miscarried: Sometimes Abounding in *Devotions* toward God, and at the same time Defective in *Benignities* towards Men. Sometimes very *Consciencious* in One Point of Religion, and at the same time very *negligent* in another. Again cry out, *Pardon me, and Preserve me, O my God.*

The Livid *Spotts* which thy *Dropsy* taints thee withal; won't they mind thee of the Sinful *Spotts* upon thy Soul? My Friend, Thou hast not kept thyself *Unspotted from the World.* Beware of that Character once given of some unhappy People; *Their Spott is that they are not the Children of God.*

The *Thirst* which parches thee and vexes thee, may putt thee in Mind of thy *Insatiable Thirst* after Satisfaction in Creatures. In thy *Thirst,* hast not thou *drunk in Iniquity like Water?* But has it not thy *Criminal Thirst* been a *Dropsical Thirst?* The more thou hast swallow'd, thou art but the more *Thirsty* Still.

Quo plus Sint potae, plus Sitiuntur Aquae.[1] My Friend, There will nothing slake thy *Thirst,* but a CHRIST. Lett that Cry be heard from thee; *O give me to drink of the Water of the Well of Bethlehem!*

Does not [thy] *Body* feel very much like a *Dead Carcase? As Cold as Death.* Certainly, This is a Symptom, that should Awaken thy Thoughts of thy *Death Approaching;* and *Enliven* thy most Sollicitous and Assiduous *Preparation* for it.

Helmont observes, That *Grief* alone will sometimes cause a *Dropsy.* The *Grief* of a Genuine *Repentance* for the Sins that may have been the Cause of thy *Dropsy;* and particularly for the *Sinful Grief,* if there has been such a Thing, that may have been a Cause of thy *Dropsy;* this *Godly Sorrow* will be no Damage to thee, no accession to thy Malady.

§ *Abstinence! Abstinence!* This Alone has done wonderful Things.

Abstine, et efficies quod Medicina nequit.[2]

Especially Abstain from *Liquids,* during the whole Cure. By This alone, how many have been cured!

For this Cause, *D'Ube* observes, The poor are oftner Cured than the Rich.

§ *Evacuations* may be useful. Not Violent Ones; But such as won't Exceed Four or Five Stools.

An Ounce of the Syrup of *Buck-thorn,* may do well.

A Vomit may not be amiss, if the Stomach heave that Way.

§ There is a *Vinum Millepedum,* or, *Sow-bug Wine,* which is thus prepared. Take *Sow-bugs* half a Pound; putt 'em alive into a *Quart* or two of Wine; After a few days Infusion, Strain them and Press them out very hard. Then putt in *Saffron,* two Drams; and *Salt of Steel*[3] one Dram; and Salt of *Amber*[4] one Scruple. After three or four Days you may strain it, and keep it for use.

The Learned assure us, This is an admirable Medicine against the *Dropsy* and the *Jaundice,* and indeed any *Ill-habit* of Body. It greatly deterges all the Bowels, and throws off Superfluous Humours by Urine. It may be given twice a day; Two Ounces at a time.

§ In the Intervals, Use Diureticks. This is a Notable one. *Garlick,* two Drams, bruised in a Mortar, with about three Ounces of White Wine. Strain it, and so drink it.

Or, two Drams of Mustard-seed, rub'd unto a fine Powder; given three times a day in a glass of Rhenish Wine.

§ Take the Juice of *Chervil,*[5] in a glass of White-Wine.

§ Some have been Strangely Cured, with Half a dram of yellow transparent *Amber,* given twice or thrice a day, in any Convenient Vehicle.

§ A Decoction of *Guajacum* and *Sassafras,* is a proper Drink in a *Dropsy.*

§ Roots of *Dwarf-Elder,* boil'd and strain'd, and a Draught of the Decoction drunk, three times a day, for a fortnight or three weeks. This has often cured a *Dropsy.*

Or, Take the green Rind of young *Elder,* an Handful; Boil it in a Gallon of White-Wine to the half. Drink a Draught of it, cold in the Morning, warm at Night.

§ Strengthen the *Lymphatic* Vessels.

Whey wherein Red hott Iron has been often quenched, is a Potent Remedy.

§ If you'l Beleeve *Pontaeus;*[6] The Best Remedy in the World, is, To take *Morsus Diaboli,*[7] and putt it over Fire in a dry Kettle, that it may wett it only with its own Juice; and of this apply a Quantity to the Belly and Reins of the Patient; Covering him up warm, and so provoke Sweat; which will come away in great Quantity.

§ Dr. *Hulse*[8] affirms, That he has known the following Pasty to cure very grievous *Dropsies.*

Take Rye-Meal, (some use Æqual Quantities of *Rye* and *Barley*) and make a Pasty, that will hold a Peck of Sage-Leaves, Having filled it with Sage, Lid it, and bake it in an Oven. When it is baked, break it into a Canvas-Bag, and hang it in a Barrel of pretty good Beer; and when it is Ready, drink it for Ordinary Beer.

§ In the *Anasarca,* there is a good Use of *Sudorificks.*[9] Take little handfuls of *Camomil-flowers:*[10] Boil them a little in a Mess of thin *Water-gruel;* strain the Gruel and Sweeten it. It has been said, This never fails to procure *Sweat.* It also provokes the Urine; Quenches the Thirst; and Abates the Fever. *Woodman* sais, Tho' this look like a Simple Medicine, Lett it be tried; and not be despised for the seeming Meanness of it.

§ In a *Tympany,*[11] there should be Carminative[12] Clysters used.

§ Tiny drops of Sweet *Spirits of Nitre,* taken three times a day. Tis a noble Medicine.

§ An *Hydrocephalus* has been cured, cheerfully with Gum of *Gamboge*[13] in Powder, one Ounce, and Salt butter enough to make it into a Mass for Pills. Take a scruple more or less every day; or Enough to give three or four Stools in four and twenty hours; Adding for the shaved Head, an agreeable Fomentation.

§ An Ointment of *Soap* dissolved in *Aqua* Vitae;[14] This applied unto the Legs, removes Hydropsical Swellings.

§ For the Thirsty Nothing better than Chaw'd *Liquorice*.

§ For a Dropsy, here is a Remedy that has been bless'd with a Marvellous and Surprizing Efficacy; Hardly Ever known to fail.

Take a Gallon of *Cyder;* then take Roots of *Dwarf-Eldar,* an Handful (Scrape 'em clean, and also throw away the Pithe of 'em) and an Handful of *Horse-Radish*; With an Ounce of *Annis-seed.*[15] Steep these in the *Cyder,* twenty-four Hours. Drink a Glass of this Liquor, Morning and Evening.

Some also that have Languished under a Sort of *Cholic,* and in Vain tried many other Medicines, have with the Use of this alone, in two or three Days been Cured; and had their Appetites notably restored unto them.

§ What need of any more?—And yett I will add, what M. *de la Hire*[16] is my Author for; That one under a *Dropsy* was Cured of his Distemper, by putting round his Loins a *Girdle* of Cloths, full of *Salt,* well dried and bruised. And that a Couple of old People were cured of the same Distemper by being under a necessity to drink *Salt-Water,* which purging them *Sursum ac Deorsum*[17] carried off the Malady.

Cap. XXIV. *Bethlem*[1] visited.

or,

The Cure of <u>Madness</u>.

A DISMAL Spectacle! Wherein the *Animal Spirits* inflamed, form Raging, or Shatter'd *Ideas* in the *Brain,* and raise in a Confused Manner, those that have been formerly there: and perhaps rush from thence into all Parts of the Body, with *Fiery Irradiations;* from whence proceeds often an Extraordinary Strength in the Limbs, with Patience of Cold, and other Inconveniences. My Friend, Thou art *it,* in some degree, if thou canst behold the woful Spectacle, and not say, *My Eye affecteth My Heart!* Tis not Easy to describe those Irregular Particles, which being fixed in the Blood, with Acid or Bilious Ferments there, do help to fire the *Animal Spirits* in this Calamity. But what shall be done upon the Deplorable Occasion?

To address the *Distracted,* were but a Sort of *Distraction.* Tis the Spectator that is to be led into Thoughts and Points of *Wisdome,* from the View of the *Madness,* which he sees his Neighbour *Unman'd* withal.

O *Sober* Spectator of the *Mad,* Think, [and so prove thyself to be *Sober-Minded.*] "How Thankful to my Gracious God, ought I to be, for the *Powers* of *Reason,* in the free Exercise thereof, Conferred upon me, and Continued unto me! The *Unreasonable Things* that I have done in *Denying the God that is above,* while I have been also Prostituting of my *Reason* to mean and base Purposes, render me worthy to be *Smitten with Madness, and Blindness, and Astonishment of Heart,* and be like the *Chaldaean* Emperour, *driven from among Men,* and *have my Dwelling with the Beasts of the Field,*[2] O my SAVIOUR, Tis Thou, who doest *Enlighten Every Man that Comes into the World;* unto thee am I Endebted for the Use of *Reason,* wherewith I am *Enlightened.* And it is owing to thy Compassionate Mediation for me, that my forfeited *Reason* is not utterly taken from me."

This Acknowledgment ought certainly to be accompanied with Supplications for the Rescue of the *Mad* now before thee. With a Soul full of Compassion, Supplicate, *O Thou who formest the Spirit of Man within him! O Thou who didst of old help them that kept wounding themselves among the Tombs! Have Pitty on the desolate Object here before thee!*

Think; "A more fearful and foaming *Madness* than what I now see in this poor Creature, and a very criminal one too, shall I be chargeable withal, if I *Sin* against the Glorious God! If I provoke the Almighty, as if I were *Stronger than He!* If I make any thing but the Serving and Pleasing of God my Maker, the *Main Scope* of my Life! If I seek *that* in Creatures, which is to be found only in the Creator! If I harken to the *Destroyer,* more than to my *Redeemer!* If I forfeit *Eternal Enjoyments,* yea, incur *Eternal Miseries,* for the Sake of Sinful *Pleasures;* which at best are not worthy to be called *Pleasures,* and which are *but for a Season! O my SAVIOUR, præserve me from it.*"

Think; "What is the Whole World but an Entire *Mad-house?* What is *Mankind,* but a People upon whom *God from Heaven looking down,* see that *they don't understand,* but, *Madness is in their Heart!*—Except some few here and there, *One of a City, Two of a Tribe,* who by the Grace of God are *come to themselves! O my SAVIOUR, Pitty a Mad World!* And in that I am in any Measure myself delivered, *Bless the Lord, O my Soul!*"

Maniacks are sometimes more or less *Dæmoniacks.* In this Case, *Prayer* with *Fasting,* is the chief Resort.

It has been a nice Observation, That *every Man* is *Mad* in some

One Point; There is at least *One Point,* wherein *Reason* will do nothing with him. He is a very wise Man, who finds out his own *Mad Point.* Man, *Know Thyself;* Study what it is; and in that *One Point,* keep a singular Guard upon thyself.

Be sure, Our *Original Sin,* has a *Madness* in it; renders us *Mad upon our Idols.* We are never brought unto a *Right Mind,* but in and by a Thorough *Conversion* unto God.

A Gentleman in his Travels, ask'd another, *Which was the Way to Bedlam?* His Friend made a *Jocose Reply,* which deserves a *Serious Review.* He said, *Which Bedlam do you mean? The Great Bedlam, or the Little Bedlam? If you mean the Great Bedlam, you are in it already. If you mean the Little Bedlam, you are to turn down such a Street.*

§ Both the *Meats* and the *Drinks* of the *Mad,* should be very *Cooling.*

Vina grievant animos, faciuntque furoribus aptos.[3]

A Decoction of *Swallows,*[4] with *Lapis Prunellae,*[5] has been found very good for them.

§ *Bleeding* often Repeted, has done Something to Extinguish the Fury of the *Animal Spirits;* Yett it must be but a little at a time, Lest it cause a *Dropsy.*

§ If any *Excretions* of the *Mad* are stop'd, they must by all means again be opened.

§ A famous Physician cries up, the Decoction of Purple-flowered *Pimpernel;*[6] as also the Tops of *St. Johns Wort;*[7] as a Specific for *Madness.*

§ The Use of *Hellebore*[8] for the *Mad,* has been considered, Even to a Proverb.

§ *Chalybeates* are sometimes Potent Remedies, for *Madness.*

§ *Opiates* have been Significant; But when Anadynes are used for the *Mad,* Some have preferr'd *Camphere*[9] unto *Opium.*

What say you, to *Meconium*[10] fermented with the Juice of *Quinces?*

§ *Madmen* have sometimes been perfectly Cured by *Salivation.*

§ The Blood of an *Ass,* drawn from behind his Ear, has a Singular and Wonderful Vertue, in destroying the *Volatil Acid,* which is the Cause of *Madness.*

§ The *Mad* allow'd no Drink, but what has an Infusion of *Ground-Ivy* in it; would probably find a good and great Effect of it.

§ To be shutt up in a Press, where the Scent of *Musk* is too strong for Ordinary Constitutions, has been found a very powerful Cure for *Madness.*

§ One cured many *Madmen,* with the Juice of Young *Swallows,* given to the Quantity of an Ounce, twice or thrice, in the Water of *Pimpernel.*

§ Living *Swallows,*[11] cut in two, and laid reeking hott unto the shaved Head, have been præscribed, as a Cure for *Madness.*

§ Concerning the Root of *Nymphaea,*[12] the *Water-Lilly,* dug up in the Month of May, the great *Sennertus* has this Remark; *Specifica proprietate Maniaerisistere Creditur.*

§ According to *Valschmdius,*[13] the gentler sort of Acids, and the Cinnabarine Powders, with Emulsions, are the Chief internal Remedies in a *Phrensy.*

§ *Willis* præscribes; Take boyling *Whey;* pour it upon Flowres of *Violets* and *Water-Lillies.* After two Hours Infusion, the Mad Person is to drink plentifully of it.

§ *Borellus,* tells of a Woman that was under *Madness* of an *Uterine Original,*[14] which was cured only with wearing a *Loadstone* on her Stomach.

CAP. XXV. De *Tristibus.*
or,
The Cure of Melancholy.

IT has been a Maxim with some, *That a Wise Man will be Melancholy once a Day.* I suppose, they mean Something more than, *Serious,* and, *Thoughtful.* Such a Frame as *That,* is to be advised for more than, *Once a Day.* I must rather say, *My Son, Be thou in it all the Day long.* I am sure, a *Dying Man,* as thou art, has Reason to be so.

But, for a *Crasy Melancholy,* or a *froward Melancholy;* For this, *Once a Day,* is too much.

There is a Malady, which goes by the Name of *Melancholy.* Tis Commonly Called, The *Hypocondriac Melancholy:* [and for Brevity, and for *Division,* sake, often called, The *Hypo':*] because *Flatulencies* in the Region of the *Hypocondria,* often accompany it. And so, the poor *Spleen* frequently, but wrongfully Enough, comes to be Charged with it.

None are more Subject unto it, than such as have had Inveterate

Headakes torturing of them; and Women who labour under *Obstructions.*

How the *System of our Spirits,* comes to be dulled, and sowred, in this Distemper, lett them, who *know,* Declare; They who can only *guess,* will be Modest and Silent.

The *Fancies* and *Whimsies* of People over-run with *Melancholy* are so Many, and so Various, and so Ridiculous, that the very Recital of them, one would think, might somewhat serve as a little *Cure for Melancholy.* The Stories might be, what the Title of some silly Books have been; *Pills to purge Melancholy.* Tho' Truly unto a Reasonable and Religious Beholder of them, these Violations of *Reason,* are a *Melancholy-Spectacle.*

These *Melancholicks,* do sufficiently *Afflict themselves,* and are Enough their *own Tormentors.* As if this *present Evil World,* would not *Really* afford Sad Things Enough, they create a World of *Imaginary Ones,* and by *Mediatating Terror,* they make themselves as Miserable, as they could be from the most *Real Miseries.*

But this is not all; They *Afflict others* as well as *Themselves,* and often make themselves Insupportable *Burdens* to all about them.

In this Case, we must *Bear one anothers Burdens,* or, the *Burdens* which we make for One another.

Lett not the Friends of these poor *Melancholicks,* be too soon *Weary* of the *Tiresome Things,* which they must now *Bear with Patience.* Their *Nonsense* and *Folly* must be *born with Patience, We that are Strong must bear the Infirmities of the Weak;* and with a patient, prudent, Manly Generosity, pitty them, and Humour them like *Children,* and give none but *Good Looks* and *good Words* unto them. And if they utter Speeches that are very *Grievous* (and like *Daggers*) to us, We must not Resent them as uttered by these Persons; Tis not *They* that Speak; Tis their *Distemper!*

The *Ministers* of the Gospel, undergo a very particular Trial on this Occasion. These *Melancholicks* will go to, or send for, *Ministers,* and with Long Impertinencies tell them *How they seem unto themselves to be;* And after the *Ministers* have spent many Hours in Talking with them, they still are, *Just where they were before.* Some Diligent and Vigilant Servants of God have observed Something that has look'd like a Sensible *Energy of Satan* operating in this Matter; inasmuch as the *Time,* which the *Melancholicks* often take, to pester them, has been, what the greatest Enemy of their more *Useful Studies,* would have chosen, to give them an Interruption at.

If I may offer my Opinion, unto those who are to *Watch for Souls,* I would say;

Syr, It will be Easy for you, to discover, whether your Patient, be really under the *Trouble of Mind,* that calls for the Skill of one who shall be, *Insignis Animarum tractandarum Artifex,*[1] to be Exercised upon it. If you do really discover, That the Patient is under *Awakenings* from the SPIRIT of God, and under Apprehensions of the *Wrath Reveled from Heaven* against the *Ungodliness and Unrighteousness of Men,* God forbid, that you should make Light of the Matter. The Profane, Baneful, *Epicurean* Folly,[2] of making such *Trouble of Mind,* nothing but a *Mechanical Business* in our *Animal Spirits,* very ill becomes a *Minister of the Gospel.* The *Pastoral Care* no better Exercised than so, would become the Men that are *Sensual, not having the Spirit.* No, All Possible and Exquisite Care must now be taken, to carry the *Troubled Sinner* thorough a *Process of Repentance;* And after a due Confession of his Guilt, and Impotency, and Unworthiness, *Lead him to the Rock:* Show Him a Glorious CHRIST, *Able to Save unto the Uttermost,* and *Willing to Cast out none that Come to Him.* Having obtained his *Consent,* that a Glorious CHRIST should accomplish all the Offices of a Mighty and Holy *Redeemer* for him, then gett him fixed in the *Resolutions* of PIETY. And now, *Comfort him, Comfort him, speak thou comfortably to him. Tell him* what the *very great and precious Promises* in the *Covenant of Grace* do now assure him of; inculcate upon him, the *Consolations of God.*

But you may often see Cause to Suspect, that the *Spiritual Troubles* of your *Melancholicks* are not of such an *Original* as is pretended for. If you trace them, you may perhaps find out, that some very intolerable *Vexation,* or some *Temporal Troubles,* begun their Uneasiness, and first raised that *Ulcer* in their Minds, which now finds *New Matter* to work upon, and the *Old Matter* is no Longer Spoken of. If this be the Case, *Wisdome is profitable to direct,* how the Patient is to be treated. A Cheerful, Courteous, Obliging Behaviour to them, with *Length of Time,* and some Notable Contrivance, if there be Opportunity, to *mend what is amiss* in their Condition, will do something towards the Cure.

If your *Melancholicks* are gott into a tedious Way, of *Complaining against Themselves,* why should not the Best Way be, to Allow that all their *Complaints* may be *True.* But then tell them, what is <u>NOW</u> to be done, that they may *do better* than they have done, and *all may be well* with them. Rebuke the *Pining, Moaning, Languid,* and *Slothful* Sort of Christians, and lett them know, that they must be rowsed out of their *Inactivity,* and abound more in *Direct* Acts, than in *Reflex* ones. Grant, that they have never yett *Repented,* and *Beleeved,* and Laid Hold on the *Covenant of Life;* But then, Demand it of them that they do all of it <u>NOW</u>; and plainly describe to them the *Acts* of a Soul Turning and Living unto God. Require them NOW to make a *Trial,* whether they can't, with the Aids of Heaven, *Do* those *Acts,* and keep at the *Repetition* of them, until they have some *Satisfaction,* that they have Heartily and Sincerely done them.

It is not without a Cause, that *Melancholy* has been called, *Balneum Diaboli.*[3] Some *Devil* is often very Busy with the poor *Melancholicks;* yea, there is often a Degree of *Diabolical Possession* in the *Melancholy.* King *Saul* is not the only Instance to be produced for it. The *Diabolical Impression* appears very Sensible, Either when *Thoughts* full of *Atheism* or *Blasphemy* are shott like *Fiery Darts* into their Minds, and so seriously infest them, that they are even *Weary of their Lives;* or, when their Minds are violently impelled and hurried on to Self-Murder, by *Starving,* or *Strangling,* or *Stabbing,* and the like. In this Case, Lett *Prayer with Fasting* be Employed; It may be the *Kind will go out no other Way.* But the astonishing Experiments that I have seen, of *Beseeching the Lord THRICE,* in this Way!—And of *Prayer* not prevailing, until the Number of THREE *Days* could be reached unto!—

As to Conferences with the *Melancholicks,* my Advice is, That if you would not *throw away much Time* to little Purpose, you would in short lett them know; That these are *Faithful Sayings, and Worthy of all Acceptation;* First, A Glorious CHRIST, is willing to make them *Righteous* and *Holy,* upon their *Cordial Consent* unto His doing so; and therefore Invites them to look unto Him for all the Blessings of His *Plenteous Redemption.* Secondly, That upon their *Looking up* to Him, with a Soul consenting to be under His Gracious Influences, it is their *Duty* to Entertain a *Perswasion,* That He has made them *Righteous* and will make them *Holy;* and so to Resolve upon always *Chusing the Things that please Him.* Lett them know, That when you have said all that you can say, *This* must be the *Sum,* and *Scope* of all. This is Enough. With This, Bestow some *Suitable Book* upon them; And so take your Leave.

Among *Melancholy Diseases,* there is one which in *Hippocrates* goes by the Name, φροντίς, or, *Care;* and he gives a very dismal Report of it. We must cure *this* as much as we can, and all the Ways we can, in our poor *Melancholicks.*

Curas tolle gravas,[4]—was a good Maxim, long before the *Schola Salerni* was in the World.

§ I will transcribe a Passage from a Treatise Entituled, *The Curiosities of Common Water;* published by one *John Smith C. M.*[5] [The Learned may please to know the Difference between A.M. and C.M. to be This; that C.M. stands for *Clock Maker!*] And if the Passage only make the *Melancholy* Reader to *Smile,* Even This may be a Little Step towards his Cure. He *Says:* "Being very *Hypocondriacal* and of a *Melancholy* Temper, I have often been strangely dejected in Mind, when under Grief for some Misfortunes, which sometimes have been so great, as to *threaten* Danger to Life.—But I have now found a *Good Remedy:* For upon Drinking a Pint, or more, of *Cold Water,* I find Ease in two or three Minutes, so that no Grief seems to afflict me. This Experience I discover for the Sake of others in the like Circumstances, being verily perswaded that the Stomach Sympathizes with the Mind."

§ *Borellus* tells of a Lady, Strangely Overwhelmed with *Melancholy,* that was cured with wearing upon her Heart, a Bag of *Saffron.*

§ The Exercise of *Riding,* wisely managed and followed:—By Degrees People have Rid away *Melancholy,* that has been growing upon them. The Wiser, and more pleasant the Company, the better.

§ Some have seen a Strange Effect, of having their *Hæmorrhoidal Veins* drawn by *Leeches*[6] applied unto them. Tis incredible, how Lightsome and Easy they have grown upon it, and for many Months free from the *Melancholy* that had besotted them.

§ Of Singular Use in *Melancholy,* is, as *Willis* tells us; The *Syrup of Steel,*[7] four Ounces; a Spoonful to be taken twice a day in a Convenient Vehicle.

§ He also mentions, *A Simple Medicine, used often with good Effect in Melancholy.*

Tis this. Take *Whey;* Infuse *Epithymum*[8] in it; And of this Drink Plentifully for Several Days.

§ See *Quincy's Elixir Hypocondriacum.*[9]

§ It is a very Odd Observation of the famous *Olaus Borrichius;*[10] in *Bartholinus,* his *Acta Medica: Sanatos Melancholicos (Convenit et hoc Deliris aliis) Medicum Suum a quo gravi illo onere levati sunt, plerumque Odisse:*—[11] Imagining it seems, that these their *Friends* retain a Disadvantageous Remembrance of what pass'd in their *Fitts;*

or that they have produced in the People a false Opinion of them, as having been whimsical, when they were not so. I hope, the Observation will not be always verified!

CAP. XXVI. *Paralyticus resuscitatus.*

or

The <u>Palsey</u>-*struck* taking up his Bed and Walking.

THERE is a *Numbness,* either *Partial* or *Total,* wherin the *Feeling* and *Motion* is diminished; which is an Essay towards a *Palsey,* and often terminates in it. There is also a *Palsey,* which is oftentimes the Result of an *Apoplexy;* when by the Strength of Nature, the Matter which caused the *Apoplexy,* is carried unto the Extremities of the Nerves; and which oftentimes returns to an *Apoplexy,* when that Matter does recur to the Brain.

The Seat of this Disease, Every body knows, is in the *Nerves.* And as the *Spinal Marrow,* thro' which they spread from the Brain, is distributed into Two Branches, the Right and the Left; when the *Right* is hurt, the *Palsey* is on the *Right* Side; when the *Left* is hurt, it is on the *Left.*[1]

Sometimes, tis only a *Particular Part,* that is affected.

And sometimes, only *Feeling* ceases, and not *Motion;* sometimes only *Motion,* and not *Feeling.* Tis what we call, *An Imperfect Palsey.*

The *Same Remedies* are proper for the *Numbness* and the *Palsey;* only the Latter will require them in *Stronger Portions.*

I am sure, the *Same Sentiments* will not be improper, or unwholesome.

Think: "Alas, Have I not a SOUL that is *Palsey-Struck!* My SOUL, Indisposed for the *Motions,* with which a Life of PIETY is to be carried on; My SOUL, Insensible of Impressions from God; Certainly, It has a *Palsey* on it. But tho' a *Palsey* be an Obstinate Malady, yett I find the Almighty Hand of my SAVIOUR miraculously, and irresistibly curing of it. *For the Cure of my palsey'd SOUL, I will hope in thee, O my SAVIOUR.*"

Think; "If my SAVIOUR will now speak to me, what He spoke once unto a *Paralytick; Child, Be Comforted, Thy Sins are forgiven Thee!* The *Sting* of my *Sickness* will be taken away. I shall Enjoy what may make me Easy under my Calamity. *O my SAVIOUR, lett my Repentance be so Sincere, so Thorough, that thy Holy Spirit may give me to Read my Pardon in it!"*

Think; "Tho' my *Body* be reduced into such a State of *Inaction,* yett lett my *Soul* be lively in the Service of God. When my *Will* cannot any Longer Dispatch the *Spirits* into Every Part of my *Body,* for the moving of it at my Pleasure, yett lett the Sanctified Faculties of my *Soul,* yeeld a Ready Obedience to the Calls of my *Will,* for Conversing with God, and with the *Things which are above. Quicken me, O my SAVIOUR!"*

Think; "The Influx of the Animal Spirits, into their Conduits, being stop'd, what miserable *Palsey* ensues upon it! what *Fetters of Death* are laid upon me! *Glorious LORD, If the Influences of thy Grace are witheld from me, I am Dead. Without Thee, I can do nothing."*

It has been unto some, a Matter of Wonder That our SAVIOUR several times, does mention unto *Paralyticks,* their *SINS,* as having brought their Maladies upon them, and never intimated any such thing unto those that laboured of any other Maladies. Lett Ingenious Minds, Expatiate on this Curiosity. I will only offer one Remark upon it, which I have somewhere mett withal. A *Paralytick* Distemper, does restrain People, from committing Abundance of *Actual Sins.* They are under a Necessity of Living so *Unactively,* that they may perhaps think themselves to live almost *Innocently.* Now, our SAVIOUR, that He might Remind the poor *Paralyticks,* of their former Sins, which they had, it may be, too much forgotten, and of the Inclinations to *Sin,* yett lurking in their Hearts, and ready to break forth, when the Chains of the *Palsey* should be taken off, He speaks very particularly about their *Sins* unto them.

§ S———h is Poison. And *Aqua Vitae* will carry *Death* in it.

§ The Internal Use of the Chymical *Oyl of Penny-royal,*[2] has releeved *Palsey's* to Admiration.

§ If the Numb'd Part *meet with Rubs,* t'wil be no Damage to you. Not only Frictions, but Nettles often applied, have done some good.

§ Or, Hold them a good While at a time, in a Decoction of *Rosemary,* kept very warm.

§ The *Baths* have done Wonders. And so have the hott Entrails of Animals.

Tho' *Oils* by themselves, and *Fatts* are not safe to be frequently used, yett the Belly of a Pullet, fill'd with Suitable Things, and roasted, the Fatt which drops from it has been very serviceable. And so has [torn]

§ *Baglivi* speaks of a Woman, Sixty years of Age, having a *Palsey* on one side, and in her Tongue, which was cured in Three Days with the following Method.

After drawing Ten Ounces of Blood, out of the Arm, on the paralytic Side, the following Mixture was given. ℞. Water of *Peony* flowers,[3] and *Carduus Benedictus*,[4] of Each, Three Ounces. Spirit of *Sal Armoniac*, Twelve Drops. Powder of *Humane Skull*, and *Diaphoretic Antimony*,[5] of Each, a Scruple; Mix, and make a Potion, to be taken off Immediately. Lett the whole *Spine of the Back*, and the *Paralytic Part* of the Body, be anointed hott, with Oil of *Foxes*,[6] mixed with the Spirit of Wine. Hold in the Mouth, a Gargarism of the Decoction of the *Missletoe*[7] of the *Oak;* and *Oxymel* of Squills.[8]—

CAP. XXVII. *Attonitus*.

or,

The <u>Apoplexy</u> considered.

A DISTEMPER that brings *Astonishment!* It is rather the Astonished *Spectator*, than the *Sufferer*, that the Admonitions of PIETY fetch'd from this Distemper, are to be address'd unto.

There is indeed a *Something*, (and they who are positive and præsumptuous Enough to speak more particularly, say an *Acid*,) that kills or stops the Spirits, and Coagulates the Blood, or sometimes forces it with an *Extravasation* into the *Brain*, in this Distemper; and *at Once* throws the Patient into the Arms of Death, from whence rarely are any rescued, without falling into a *Palsey*.

A *Narcotic Sulphur*,[1] drawn in with the Air, by that *Respiration*, wherewith we are Continually Struggling for Life, may Cause this Distemper.

But, O *Stander-by*, Canst thou Behold, the Sudden, and the Deadly Arrest here served upon thy Brother, without some such Thoughts as these upon it?

Think; "How true is that Word, *Man knoweth not his Time!* Little was my Neighbour aware, a few Hours before, what a *Stroke* was going to be given him. He is like one *Thunderstruck*. Nothing but a little *Breath* and *Pulse* discovers the Remains of some *Life* within him. The *Lamp of Life,* how Suddenly, how Speedily, how Easily Extinguished! *Lord,* with what Sollicitude, with what Expedition, ought I to *make Ready,* for the Stroke of *Death!* O Quicken and Assist me, Immediately to *make Ready* for it, by such a Process of a *Repenting Faith,* as will bring me into Good Terms with Heaven, and then *Do with my might what my hand finds to do,* of Every thing that it will be a Grief to have left undone, when I come to dy."

Think; "In what a forlorn Condition does my Neighbour ly! How unable to speak, unable to stir, unable to help himself! Tis the Condition of my Soul, *O my SAVIOUR,* Till Thou help and heal me with thy *Enlivening* Influences. *Enliven me, O my God, and Enable me, to Rise, and Move, and Work, and Live unto thee!"*

If the Patient Recover in any Measure, Lett him come into such Sentiments. But, *My Friend,* Without any *Delay,* do thou *Redeem* thy Time; gett the *Tokens of Salvation* to become very *Evident* and Legible upon thee. *Dispatch* Every thing that a *Dying Man* has to do. For, the *Time of thy Departure is at hand.* Thou hast Reason to keep in Hourly Expectation of a *Second Attack.* It won't be very long before the *Clouds Return.* No Time should be Lost. Every Moment of Time, should now be precious to thee, husbanded with thee.

§ Old *Hippocrates,* whose *Aphorisms* it seems, are *Oracles,* tells us, *To cure a Violent Apoplexy is impossible; To Cure a sleight one, is not Easy.*

Be sure, if *Blood* be extravasated upon the *Brain,* I don't see, but the Case is Desperate. However sometimes, the *Apoplexy* is of a more *pituitous*[2] Original; the *Brain* is oppress'd with an heterogeneous *Phlegm.* Wherefore, Lett us Try a Little.

§ *Bleeding* in all Ages, is the first chief Refuge, under an *Apoplexy.* But tho' it may be proper in what they call the *Sanguine Apoplexy,* it may be pernicious in the *Flegmatic,* which is unobserved.

§ *Vomits* do a deal of Good.

§ *Clysters,* are seasonable. They must be sharp ones. *Emetic Wine*[3] has been used this Way.

§ *Blisters,* as well as *Cupping,* on the Crown of the Head, are not now out of their Place.

§ The Soles of the *Feet,* are to be rub'd with Vinegar and Salt.

§ While other Things are doing, lett the Nose and the Temples be rubbed with Spirit of *Hartshorn,* Tincture of *Castor,* and Oyl of *Amber.* Give Thirty drops of this Mixture, in any proper Liquor. And lett Spirit of *Sal Armoniac* be now and then held to the Nose.

§ *Mustard* is a sort of *Specific,* in *Apoplectic* Maladies; diverse wayes prepared and applied.

§ A *Salivation* has cured an *Apoplexy.*

§ An Issue at the Meeting of the Sutures[4] kept open for a good While; This is in the *Boylaean* Receits called, *A Powerful Application.* It is added, If the Case admit not a Delay, clap on a good *Cupping-glass* at the same Concurse of the Sutures.

§ *Sneezing* is one of the Things commonly attempted on the assault of an *Apoplexy.* But Mons. *Dube* finds fault with *Sternutations,* and had rather have *Castoreum* with *Rue*-leaves, thrust up into the Nose.

§ *Castoreum* and *Rue*-leaves, putt into a Strong Vinegar, and Cast upon a Red-hot Stone or Tile; the Exhalations received, have been serviceable.

§ *Cauteries,* (Especially *Moxa* burnt on the Top of the Head,) have done considerable Service.

§ In *Apoplectic Fitts,* fix a *Cupping-glass,* to the Nape of the Neck, and another to Each of the Shoulders. Lett 'em stick on a Time Convenient.

§ If the Enemy begin to fly, then the use of Saline and Volatil Spirits, may be seasonable. Among which, the *Spirit of Soot,*[5] has been so Considerable, that our *Dolaeus* tells us, *If the Virtues of that plain thing were better known, we should not fetch Drugs from the India's.*

§ *Issues* and *Setons* are of great use to prevent a Relapse.

Cap. XXVIII. *Caducus.*

or,

The Falling-Sickness considered.
With a New Discovery of a most unfailing Remedy,
for all Convulsive Diseases, in old or young.

THE *Spectator,* beholding one arrested with an *Epilepsy,* thrown down on the Ground with a Sudden Abolition of Sense, the Eyes distorted, the Mouth perhaps foaming, the Face with an Aspect full of Agony, and *Convulsive Motions* of the Limbs, from a depraved *Lympha* mixing with the Animal Spirits in the *Brain,* and thence issuing forth with an Irritation of the Nerves, the Involuntary Contraction whereof draws the Tendons and their dispersed Fibres, into a Consent with them; How can he but say, *Mine Eye affecteth mine Heart!* And, *Lord, what is Man, when thou layest thine Hand upon him?* And, *Lord, How Thankful should I be, in that I am Spared!* When we read, in the Divine Comminations, *I will appoint upon you TERROR, and Consumption and the Burning Ague,* the *Jews,* while under the Term of, *Consumption,* they understand all *Chronical* Diseases, and under the Term of *Burning Ague,* all *Acute* ones, by *TERROR,* they understand the *Falling Sickness.*

Will the *Spectator* be perswaded unto Gratitude and Piety, *Knowing this Terror of the Lord.*

But the *Patient* also, Coming out of his Fitt, will have Opportunity to Entertain some affecting Thoughts upon his own Deplorable Condition.

At least, if he be not so far gone, as to become a meer *Ideot,* which is often the unhappy Consequence of this Distemper, when it has Long Prevailed.

Epileptic, Thou are already worse than an *Ideot,* if thou hast no *Religious Thoughts,* upon thy grievous Calamity.

Think; "I dread my *Falls* into those *Fitts,* which are so horrid, so painful, and which leave me so very feeble. But oh! Lett all *Falls* into Sins be more dreadful to me! O *Lord, I Beseech thee deliver my Soul.*"

Think; "Tho' I have now some Command of myself, yett when my *Fitts* come upon me, I Cannot Command any of my Members and their Motions. But much more miserable am I, when I fall into any criminal Passions, of *Anger,* or of *Avarice,* or of *Unchastity.* O *Lord, Lett no Iniquity have Dominion over me!*"

Think; "There has hitherto been a merciful Providence watching over me, in that my *Falling* into my *Fitts* has not thrown me into the *Fire,* or into the *Water,* or down the *Stairs,* or so as to give sad Wounds unto me, or over some deadly *Præcipice. O my SAVIOUR, I Bless thee for my Præservations. But, O Thou Præserver of my Soul, keep me from falling down into the Horrible Pitt!*"

Think; "*Epilepsies* do sometimes anon, so affect the *Brain,* and the *Spirits* there, that the *Rational Spirits* of the *Invisible World,* Strangely Insinuate themselves into the Malady. *Spirits* of an unknown Quality, gett their Operations into the Malady. Some of the *Dæmoniacks* in the Gospels, were *Epilepticks.* Hence follow marvellous *Visions;* and many Things that look very *Præternatural. My God, Save me from Diabolical Illusions. Lett no Devil now Play and Prey upon me!*

If thy *Tongue* has been Bitten in any of thy *Fitts;* Poor Sinner, Lett a *Repentance* for the *Sins* of that *unruly member,* have a *perfect work* upon it.

The Disease has been called, *Morbus Sacer.*[1] By these Methods it may become Emphatically *such.*

§ If an *Epilepsy,* be Hæreditary; or if it come after Thirty years of Age; tis very hardly curable.

§ *Barbette*[2] wrought a Wonderful Cure of an *Epilepsy.* After Once purging, he gave the Patient, the Following Draught Twice a Day. Take *Venice-Soap*[3] half a Dram; Boil it in Milk to three Ounces. Then strain it out for one Draught. The Cure was Entirely Wrought in Thirty Day.

§ In the Time of the Fitt, all possible Means must be used for the Releef of the direful Symptoms; Volatile Spirits, as of *Harts-horn,* or *Sal-armoniac* held unto the Nose; the hands unclinched; the Mouth kept open with a stick that the Tongue may not be bitten; the Temples anointed with Oil of *Amber;* the Head and Limbs rubbed with a Coarse Cloth—But these things Every body knows!

§ *Fuller* mentions an *Epileptic Ale.* Take *Male-Peony* Roots fresh gathered, four Ounces; *Peacocks Dung* half a Pound; *Raisins* Twelve Ounces; prepare it for a Bag, for Two Gallons. It is held a Specific, against an *Epilepsy,* and a Vertigo. You had best only take that Part of the Dung, which is white and uniform.—

§ *Borellus* cures an *Epilepsy,* with only *Peacocks* Dung, a Dram, taken in Wine.

§ A Necklace made of *Peony* Roots, till Dry; then powdered, and the powder taken in Sauces; and another moist Necklace at the same time substituted, has been found a good Remedy.

§ In the *Acta Medica* of *Bartholinus,* it is affirmed, that for an *Epilepsy,* the *Gall of a Dog,* is, *Infallible Euporiston.*[4]

§ Swallows dried and powdered, a Dram every Morning, before the New and Full Moon, has cured many.

§ I have read, a Girdle of *Wolfs skin,* præscribed for to be worn, with much Expectation.

§ *Issues* and *Setons,* are very good.

§ *Willis* proposes a Cure by this Bag, worn on the Pitt of the Stomach. Take Roots and Seeds of *Male-Peony,* of Each Two Drams; *Missletoe* of the Oak and *Elks*-hoof, of Each a Dram. Slice them, and bruise them; and sow them in a fine Linen Bag; to be hung about the Neck.

§ *Epilepsie*s have been cured by the Cure of *Worms.*[5]

§ *Baglivi* says, In Convulsive and Nervous Diseases, *Violets* are a specific.

§ Ingenious *Woodman,* affirms, That this Ale has done Wonders, in totally curing this fearful Disease. Take Oak,[6] Fern,[7] and Male-Peony Roots fresh, of Each Four Ounces; Missletoe of the Oak, cutt small, and Sassafras Wood, of Each two Ounces; The Dung of Peacocks, and of Pigeons, Each one Ounce and an half; Raisins of the Sun Stoned, ten Ounces. All being cutt small, putt it into a Bag, and hang it in Three Gallons of New Small Ale; After it has done working: Lett this continue Eight or Ten Days; Then lett the Party drink a Quarter of a Pint, Every morning Fasting, and about Eleven a clock, and at going to Bed.

§ The Grand *Epileptic Electuary.*

Take the poudered *Peruvian Bark,* Six Drams; *Virginia Snake-root,*[8] Two Drams: *Syrup of Peony,* as much as needs. Mix it up into a soft Electuary.

If (after due Evacuations) there be given One Dram to Adult Persons (and a Less Dose for others,) Morning and Evening, for three or four Months and afterwards for three or four Days before the Change and Full of the Moon, an Eminent Physician sais, *It absolutely* Eradicates *Epileptic* and *Hysteric* Diseases.

§ A Good Neighbour of mine, releeved an *Epilepsy* on himself, by the frequent use of *Mullein-Water.* His Wife also commonly cures *Convulsions* in Children, with the simple *Mullein Water,* Sweetened with a Little Syrup of *Saffron.* Some affirm that both in old and in young, it hardly ever fails.

§ *Willis* mentions, A *Simple Medicine, that has Cured many of the Falling-Sickness, when other Remedies proved Ineffectual.* Take of the simple Decoction of *Guajacum,* Six or Eight Ounces, twice a day. Drink a second weaker Decoction for Common Drink.

§ Sometimes *Worms* are at the Root of the *Falling-Sickness.* Then, I need not say, Strike at the *Root,* with potent *Worm-killers.*

§ In some *Women,* troubled with the Epilepsy, Bleeding in the Foot, may give Releef.

§ Tis among the *Boylaean* Receits.

For the *Falling-Sickness* in Children; take half a Dram of Choice *Amber,* finely powdered. Give it once a day for several Weeks together, when the Stomach is Empty; in about four Ounces of *Good White Wine.*

§ They often præscribe something of an *Humane Skull* pulverised. But our Dr. T. *Fuller* sais, "I declare, I abominate it. For I take *Mans Skull* to be, not only a meer dry Bone, void of all Vertue, but also a nasty, mortified, putrid, carrionish piece of our own Species; And to take it Inwardly, seems an Execrable Fact, that Even the *Anthropophagi*[9] would shiver at. And therefore, in my Opinion, it would be decent; and almost pious, to carry them all out of the Shops, and, *Ossa Sepulchrali Continulate Domo.*"[10]

A Communication

of a Specific and Victorious

REMEDY,

in *Epilepsies,* and all <u>Convulsive Diseases</u>:

particularly <u>Convulsions</u> in *Children.*

Tho' *Epilepsies,* and Convulsive Diseases, are in the Tragical Effects and Symptoms of them some of the most formidable, that Mankind *Fallen* from God, is Arrested and Afflicted withal; yett it is very Surprising how many *Earthly Tabernacles* are *shaken* with them, and Even totally Demolished. In the *Bills of Mortality* for the City of *London,* the Article of <u>Convulsions</u>, is by much the largest of any, and no less than the *Fifth Part* of the whole; Yea, double to that of the *Fevers,* in the Greatest, and Hottest, and most Mortal Raging of them. A Generous and an Effectual <u>Anti-Convulsive Remedy</u>, would therefore be a Marvellous *Blessing* unto the World; and the more Plain, and Cheap, and Easy to come at, the *Remedy,* the most Conspicuous and Considerable would be the Blessing. A gracious God having directed that Eminent Physician, and Ornament of his Profession, Sir *John Colbatch*[11] to such an one, has also disposed him charitably to publish it unto the World, and invite the most indigent, and instruct the most Ignorant, unto the using of it.

The Honourable and Admirable *Boyl,*[12] mentions a Lady of Great Birth, long troubled with an almost Hæreditary *Epileptical Distemper,* and unreleeved by the most famous Doctors, who was Cured only by the Powder of the true *Missletoe of the Oak,* taken as much as would ly on a Sixpence, Either in Black-Cherry Water, or

Even in Common Beer, for some Days near the full Moon. The ingenious Dr. *Cole*[13] mett with somewhat of the Like Success.

From such Hints, this Meritorious Gentleman, was animated, unto Experiments, with *Missletoe* growing on the *Lime*-tree; because that of the *Oak* was rarely to be gotten, and what grows on the *Lime,* or the *Crab,* or the *Pear,* or any other Tree, he did with good Reason Judge might be of æqual Vertue. And anon, his Experiments Enabled him to publish *A Dissertation Concerning Missletoe;* wherein he declares: "I have known so many Instances, both in Young and Old, in Rich and Poor, of both Sexes, some of whom have been many Years afflicted with *Epilepsies* and other *Convulsive Disorders,* that Either have been Cured, or have received Benefit, from this Divine Remedy, that I think myself *Bound in Conscience to divulge the Use of it to the World;* Since, it is Capable of doing *greater Things than ever I knew perform'd by any One Remedy,* and, I think it, uncapable of doing any Hurt:—And this, *for the Sake of the Poor;* the Meanest being able to procure it, as well as the Rich; and it wants little or no skill in the administration of it." Yea, he Suspects, That the Veneration paid by all Ranks of People, to the *Druids* of old, who Esteemed not any *Oaks* to be Sacred, which had not *Missletoe* upon them, did proceed partly from the Cures they wrought by the *Missletoe* growing there.

He observes, That a *Seed* of the *Missletoe,* stuck into a Slitt of the Bark on any Tree, produces it; and makes the Tree look Delightfully in the Winter-Season. Its Berries are full ripe, about the Latter End of *December;* and *then* is the Time to gather it. Gather the Leaves, Twigs, and Stalks, and Berries, and all. Dry it over a Bakers Oven, where it may Enjoy a Gentle and a Constant Heat. Reduce the dry'd Plant into a very fine Powder; putt the Powder into a glass. Cover the glass with Bladder or Leather. Keep it in a Dry Place. If it be Scorched in the Drying of it, it will be Spoiled; If it be not kept where its Dryness may be preserved, it grows mouldy, and good for nothing. He finds A Dram of *Assafoetida*[14] added unto an Ounce of the *Missletoe*-powder, and made into an Electuary, makes it yett more powerful.

The Greatest Article of *Convulsions,* is that of *Infant-Children;* and this is the Doctors way of giving them the *Missletoe.* He sais, *Most prodigious Things I have seen done by it.*

"Take of the *Powder of Missletoe,* Two Drams, *Rue* and *Penny-*

royal Water, of Each Two Ounces; Syrup of *Pæony,* half an Ounce. Mix them; and give half a Spoonful, as oft as you can gett them to take it."

If you can't get the Children to take it, mix the Powder, with their Panada.

If they are Exceedingly Grip'd and Loose, apply also this *Plaister* to their Bellies.

Venice-Treacle, and *Oil of Nutmegs* by Expression; of Each, Two Drams. Mix them, and spread them upon Soft Leather.

If the Looseness continues, give this *Clyster. Diascordium* made with *Diacodium*[15] instead of Honey; a Dram. The Powder of *Missletoe,* half a Dram. *Penny-royal* Water, three or four Ounces. Mix; and give it warm.

If they are Bound, which they rarely are, when they are convuls'd, give them a little *Manna,*[16] in some of the *Missletoe-Julep.*

To Children of Ten or a Dozen years of age, may be given, Half a Dram of the *Powdered Missletoe,* with three Grains of *Assafoetida,* three times a day; and a Draught of the Infusion after it.

Men and *Women* may take a Dram of the Powder, with Five or Six Grains of *Assafoetida,* three or four times a day according to the urgency of the Case; Drinking a Large Draught of the Infusion after it; and betwixt whiles.

A *Tincture* may be made of the *Missletoe,* in Spirit of Wine, which may after all, prove one of the Noblest Ways to convey its Vertues.

If *Worms* cause the *Fitts,* the *Missletoe* will be yett of good Use. But further *Anthelminticks* must accompany it.

The Case may be such, that the Use of the *Missletoe* must be continued some Weeks together. It generally keeps the Body Open; But if it fails of doing so, in three or four days give some Small Opener; Never any *Strong Purge,* which always does mischief in *Epileptical* Troubles.

The *Berries* of the *Missletoe,* Ten or Twelve, taken Green or Dry, and a Draught of generous Wine drunk after them, Every night at going to bed, are by Sir *John Colbatch,* Esteemed the *greatest Restorers of Decay'd Nature* that can Easily be litt upon.

He thus cured, a *Convulsive Asthma* (which is by *Helmont* called, *Caducus Pulmonum,*)[17] in a Gentleman who was *in as Distress'd a Condition* (he sais) *as an human Creature could possibly be:*

and had not been able to keep his Bed a whole Night for many Months; and was forced sometimes to sitt up the Whole Night with Windows open upon him.

"I ordered four Ounces of bruis'd *Missletoe,* to be infused in a Quart of Boiling Water, for an Hour; Then to be Strained out; When perfectly cold, to add half a Pint of *Lisbon-White-Wine:* Afterwards, with two Ounces of blanched Almonds to make an Emulsion; and to be sweetened with a sufficient Quantity of fine Sugar. I ordered him a Large Draught of this Emulsion Every Night before he went to Bed; and at times to drink the whole Bottel before he rose, if Sleep did not prevent. To the best of my Remembrance, he never had one Fitt of the *Asthma* afterwards."

Indeed, it may be so, that the Texture of the *Brain* may be so destroyed, as never to admitt of being repaired. And then, there's no more to be done! We won't please ourselves That the *Missletoe* was the *Golden Bough,* which *Æneas* made use of, to introduce him into the *Elysian* Regions. It has done a more Creditable and Valuable Thing in bringing Sir *John Colbatch* into the Way Encountring a formidable Adversary.

This Benefactor to the World, rejoices in his having an Opportunity of introducing into the World, (as he Expresses it) a *most glorious and useful Medicine,* Capable of doing the greatest Good, in one of the most formidable Diseases; and in this differing from the *Peruvian Bark,* that it will never do to any one, the least Hurt in the World. Even to *Infants,* there can be no Error in giving too much. The more they take, the better; so far is it from causing a *Fever,* that it is a curious *Febrifuge.*

And, he adds, concerning *the Redeemer of the World, the Eternal SON of God,* who of old miraculously cured *Epilepticks* with a Word; *Glory be to Him, that in the Absence of Himself has created such Medicines* as this *for the Releef of the Distressed!*

CAP. XXIX. *Vertiginosus.*
or, How to Steer under
<u>Dizziness.</u>

WHEN a *Vertigo* takes People, the Animal Spirits take not a Right Course, and things are not as they should be in those Parts of the *Brain,* where the *Common Sense* resides with the Powers of the *Im-*

agination. Sometimes a *Paucity* of the *Spirits,* and Sometimes a *Disturbance* of them, is that which gives the *Irregular Turn* unto them; wherein the *Swimming Head* of the Patient is unable to look down from an *High Place;* and in his *Walking,* or on his *Rising,* there will be danger of his *Falling* to the Ground, if there be nothing at hand, that he can take hold upon.

The great Physician and Philosopher *Bellini*[1] demonstrates, That a *Vertigo* is not accasioned by a Circular Motion of the Animal Spirits, but by a Removal of the *Retina,* or Nerve, through a Distention of the Arteries in the Eye. For which Reason, *Pitcairn,* advises not Volatile Salts to be used for it, but such things as hinder the Rarefaction of the Blood, after Necessary Evacuation.

It is a little *Epilepsy:* and so often a Forerunner of the *Falling Sickness,* that it should not be neglected.[2]

But in the first place, the mischiefs of a *giddy Soul,* are those from which the Patient should seek to be delivered.

Inconstancy is the *Vertigo* of the Soul. 'Tis a *Giddy Soul* that is Easily drawn from Good *Principles,* or from Good *Purposes;* or from Good *Practices.* A Soul *given to Change;* Or unreasonably *Inconstant* in Points that ought stedfastly to be *Adhær'd* unto; has a Crazy *Dizziness* attending of it. My Friend, make thy Supplication to thy God; *Lord, Leave me not unto the Follies of a Giddy Soul; But lett me Stand fast in all the Good which thou dost bring me to!*

'Tis a Good Wish; "*Lord,* Lett me never *Stagger* in my *Faith* of a Glorious CHRIST, and of the *Mysteries* and the *Promises,* of which His Gospel has assured me."

'Tis a Good Thing for thee to keep a perpetual *Hold* of thy SAVIOUR; For thou hast at the very Best, such a *Staggering Soul,* that if thou lett go thy *Hold* of Him, thou wilt certainly fall into Mischief. Happy Soul, No Safety for any but that Soul that can say; *Lord, I am Continually with thee; Thou hast holden me by my Right Hand.*

Be not ambitious of too *High Stations.* They may make thy *Head Swim.* They may throw thee into Wondrous *Inadvertency.* T'wil be well, if thou canst bear them, and with *Decency* go thro all the *Duties* of them.

If thou art brought into *Prosperity;* by an Affluence of *Wealth* or *Power;* or a Confluence of many Comfortable Circumstances; Be sensible; "There is danger lest I grow *Giddy* in this Condition: Danger, Lest I lay aside the *Humility* which my Whole Conduct should be beautified withal; Danger, Lest in a vain security I become unapprehensive of the Changes that may be near unto me. *Deliver me, O my God."*

§ The *Dizziness* which comes from *Drunkenness;* the Best Cure for it, is, *Repent Soberly and Seriously; and be not like the Dog returning to the Vomit any more.*

§ Medicines good for the *Epilepsy,* are good for the *Vertigo.*

§ *Gentle Vomits* are often very profitable and very necessary. *Bellini* gives weighty Reasons for it.

§ Some have been cured by a Pipe of *Tobacco* in the Morning, on an Empty Stomach.

§ *Dolaeus* will tell you, That the Juice of *Chervil* taken in Broth, is a Specific in this Distemper.

§ Burning the Top of the Head, with *Moxa* or *Touch-wood,* has been found Successful, when the *Vertigo* has been look'd upon as desperate.

§ An Issue there, has been found a Powerful and Wonderful Remedy.

§ Great Cures have been wrought by a *Sinapism,* Laid and Worn between the Two Shoulder-Blades. The *Sinapism* is prepared with powdered Mustard-seed, and Figs, and Olibanum,[3] in Convenient Quantities, beaten up well together.—Some add, Burgundy Pitch.

CAP. XXX. *Dormitantius.*

or,

The Lethargy;

and other Sleepy Diseases.

WE sometimes behold our Friends falling into a Necessity of *Sleeping;* with a perfect Oblivion; arising, as they who think they must say *Something* will think fitt to say, from the Animal Spirits unhappily Sticking in a Viscid and perhaps *Acid,* and glutinous Matter, and so forgetting their Offices.

If the Patient have something of a *Fever,* and open his Eyes at Loud Noises, and attempt impertinent *Answers,* tis called, A *Lethargy.*

If the Patient have no *Fever* at all, but opens his Eyes on a Call, answers to Quæstions Rationally and soon drowses again with a falling Jaw; this is called, A *Coma.*[1]

If the Patient have no *Fever,* and yett never opens his Eyes, nor speaks, nor stirs, but lies as one dead, in almost all Points but Breathing, this is called, A *Carus.*

Upon the Beholding of such Maladies, how can it be, but such *Thoughts* as these must be *Awakened!*

"*Lord,* Is not my Soul, miserably lock'd up, under a most grievous *Lethargy?* What a miserable *Sleep,* and how Distempered an one, has fettered my Soul, when I so *Forgett* all that I have to do! When I ly in such a State of *Inaction,* for all that I have to do in living to God! When I take so Little Notice of all that the Glorious God *Speaks* unto me, or *does* unto me! *O Thou Eternal God, my God, Look, Listen unto me; Enlighten thou mine Eyes, Lest I do fall asleep in Death.*

O my SAVIOUR, whose Quickening Voice will one Day *Raise the Dead;* even those that are fallen into the *Great Sleep;* Do Thou *Awaken* my Soul; make me a *Wakeful Christian;* and always well *Aware* of my Duty and of my Interest. How sad is the [portion] of those, that must have this Account given of them; *At thy Rebuke, O God, they are Cast into a Dead Sleep!*

It was of old said, *Lord, If he sleep, he shall do well.* But if I *sleep* in a senseless unapprehensiveness of my own Circumstances; a Criminal Negligence, and Stupidity, and Security; I shall be far from *doing well.* O my SAVIOUR, Cause me to *Awake unto Righteousness.*

It will not be Long, before the *Long Sleep* of *Death* will come upon me. Oh! Lett me be so *Awake,* as to prepare for that *Grand Sleep.* No greater Proof of a *Soul Awake,* than an Effectual and a Seasonable Preparation for the Time, wherein Man is to *fall Asleep.* O my Soul, *Awake; What meanest thou, O Sleeper? Arise, and Call upon thy God.*"

§ These *Sleepy Diseases* are fatal to old People. But it is possible, by Vomits, and Purges, and Sweats, with Blisters, and Irritating Clysters, they may find some Releef. Try them all.

§ Volatile Spirits must be held unto the Nose; and the Nostrils and the Temples be rubb'd with them.

⫯ But then there is an Excessive *Want of sleep,* or, a Waking *Coma,* wherewith some complain, I *am very much Afflicted.*

It Exceedingly dries the Body, and brings on great *Weakness,* and perhaps *Madness* at the Last.

The Spirits that are sent by the Brain, into the distant Parts, tarry too long there, and becoming too sharp don't return as they ought to do.

I know not whether *Thoughts of Piety,* will be powerful enough, to bring on *Sleep* in this Case, as they will in the Ordinary Course of Life; But I am sure, there are some such that will now be very Seasonable.

Think; "Have not I *Slept,* when I should have *Wak'd?* Not only with a *Moral Sleep* upon the Faculties of my Soul, but also with a *Natural Sleep,* when I should have been Engaged in the *Worship* of God, or in the *Business* of my Calling? A Want of *Sleep* now Chastises the Faults of too Indulged *Sleep. O my God, Pardon me, for the Sake of the Expiation made for my Offences, by a SAVIOUR, who in suffering for me, said,* Thou holdest mine Eyes waking."

Think; "I am now of the Tribe, that saw, *Rest is Good.* If the Want of *Rest* be so grievous and so Threatening to me, how lively should be my Addresses to a dear SAVIOUR, whose Invitation is, *Come unto me, and I will give you Rest?* O my SAVIOUR, *I come unto Thee; Thy Rest will be Glorious!*"

§ *Anodynes! Anodynes!* Gentle Purges may be also necessary.

§ A Bath of Anodyne-Herbs, (as *Lettice,*[2] *Poppy, Water-Lillies, Camomil-flowers,*) for the *Feet,* yea, and for the *Head* also, may be very useful.

§ A Bath made only of *Rain Water* does good. And so does the Q. of *Hungaries Water,*[3] applied unto the Mould of the Head.

§ The Head Shaved, and a Napkin dipped in a Mixture of *Water* and *Vinegar* and a little *Spirit of Wine,* is of great Efficacy. If the first Application don't answer the Intention, Renew it.

§ Tho' *Opiates* must not be given too freely to *Old Men,* yett ordinarily *Opiates* (and *Opium* itself) moderately given, rarely do hurt, when due *Evacuations* accompany them. Always mind, that you keep the Body open, and *Opiates* may do very well in This, as well as in other Cases.[4]

§ Give the Patient, at going to Bed, a Decoction of the Leaves of Lettice, and of White-poppy-seeds.

§ Take Oil of Roses,[5] mixed with some Rose Water, and apply it unto the Forhead.

Or, a Rose-Cake, Sprinkled with Vinegar.

§ A Mixture of Rose-Water and Saffron may be laid unto the Temples.

§ In young Children, the Nurses commonly venture on a Little *Diascordium.*

Cap. XXXI. *Ephialtes.*
or,
The <u>Night-Mare</u> beaten off.

PEOPLE are sometimes in their Sleep Siezed with an Obstruction of the Animal Spirits, which Enter the Nerves, and carry Motion to several of the Muscles, especially those that Serve the Respiration; which Obstruction is usually accompanied with a Pressure on a *Diaphragm,* from a Vapour, which is the Effect of Some Ill Digestion in the Stomach.

Usually, the Person assaulted with this *Incubus,* has the Exercise of his Reason awakened at the First Assault; He knows where he is, and who is near him; he Groans, he Strives, he Cries for Help; a Jog of a Neighbour delivers him. Could he then with the Mechanism of *Ructation* fetch up the *Wind,* which an Ill Digestion fill'd him withal, he might safely go to sleep again; and, *in utramque aurem domire.*[1]

The Nations of the North, had a Whimsy of One *Mara,*[2] a famous and a mighty *Dæmon,* who is the Death of all them who dy by *Suffocation.* Our *Night-Mare* has its Name from this Northern *Dæmon.* And it has been too Common a Thing, for People under the Invasion of this Malady, to imagine a *Witchcraft* in the Case; And anon perhaps the Folly proceeds unto the Accusation of a poor, mean,[3] ill-beloved old Woman in the Neighbourhood. *Away, Away,* with such Idle Fancies. Tis one who has another Name than that of *Mara,* who inspires 'em! My *Dickinson*[4] observes, that *Inuus* was with the Latins, the same that *Ephialtes* is with the Greeks. And *Artemidorus* will tell you that it is the same with *Pan.* But lett us have no more *Dreams* upon it.[5]

A Fitt of the *Night-mare* is often introduced, with a *Dream* that we are Conversing with the *Dead.* The Malady comes to call us away unto the *Dead.* Yea, some have *Died* of the Malady. A *Sudden,* and an *Easy* Death! How Desireable for a *Man in CHRIST!*—One can scarce forbear saying, *Sic mihi contingat!*[6]—

But then, *O Man afflicted with the Malady,* How much ought thy *Præparation* for thy own *Death,* to be Quickened by thy Malady! *Immediately* Renounce thy Idols; *Immediately* Embrace thy SAVIOUR with all His Proposals; *Immediately* come into the Fixed Resolutions of PIETY; Be not satisfied, until thou find thy Soul truly and strongly Bias'd for God; That so, if the Next Assault of the *Night-mare* carry thee off, thou mayst be carried *Where to be is by far the best of all.*

The *Load* that lies upon thee, in the *Night-mare,* will it not mind thee of the *Sin* which lies upon thee, and renders thee an *Heavy-Laden* Soul, and Causes thee to Cry out, O *Wretched one that I am; Who shall deliver me?* What will become of thee, O Soul, if the *Load* should not be taken off?

Upon thy Ejaculations under the Oppressions of the *Night-mare,* a Friend at hand will presently help thee; *One Touch,* of his Hand will help thee. Whatever *Distresses,* of a Spiritual or a Temporal Importance, thou hast lying upon thee, thou hast a SAVIOUR, who is a *Friend at Hand.* He is *able to succour the Tempted;* will *Come in at the Cry* [βοηθειν] they make unto Him. *One Touch* of His Almighty Hand will releeve thee. Thy Course must be to make that Groan, *Lord, I am oppressed, undertake for me.*

Methinks, I see the Condition of People under a *Night-mare,* in a *Struggling Heave,* which is made by Millions of People among the Nations, to shake off a Religion which lies in carnal *Ceremonies,* in useless *Formalities,* in Rites, with which their *Spirits* are not improved, and Bettered and Edified; and gett into a *Religion,* which will Suit and Serve the *Life of God in the Soul of Man.* At present, this *Conatus*[7] of a Groaning World, is miserably Suppressed, with Various, and Powerful Encumbrances upon it. But it will ere long produce tremendous Convulsions. And the Best Thing that you can do, O You that wish well to Mankind, will be, to study what Assistences you may give unto it. A Few Men, well instructed and spirited this Way, may *Do Wonders;*—if God be with 'em!

§ *Anxieties of Mind,* must be mightily avoided, by them that would avoid the *Night-mare.* An Advice much Easier given, than taken!

§ The *Stomach* may sometimes require to be Emptied of its Viscidities, by a gentle Vomit. Be sure, such Things as will not be well-digested in the *Stomach,* will be a Fuel for the *Night-mare.*

§ Correct and Prevent *Flatulencies,* and you do the best Thing that can be done to defeat your Enemy. A plentiful Pumping up of the Wind in the Way of Ructation, by them that have the Knack of it, made at their going to Bed, when flatulent Symptoms warn them of a *Night-mare* approaching, [torn].

§ *Pæony,* used Every Way in the World, is a Grand Specific, in the Case now before us. The *Syrup* taken in a glass of Wine, is the most pleasant way of using it.

§ When you fear the Approach of the *Night mare,* a few Drops of Spirit of Lavender,[8] or Spirit of *Harts-horn,* or Spirit of *Sal Armoniac,* may defend you from it.

§ A Decoction of *Guajacum* has been admired.

§ *Dolaeus,* is of the Opinion, and, I suppose, had made the Experiment, That *Cinamon* Water, adding a Little *Amber,* will *Do the Business,* in this Disease.

At least, it may do as well, as a *Swallows Head,* worn about the Neck, which has been communicated, as a mighty Secret.

CAP. XXXII. The *Oculist.*

considering,
Diseases of the *Eye,*
Especially, <u>Blindness</u>.

THE EYE! An Astonishing *Organ!* Can any thing in the World be shown so *Curious?* Our Excellent *Ray*[1] very truly sais, *Not the Least Curiosity can be added unto it!* What a Just Remark do all Examiners of this *Organ,* as well as our *Derham,*[2] unavoidably and Immediately make upon it, *None less than an Infinite God could contrive and order and provide such a thing! Sturmius*[3] could not imagine it possible for any Man who survey'd the *Eye,* to abandon himself unto *Speculative Atheism.* Tis a most æqual Sentence passed by Dr *Cheine;*[4] *He certainly deserves not to Enjoy the Blessings of his Ey-sight, whose Mind is so depraved, as not to acknowledge the Bounty and Wisdome of the Author of his Nature, in the ravishing Structure of this noble Organ.* Tis impossible for me to go any further without Entreating my Reader to join with me, that we may together *Lift up our Eyes* unto our God, with our Acknowledgments. *O Thou glorious Maker of the EYE: With what Astonishments is thy Power and Wisdome and Goodness to be adored! Certainly the GOD that made the Eye must Himself see me, and all the Works of His Hands. Oh! May I always behave myself as having His Eye upon me!*

The Diseases whereto this Tender *Organ* is obnoxious, are, how many! And some of them, how very *Grievous!*

You that have your *Eyes* continued unto you, *Easy,* and *Lively,* be humbly Thankful to the Glorious God, and Thankfully admire His *Mercy* and His *Patience.* And while you deprecate and escape a Diseased Eye, be sure as much to deprecate and avoid the *Moral*

Diseases of the *Eye*. Reckon an *Envious Eye,* to be one that has the *Chrystallin Humour* in it, poisoned. Reckon an *Haughty Eye,* to be a Distorted one. Reckon an *Unchast Eye* to be an Inflamed one. An *Eye* that *Covets* what it sees, reckon that it has *Dirt* thrown into it. An *Aim* at low and base *Ends* in what we do is a *Squinting Eye.* Be studious of a *Pittiful Eye,* that shall *affect your Heart* when Miserable Objects are before you; A *Bountiful Eye,* that shall be on the *Look-out* for Objects which you may do good unto. Employ your *Eye* on the *Book* which will feed it well. Have your *Eye* in the Season of it, on a CHRIST at His *Table, Evidently sett forth as crucified before it* there. Above all, make it your Study to reach unto that Attainment; *My Eyes are Ever towards the Lord.*

But if you find any Distempers beginning to fall into your *Eyes,* now *Look Backward,* and with a *Sorrowful Reflection,* mourn for the *Moral Diseases* of the *Eye,* which you may find yourself to have been guilty of.

Yea, The *Sins* of the *Eye* have been so many, that if our *Eye* were a *Fountain of Tears,* and if *Rivers of Water* should *run down our Eyes,* all were too little to bewayl them. Here the *First Sin* came in, *She SAW;*—And Then!—Alas, the Rest.

How Many, and how Heinous are the Faults, which the *Lust of the Eye* does involve us in! Man, Lett thy *Distempered Eyes* lead thee to the Bewayling of them.

Lord, How much have my Eyes been the Portholes of Wickedness! How often has Death gott into my Soul by these Windows!

Man is furnished with *Tears* above any *Animal.* And many Distempers of the *Eyes,* are attended with, and productive of, an Immoderate Flowing of them. The Occasion which our Sins have given for our *Weeping Bitterly,* are now to come into Contemplation and Operation with us. It was an Ancient Problem, *Cur Deus oculos Fletus esse Instrumentum voluit?* And the Answer to it, was; *Ut quo Sordes Peccatorum hauriuntur, Eodem per Lacrymas deluantur.* Why must our *Eyes* be a Spring for our *Tears?* The *Sins* which defile us enter there. The *Tears* of *Repentance,* which are of use in washing away the *Defilements,* are properly to be expected there.

I remember, *Tympius*[5] has an odd Quæstion; *Why the Eyes are the Last Things that are Quickened with us, and the First Things that are decayed?* It is answered, *Ut quo majus est ipsorum periculum, Eo minus sit nocendi Spacium.* It seems, our *Danger* of Hurt from our *Eyes,* being so great, the *Time* for them to do it, must be the Less. My Friend, It will be well, if *Distempers* falling into thy *Eyes,* may præserve thee, from the Hurt, which those *Inletts of Sin* often bring in to the sinful Children of Men. There was a famous Dispute before King *Alphonsus,*[6] on that Problem, *What was the Best Thing to Sharpen the Sight.* An Humoursome Gentleman maintained it, for *Envy.* To Employ, or to Suffer, such a *Sharp Sight,* Reader, Thou wilt not be ambitious of it.

SPECTACLES!*[7]*—Mankind is prodigiously Inexcusable in that the Name of the *First Inventor* is entirely Lost: That Statues of *Corinthian Brass*[8] have not Immortalized it.—But indeed, it is fitt that none but the Glorious God, should be considered in the Grant of so vast a Benefit. *Lord!* What would have generally become of us *after Fifty* (and many of us *Before!*) if such *Glasses* of a *Modern Invention* had not Supplied our Necessities? Christian, very often, when thou art going to putt on thy *Spectacles* (or use thy *Hand-glasses*) Lift up thine *Eyes* unto the Glorious God, and lett thy *Heart* form some Acknowledgement of this Importance; *Great God, For this Blessing to the World, I give Thanks unto thee!* Or, *O SAVIOUR of Men, How graciously hast thou favoured us.*

§ Præservatives of the *Eyesight.*

§ Have you never seen a very Common Plant, call'd, *Eyebright?*[9] It forever sais to the *Eye* that looks upon it; *Make use of me, and I will do thee Good and not Hurt, all the Days of thy Life.*

A plain *Eye-bright* Water constantly or frequently used, will continue to the *Eye-sight* a *Brightness* to be wondered at!

Inwardly, an *Eye-bright* Tea, has Efficacy.

Manlius was by a Dream directed unto the Use of *Eybright* for a Defluxion on his Eyes, and found a Cure by it.

§ *Ask now the Fouls*[10] *of the Air, and they shall tell thee.* The *Swallows* will carry thee to the *Celandine.*[11] Feeble *Eyes,* will not find a greater Friend, in the whole *Vegetable Kingdom.* Drop the Juice of it into the *Eyes.* It may be diluted with *Fair-Water.*[12]

§ A Lye, made of the, *Vine-branches,* has been by some counted the most noble and potent *Eye-Water* in the World.

§ Take a Little *Coperas*[13] and *Bole-Armenick*[14] finely powdered, and putt it into a Convenient Quantity of Water. (If the Mixture be too sharp for the Eyes, increase the Quantity of the Water.) Tis a notable *Eye-Water.* It preserves and strengthens the Sight, unto Admiration.

§ Take *Eye-bright,* three Drams; *Mace,*[15] one Dram; and make a Fine Powder.

§ *Montagnana*[16] sais, "I have seen decrepit old Men, almost blind, which have been restored unto their *Entire Sight,* by the Help of this Powder."

Take half a Spoonful before Meals, in a glass of Sack.

§ *Raw Oysters* Eaten Three or Four Every Morning for some time, have a Strange Vertue, to Restore an Impaired *Eysight.* Some struck *Stone*-blind, with the Lightening have been Strangely Recovered by this Remedy.

§ This Powder has done great Cures, in *Dimness of Sight,* and *Rheums*[17] in the Eyes.

Take Powder of *Eye-bright,* one Ounce: *Fennel-seed*[18] in Powder, half an Ounce: double-refined *Sugar,* two Ounces. These Powders, well sifted, are to be Mixed: (and kept in a Dry Place) are to be taken, as much as may ly on a Shilling, as often as you please.

§ Sir *William Temple*[19] sais, *Betony* often putt up the Nostrils, has præserved the *Eyes,* to a great Age.

§ A Syrup of *Betony-Water,* and *Honey;* A Spoonful taken two or three times a day, is a mighty Strengthener of *the Ey-sight.*

§ Some very Decay'd and Aged *Eyes,* have been Strangely recovered, with *Fennel-Water.* The Internal Use of the *Fennel* at the same time, has added unto the Efficacy of the *Collyrium.*[20]

§ Even *Cataracts* in the Eye have been cured, by the Internal Use of *Millipedes.*

§ Here's a famous *Eye-water.* My Lady *Fitz-hardings.*[21] Take three Spoonfuls of white *Rose Water;* as much *Eye-bright* Water; and as much sifted white *Sugar-Candy,* as may ly upon a Threepence; and the same Quantity of fine *Aloes* sifted, and putt to the Water, and shake them together. A Few drops of This, at going to Bed.

§ Sometimes, a Distemper of *Sore Eyes,* even with painful and grievous Inflammations, comes upon People; yea, becomes a Little Epidemical; or at least so, that very many together are troubled with it. In this Case, there are several *Poultis's,* which being applied unto the *Eyes,* have had Notable Successes. A Poultis of *White-bread* and *Milk* is one of them. A Poultis of *White-Beans* and *Milk,* is another of them. A Poultis, of a *Rotten Apple* is another. *Blisters* drawn in the Nape of the Neck, have been of Good Consequence.

But the Best Thing that I know, is a Lotion, of *Saccharum Saturni,*[22] three or four Grains, dissolved in an Ounce or two of *Rose-Water.* Add, Powder of *Tutty,*[23] the same Quantity. If the Inflammation be very Violent, add three or four Grains of *Camphire.*

The Sad Case of
Total Blindness.

Very Grievous is the Hand of an *Holy* and *Righteous* God,
[*O Sufferer, Still Confess Him so!*] upon those among the Children
of Men, who are making these Lamentations, *The Light of my Eyes
is gone from me.* And, *He hath brought me into Darkness and not
into Light.* And, *Lord, Thou hast Laid me in Darkness.*

But, *My Friend in the Dark,* Thou mayst *See Cause* to be Thankful for the Senses that are yett left unto thee. Tis a Remarkable Instance and Effect of the Divine Compassion unto Mankind. Tho many
have been born *Blind,* and many have been born *Deaf,* yett it was
never known that any one was born *Both* of these. They must soon
have perished, if they *had.* Tho' thou canst not *See,* still thou canst
Hear, And be Thankful for *That!*

One Cannot well without Astonishment Consider; the Strange
Performances of Some that have been *Totally Blind;* Especially, when
they have been so from their *Nativity,* or their Early *Infancy!* How
Strangely what has been *Defective* in One Sense, has been Supplied in
another! The Glorious God in such Things takes Pleasure to convince
us, *That HE is the Doer of all the Good that is done by the Children
of Men, and can do by whom He Pleases! Blind Men* have been
famous *Preachers,* yea, famous *Writers,* in the Church of God. But
tho' many have *done wondrously* this way, Thou Master *William
Jameson,*[24] Professor of History in the Renowned University of *Glasgow,* hast Excelled them all! This wonderful Man, tho' *Born Blind,*
what Books has he written, in the *Latin* as well as the *English*
Tongue: *Books* which none but one of a vast Reading ever could have
written: *Books* which discover him an uncommon Critic, in the
Oriental, as well as the *Latin* and *Græcian* Languages; and a most
intimate Acquaintance with Antiquities; *Books* wherein many Mistakes of our greatest and most *Gigantic* Literators, are with a most
nice Erudition refuted and corrected!—Every Page of this my dear
Friends late, *Spicilegia Antiquitatum,* gives me an Amazement in
the Perusal of it. *Since the World began, it has not been heard that
any man that was born blind has performed such things as these!*

Tis probable the Person that has these things Readd unto him,
does not propose any such *Attainments* and *Atchievements.* However,
I will show unto him a More Excellent Way!

My Friend; Thou mayst Come to *See Him who is invisible,*
in thy Realizing Apprehensions of a Glorious God.

Thou mayst come to have a deep *Insight* into the *Mystery of CHRIST,* and those Things which the *Angels desire to look into.*

Thou mayst come to have a True *Sight* of thy *Own Heart,* and notably discover the *Mystery of Iniquity* working there.

Thou mayst come to see, the *Evidence of Things not seen,* in thy *Faith* of what is in the *Invisible World,* and of the *Things which are not seen and are Eternal.*

Thine *Eyes* may be so *opened,* as to see *Wondrous Things* in the Law of thy God.

If thou dost arrive to such a *Sight* as this, thou mayst Esteem it an Abundant *Compensation* for thy Want of that *Bodily Sight,* which might have been abused, if thou hadst Enjoyed it, so as to carry thee away from the *Best of Objects.*

My Blind Friend, what are the Best Objects which thou hast lost the Sight of? The Old *Persian* Physician who commonly is quoted as an *Arabian,* under the Name of *Razis,*[25] (tho' his true Name was *Mehemmed,* Son of *Zekeriah*) when he was grown *Blind* with Old Age, would not accept the Operation of a *Quack,* who pretended and offered a Cure for him; And when his Friends urged it, he still refused it, and gave this Reason for his Refusal; *I have Seen the World so long, that I desire to see no more of it!* O *Christian,* Lett not a *Mahometan* go beyond thee, in *Mortification. Cicero* reports it, even of his Brother-pagan, *Democritus:* That he comforted himself, under the Loss of his *Eysight,* With this; That if he was not able to distinguish *Black* from *White,* yett he could readily Distinguish *Good* from *Evil, Right* from *Wrong.* O *Christian,* Thou hast yett *Greater Consolations.*

And thou mayst comfortably wait for that *Resurrection from the Dead,* wherein thou shalt *see for thyself,* and *thine Eyes behold,* thy *Living* REDEEMER.

Cap. XXXIII. *Colaphizatus.*[1]
or Diseases of the Ear:
Especially <u>Deafness</u>.

THE EAR! A Constellation of *Miracles!* Consider, O Man; The Scituation of the *Ear;* The *Substance* as well as the *Figure* of the *Outward Ear;* The Artful *Tunnel* that Leads to the *Inward;* The

Four Little Bones, and the *Three Little Muscles* about them, in the amazing *Labyrinth;* and the Hitherto-undiscovered Nature of *Sound:* And lett the God, who *Planted the Ear,* have thy *Praises.* But conclude, *This GOD must Himself hear all thy Praises, and all that passes;* and Lett thy *Speech* be that of one who Remembers, *Each Word that I shall speak; While it is not yett in my Tongue Behold, O Thou Eternal God, Thou knowest all of it!*

There is an Instance of the Divine Compassion, which under *Diseases of the Ear,* we may take a particular Notice of. Many have been born destitute of *Seeing;* many born destitute of *Hearing.* It was never known that any Child of Man was born destitute of *Both Senses:* the Condition of such an one would have been too forlorn; the wretched Creature would have been too uncapable of being provided for. *Friend,* if thou dost not Enjoy thine *Ears,* be thankful, that the Enjoyment of thine *Eyes* is allow'd unto thee.

Whether thy *Ear* be *pain'd,* or be *Deaf, Hear* thou the *Voice* of the Glorious God therein *Speaking* unto thee, and Calling thee to *Repentance,* for thy having thy *Ear* too open unto things that should not have been received there; *Blasphemies,* or *Calumnies,* or *Obscænities:* And thy turning a *Deaf Ear* to the *Doctrines* and *Lessons* of Goodness. And having obtained a Pardon for the *Sins of the Ear,* by pleading for it, the Great Sacrifice the SAVIOUR who could say, *Thou for thy Service borest the Ears thou'st given unto me:* Now Resolve, to shutt thine *Ear* against Every *Evil Thing,* and upon all thy *Tempters;* but with an *Attentive Ear* to *Listen* unto such Things as GOD requires thy good Attention to.

The *Ear-Wax* is a Marvellous Provision: But Some Disorder in *That* sometimes renders the *Ear* to be otherwise than it should be. I will make One Remark upon it. I suppose the Gentlemen Physicians, are well-enough pleased, That they be not obliged, by Customs now, as they were in the Days of *Hippocrates,* to taste ever now and then the *Ear-Wax* of their Patients. But *Pliny* affirms, That *Sordes Ex Auribus,* the *Ear-Wax,* would Cure the Bites, not only of *Serpents* and *Scorpions,* but also of *Men,* which [*inter asperrimos numerantur*)[2] are the worst of all. And Modern Experience informs us and Confirms it, that it is a Notable *Balsame.* Truly, In the *Hard Words* that Men Speak of us, we suffer the *Bites* of *Men;* And we have a Remedy in our *Ears* themselves for these *Bites.* If the *Ear-Wax* won't help us, yett we may be *Deaf* unto them: *That* will help us. Here *Deafness* will be no Distemper.

As the *Ear* is a very *Noble* Organ, so it is a very *Tender* one. Certainly, People need not be told, that they should be *very cautious, how they tamper with it.*

For *Pains* in the *Ear.*

℔ For the *Ear-ache,* we commonly apply a Roasted *Turnip* as hot as we can bear it. Or, putt a warm Clove of *Garlick,* dipp'd in Oyl into the *Ear.*

§ The Dirt gathered on the Stairs of a *Bruers Cellar,* Laid warm in a Linen-Cloath, to the *Ear;* Tis an odd Remedy, and one would wonder how it came to be first litt on. But they say, Twil cure a *Pain in the Ear,* to Admiration.

§ A Pain of the *Ear,* with *Deafness,* (proceeding from a Cold Original,) is marvellously releeved, by *Juice of Onions* injected into the Ear.

Or, Take *Juice of Onions,* and a Third Part as much *Spirit of Wine;* mix them, and Either drop into the Ear, or throw in with a Syringe.

§ *Sheeps Urine* does good. Or, A *Boys* new-made *Urine,* with some Spirit of Wine, wherin a Little *Camphire* is dissolved. *Salmon*[3] sais, *It seldom fails.*

§ The *Ear-ache* proceeding from Windy Vapours, distending the Membrane, is helped by a Little Oyl of *Anise,* or, *Fennel,* or *Camomil-flowres,* dropt into the Ear. Or, Make a Decoction of *Camomil-flowres,* with *Milk;* and in a *Bladder,* hold it Warm to the Ear.

§ The *Ear-ache* proceeding from an Inflammation, may require *Blood-Letting.*

§ For an *Ulcer* in the *Ear; Marcellus* tells us, Two Ounces of *Cows Milk,* mixed with an Ounce of *Honey,* being dropt into the *Ear,* and the *Ear* stopped with Wool upon it; This will wonderfully heal the Ulcer, yea, tho' it were a cancerous one.

For Deafness.

℔ The *Syringing* of the *Ear,* with Warm *Water* or *Beer,* or, *Urine,* does Wonders for the Help of Curable *Deafness.*

After the Syringing, Stop the *Ear* with *Wool;* tinged with a Drop or two, of the Oyl of *Rose-mary.*

§ Tho' Oil of *Bitter Almonds* be commended for *Deafness,* and a Noise in the Ears; yett *Simon Paulli*[4] sais, it should be used Sparingly, by reason of the Winding Passage, for when it getts up to the *Tympanum,* and cannot Easily be thence deterged, it will relax that

Membrane, and the Thickness of Hearing will be turned into *Total Deafness.*

§ Make a Decoction of *Camomil-Flowres* (or *Wormwood;*) The Hott Steam of this taken thro' a Tunnel into the Ears; This wonderfully helps *Deafness* in many Cases.

§ One of the *Fabers*[5] tells us, That *Nitre* dissolved in Strong *Vinegar,* and often dropp'd into the Ears, quickly cures the Noises and Ringings in them.

§ To wear a Bitt of *Negroes* Wool in the Ears, has been often found a Strange Cure for *Deafness.*

§ A Green Stick of *Black Ash* Wood (Cutt in *May*) being Laid on the Fire, a Sap will be forced out at the Ends of it. A little of that Sap drop'd warm into a *Deaf Ear,* has releeved the Deafness to Astonishment.

§ Mr. *Martin*[6] in his Ingenious *Description of the Western Islands* of Scotland, mentions divers Instances of Even Aged People, Cured of *Deafness* in a Day or two, by Powder of *Tobacco* poured into the Ear.

§ Flay a Large *Eel;* cutt it into round Pieces of the Length of a Finger; Stick them full with *Rose-mary* and *Sage.*[7] Then take an Earthen Pan, wherein putt three or four Little Sticks of Wood Cross-Wise: Lay the Pieces of *Eel* upon them so that they touch not the Bottom of the Pan: Bake This in an Oven. Then take the Fatt of the *Eel* that is in the Pan; Strain it thro' a fine Linen-Cloath; and add as much *Spirit of Wine*[8] unto it. Then take Juice of *Onions,* and Juice of the White Ends of Leeks, an Ounce of Each; and mix it with two Ounces of the first Mixture. Putt them into a close Vial, and shake them well for an Hour. Drop three or four drops of this into the Ear, and ly for a while in a convenient Posture: continue it for a proper Season so, Stop the Ear with Black Wool.

This is in Sir *Kenelm Digbys*[9] Chymical Receits. And *Hartman*[10] affirms Wonderful Cures to have been wrought by it.

Old Man, Make sure of Good Terms with Heaven; And at the *Resurrection of the Dead,* thou shalt have thine *Ears* again.

Appendix.
Advice to the LAME.

We have been Thoughtful for the *Blind,* and the *Deaf.* But will our Charity allow us to Cast the *Lame* out of our Thoughts? No; Our Compassionate REDEEMER, in the Days of His *Humbled Goodness,* when the *Eyes of the Blind were Opened,* and the *Ears of the Deaf were Unstopped,* that *Good One* took notice of these also, and He made the *Lame Leap as an Hart.* Yea, Even in *this* Point, *His Mercy Endures forever:* And in *Our* Days, the *Lame* looking up to Him, have had *Miraculous Cures* wrought for them;—*Their Feet, and their Anclebones have received Strength.* O poor *Creeple,* as *Lame* as thou art, yett make thy *Flights* unto thy SAVIOUR: And if He will not release thee from thy *Bodily Lameness,* but oblige thee to *Wait* for the Amendment of thy Condition *all the Days of the Appointed Time,* until the Happy *Change* of *Body,* which thou shalt see at the *Resurrection of the Dead,* When *Agility* shall be one Desireable Quality of thy *Raised Body,* and thou shalt be able to *mount up as with the Wings of Eagles* [Oh! Lett thy *Lameness* among the other *Sufferings of the present time,* Cause thee to Look and Long for that *Glory!*) yett thou shalt find thy Account in doing so.

I can præscribe nothing for thy Cure: *No Remedy but Patience.* And by *This,* how much wilt thou *Glorify God!*

But under so *Humbling* an *Inconvenience,* wilt thou not mightily Labour to *Walk Humbly with thy God!* Reconciled unto *Abasing* Circumstances; *Loathing* and *Judging* of thyself, as One *Marked* by Him with a *Token* which He would have with thee with an *Abased Soul* to look upon: And Labour to *Walk Softly* among thy Neighbours; *Humbly* maintaining Low and Mean Thoughts of thyself: Sensible of thy Imperfections; Not falling into fretful Murmurs, if the *Proud ones of the Earth* Cast Contempt upon thee?

Take the *Wormwood* and the *Gall,* of thy *Confinement,* and lett thy *Soul be Humbled in thee.*

How Reputable, How Honourable, a Compensation of thy *Lameness,* wilt thou have in it, if it quicken thy Cares to *Walk Uprightly? No Good Thing* shall be *Witheld* from thee, O Thou *Upright Walker* before the Lord! Be sollicitous to take *Right Steps* forever. A Course of Exact PIETY will render thee, *Stately in thy Goings.*

If I be not misinformed, the *Greatest Conqueror* that ever was in the World, was *Lame* in one of his Feet. Thy *Lameness* need not hinder thy being a *Great Man,* if there be a Wise and Strong Application of thy Studies. I am sure, it should quicken thy being a *Good Man;* Then thou art a *Conqueror, and more than a Conqueror.*

Lett thy Continual *Prayers* therefore be these; *My Goings, O do thou uphold* / / *in thy well-tending Pathes:* / / *When thou hast done this thing for me* / / *my Footsteps have not slipt.* / / And, *The*

Steps I take, O give to them / / Direction in thy Word: / / And grant to no Iniquity / / Dominion over me. / /

But lett thy *Faith* be therefore Continually Exercised, in a *Dependence* on thy SAVIOUR, to *Lead* thee along, thro' all the *Motions* and *Removes* of thy *Pilgrimage.*

When any Friend goes to take thee by the *Hand,* Lift up thy *Heart* unto thy GOD, and think; *Still Closely following after thee / / my Soul does cleave to thee: / / Thy Right Hand doth Sustain me, so / / that I am kept from Falls. / /*

When thou art going to take a *Staff* or a *Crutch* into thy *Hand,* with an *Heart* then leaning on the *Promises* of thy God, say, *Thy Testimonies I have took / / for my Inheritance; / / Forever so; Because they are / / the Gladness of my Heart. / /*

Be thou never so *Lame,* yett be *Quick,* be Speedy, be Nimble, in thy Obedience to the Call of God, and Compliance with the Voice of thy SAVIOUR. Be so disposed. *I with a quickened Pace will run / / the Way of thy Commands, / / when thou upon my Straitned Heart. / / Enlargement hast bestow'd. / /*

I have read of One, Struck with *Lameness,* who yett *ran* away with a *Blessing.* O Child of *Jacob,* O *Israelite* indeed: Arriving to this PIETY, Thou hast with thy *Lameness* gott a *Blessing,* which may bring thee, even to *Leaping* in thy *Praising* of God.

CAP. XXXIV. *Stiptica.*[1]
For <u>Bleeding</u>,
[at the Nose.]

THE *Blood* of People, becoming too *Sharp* or too *Thin,* they are sometimes taken with a *Bleeding* at the *Nose;* And the *Hæmorrhage* becoming Excessive, they are Extremely Enfeebled; And their *Depauperated Blood,* becomes a Seat of Diseases by which their Lives are sadly Embittered and Abbreviated.

O *Bleeding* Patient; If thou hast by any *Incautelous*[2] or *Intemperate* Conduct, brought this Mischief upon thee, Confess it, Bewayl it, obtain thro' the *Blood* of thy SAVIOUR *Sprinkled* on thy Soul, the *Pardon* of it.

Yea, Acknowledge, That for all thy Sins, if thine *Eyes* were a *Fountain of Tears,* and these were all *Tears of Blood,* it would not bee too much for the Sad Occasion.

Thou art Sollicitous to gett thy *Blood in Good Order,* that it may not thus leak away. But shall not thy Sollicitude be as great for a *Soul in Good Order* too?

With an *Humble* and a *Contrite* Heart, Think; *Lord, Must my Blood be shed for my Sin? Must my Life swim away in my Blood? Must the Blood of the Criminal be called for? Tis no more than what I am worthy of. My Sin has had a share in shedding the Blood of my Blessed SAVIOUR.*

It was a Savoury Speech of one *Bleeding* to Death; *One Blood kills me; But I can tell of another Blood that Saves me.* Lett the Sight of thy own polluted *Blood* carry thee away to the precious *Blood* of thy SAVIOUR. If thou Behold thy own *Blood* with *Horror,* yett behold that *Blood* with *Comfort.* Behold it as a *Fountain sett open for Sin and Uncleanness;* behold it as *Purchasing* for thee all the *Blessings of Goodness.*

§ *Bleeding* [at the Nose] is often to be stopt with *Bleeding* [in the Arm.]

§ Heres a Noble *Hæmoptoic Draught.*

Take *Plantain-Water,*[3] four Ounces; *Wine Vinegar,* and Syrup of *Comfrey,* Each half an Ounce; The White of one Egg beat up. Mix. It mightily Quiets and Thickens the Blood; and Constringes and Consolidates the Apertures of the Vessels. This is for all *Bleeding.*

§ Every body knows the use of the *Blood-Stone.*[4]

§ A Cloth dipt in *Cold Water,* [Better, in *Vinegar*] and applied unto the Bottom of the Belly, [especially the *Ventra,*] Stops *Bleeding at the Nose.*

§ Take *Vinegar,* half a Pint; *Sugar of Lead,* one Ounce. Dissolve. Dip a folded Linnen Cloth in this Liquor, and apply it absolutely Cold unto the Region of the Heart; and as often as it Waxes Warm, repeat it Cold again. *Fuller* mentions it, as a *Miraculous Experiment against Bleeding at the Nose.*

§ A *Toad* well-dried, held in the hand, or worn about the neck; a common Remedy for Bleeding.

§ Blow powdered *Bole-Armenic* up into the Nose.

§ *Borellus* mentions an Eminent Person cured by Clothes dipt in a Mixture of Water and Vinegar applied with Repetition, to the *Backbone:* When all other means failed.

§ On the failing of all Remedies, this has done Wonders. Lett the *Blood* of the Patient fall on an Hott Brick, or Tile, or Iron Plate.

Then pulverize it; and lett it be taken inwardly in Conserve of Roses.

§ If the Blood be fired with a *Fever,* there will be no total Cure of *Bleeding;* without Extinguishing of the *Fever.*

§ Of all *Stypticks,* will any pretend to be Equal with the *Stypti-cum Regis?* The Process is this, "Unto *Vitriol*[5] dissolved, filtrated, præcipitated with Vinegar, edulcorated[6] and dried, affuse Oyl of *Vitriol,*[7] and distil by a Retort to drieness. The *Caput Mortuum*[8] digest with Spirit of Wine, filter, warm, and abstract; Dissolve the Salt remaining in the Bottom, with four times its Weight of Water, by Digestion." The short of it is, Extract a Salt out of the *Caput Mortuum* of *Vitriol,* with Spirit of Wine. Then Dissolve the Salt in Four Times the Quantity of Water.

One of our Kings gave a Vast Sum of Money for this great *Styp-tick.*[9] It not only stops all *Hæmorrhages,* but is one of the best Vul-neraries[10] in the World. It may be used Inwardly as well as Out-wardly. The Dose, from Ten to Twenty Drops. For Spitting and Pissing of Blood, and Bloody Fluxes, (universals being præmised) *Salmon* sais, *Tis worth a whole Apothecaries Shop.*

§ *Vitriol* Calcined[11] in the Sun beams (the Sympathetic Powder) this dissolved in Water, powerfully stops Bleeding at the Nose.

CAP. XXXV. *Suffocatus.*

or,

A *Sore Throat;*
and, Quinzey.[1]

WHAT we call, a *Sore Throat,* is a frequent Malady. Sometimes, after much misery undergone, it comes to a *Suppuration.* Sometimes grievous *Ulcers* are produced there which continue a long while to terrify those that suffer them. And sometimes, the Inflammation rises to a *Quinzey,* which threatens the Patient with a Speedy and a fearful Suffocation.

Certainly, They that are thus afflicted, have Cause to reflect on the Sins, which find a Passage thro' the *Throat.*

The *Meats* and the *Drinks,* which have with an Intemperate Ingurgitation gone down the Throat, ought humbly to be Repented of.

The *Words* trespassing on the Holy Rules of Speech, coming up thro' the *Throat*, as with the Stench of an *Open Sepulchre*, make yett more work for a Serious Repentance.

Patient, Examine thy Self, and obtain a *Pardon*, by pleading the Sacrifice of thy SAVIOUR; who Suffered for us what obliged Him to cry out, *My Throat is dried*.

Resolve, that being Restored, Thou wilt *putt a Knife to thy Throat*, when thou shalt find thyself *given to Appetite*. And that the *High-praises of God* shall be heard warbling in *thy Throat;* and no Sinful Thing be allowed a Channel there.

§ For an Ordinary *Sore-Throat;*

Columbine²-Leaves, boil'd with Milk and Water, Sweetened with Honey;—Gargled and Swallow'd; This has been found a Notable Remedy.

§ Common *Mallows* the like.

§ For the falling of the *Uvula*, or, what they call, The *Almonds of the Ears come down*, what is better than Juice, or Syrup of *Mulberries?* Or, Touch them with *Terra Sigillata*.³

§ Take a Piece of greasy Linen-Cloathe, of such a Bigness that being doubled, it may make a Bag in form of a Stay to reach from one side of the Throat unto the other, and Contain as much matter as may make it of the thickness of an Inch, or more. This Bag being filled with Common Salt, is to be heated thoroughly and applied unto the Part affected, as warm as the Patient can conveniently [bear]; When it begins to grow cold, another like it, well-heated is to be Substituted: And while it is cooling, the former may be getting ready again.

For a *Sore Throat*, Among the *Boylaean* Receits, this is called, *A Choice Medicine*.

§ A Gargarism of *Urine* made by a Boy: (Some fancy, a Mixture from diverse Lads:) has done Wonders, upon the failing of all other Medicines.

§ A Draught of warm *Urine*, with Little *Honey* on it, has been found an Admirable Thing.

§ Here's a powerful Topical.

Take two new-laid *Eggs,* roasted moderately hard; and the Pap of two well-roasted *Pippins*. Beat 'em well together; and add as much Curds of Posset⁴ made with Ale. Having well incorporated them, apply the mixture very warm, to the Part affected; Shifting it, if need be, Once in five or six Hours.

§ An Old Woman in my Neighbourhood, in this Manner, makes all Ordinary *Sore-Throats* fly before her; Boil *Pepper* in *Milk;* and then thro' a Tunnel that shall cover the Milk, take the Steam of it into your Mouth and Throat, as Hott, and as Long as you can bear it. When you have done this, then drink the Hott Milk itself.

§ Take the White of a *New Laid Egg,* and by beating it, reduce it into Water. With this Water mix as much *Conserve of Red Roses* as will reduce it unto a Soft Mass. Lett a Little Bitt of this at a time, dissolve liesurely in the Mouth.

§ Take *Houseleek,*[5] and having lightly beaten it in a Glass or Stone Mortar, press out the Juice hard between Two Plates; To this Juice, putt almost an æqual Quantity of *Virgin Honey;* Mix them well, and add unto the Mixture a Little Burnt Allum. Take a little of this from time to time, with a Liquorice Stick, or some such Thing.—

§ Take *Sow-bugs,* alive; Sew them up in the Foldings of a Peece of Linen; Apply them to the Throat in Form of a Stay; which is to be kept on all night.

§ The Foot of a *Worsted Stocking* Long Worn, with a sufficient Quantity of *Salt,* putt hott into it; Lett this be tied about the Patients Neck all night.

§ For a *Quinzey,* I remember *Batholinus* apprehends the Distemper which threatened the Life of the Celebrated King *Hezekiah,*[6] to have been a Malignant *Quinzey.* If it were so, we know of an ancient *Cataplasm* directed for it. Concerning *Figs,* a *Dioscorides*[7] will tell you, *Durities discutiunt parotidas et furunculos emolliunt.*[8]

§ Dr. T. *Fuller* mentions a *Quinzey-Plaister.*

Take *Diachylon* simple, Three Drams; Chymical *Oil of Wormwood,*[9] Eighteen Drops—Mix. Lay it unto the Throat from Ear to Ear. But my Doctor adds, *Trust to no Inward nor Outward Remedies, without good Bleeding.*

.   .   .

§ Children Subject to a *Quinzy,* and Siezed with it so as to Ly in the very agonies of Death have had Immediate and Astonishing Releef by nothing but this. Take a Little Clove of *Garlick,* and Slice it, and in a Little Hott *Honey* give it unto them.

§ When Children have been taken, with a *Sore Throat,* and *Quinsey,* and what they call, the *Bladder in the Throat,*[10] the Flight is usually and successfully made unto a *Blister,* and a *Purge.*

But Strange Cures have been wrought, by a Mixture of *Urine, Molosses,* and *Oyl,* and a Little *Nutmeg.*

Cap. XXXVI. *Adjutoria Catarrhi.*[1]

A <u>Catarrh</u>: And what we Call,
A *Cold:* How to Stop it!

WITHOUT falling into the *Deliramenta Catarrhi,*[2] and the old Fancy, of the Brain being in the Nature of an *Alembic,*[3] the Source and Seat of Every *Catarrh,* We will rather look on a *Catarrh,* as a Copious Defluxion of the Lympha from any of the Glands, into some Cavity near to which the Glands are scituated. The Glands undergo a Relaxation, their Pores are widened, usually by some External Assault from the Air.[4] The *Lympha* and *Serum* of the Blood, is considerably augmented by an Obstruction given to the Pores of the Body, and so it forces its Way thro' the Glands: with a Various Disturbance, whereof lett *Franc du Porta*[5] give Some Account;

—*Quum pituita movet malesana Catarrhum, Frigus inest Capiti; Facies fit Pallida; Murmur Vox cret; et sapor est; Urinaque Crudior exit; Mens stupet, et sensus; Motus torpore tenetur.*[6]

But one Special Instance of a *Catarrh,* and that which is most Commonly Complained of, is, what we Call, *A Cold.* The *French* hath an agreeable Term for it, whereof the *Latin* seems destitute; That is, *Enrumer.*[7]

Under a *Cold* (and Every *Catarrh,*) certainly it may not be unseasonable or unreasonable, to think; "Lord, Have I not, by breathing in the Air of this World, admitted such *Frames* and such *Thoughts,* as have brought me into *Disorders?*"

Again. Think at this Rate; "I complain of a *Cold;* the *Cold* has hurt me. But how much Cause have I to mourn under my Share in that Unhappiness; *The Love of many waxes Cold!*"

Of our Excellent *Mitchel,*[8] it is recorded, in his *Life:* that being a little kept from the Labours of his Ministry, by an *Hoarse Cold* arresting of him; he wrote this Improvement of it. *My Sin is Legible in the Chastisement. Cold Duties, Cold Prayers, (My Voice in Prayer, that is, My Spirit of Prayer, fearfully gone;) my Coldness in my whole Conversation chastised with a Cold. I fear, that I have not improved my Voice for God as I should have done, and therefore He now takes it from me.*

§ Dr. *Keil*[9] has cleared it, That *Catching of Cold,* is nothing but sucking in, by the Passages of *Perspiration,* Large Quantities of

Moist Air, and Nitrous Salts, which by Thickening the Blood and Juices, and thereby Obstructing both the *Perspiration* and all the other finer Secretions, raises immediately a Small Tumult and Fever in the whole Animal Œconomy; and Neglected, Lays a Foundation for *Consumptions,* and *Obstructions,* and Universal *Cachexies.* Whereupon Dr. *Cheyne* remarks, The Tender and Sickly ought Cautiously to avoid all Occasions of *Catching a Cold;* and if they have caught one, to sett about the *Cure* of it Immediately. The Remedy, he says, is obvious: To Ly much abed; plentifully Drinking a Small Warm *Sack Whey;* with a few Drops of Spirit of *Harts-horn;* *Posset-drink; Water-gruel;* or any other such Small and Warm Liquors; a Scruple of *Gascoin Powder*[10] Morning and Evening; *Living Low,* and in Every thing treating it, at first, as a Small Fever. And afterward, if any *Coughing* or *Spitting* remain, Soften the Breast with a little *Sugar-Candy* and *Oil of Sweet Almonds.* Go cautiously into the Air afterwards.

§ There is a World of Medicines for a *Cold.* Every Good Woman is Mistress of them.

Among the rest, a Draught of *Cold Water* in the Morning, has been found a notable Remedy. Rather take it at going to Bed. It will make you sweat; it will digest your Cold; it will hasten a Good Order of all things upon you.

§ *Soothing Things,* are much Commended, especially, your *Mulls* of all Sorts.

Here's one, that many People won't need much Perswasion to. A Pint of good *Ale;* a Glass of Sweet *Wine;* an Ounce of Loaf sugar; Two yolks of Eggs; and a good Quantity of grated Nutmeg; mull'd and warm'd.

§ Moderate *Opiates,* prudently administred, (if they don't shutt up a *Wolf* in a *Sheeps* Pen,)[11] have been highly commended in *Catarrhs.*

D'Ube commends a Decoction of the Leaves of *Lettuce;* and the Flowres of Red *Poppy;* at going at sleep.

If this prove insufficient, then, Two or Three Grains of *Laudanum,* in Conserve of Roses.

A Safer Medicine than these, may be *Venice Treacle,* mixed with powdered *Olibanum.*

§ There is a Remedy for a *Cold,* Especially when it affects the *Breast,* that is a Very Vulgar One.

Take half a sheet of Brown *Paper;* anoint it very well, with

Candle-grease, the Oldest you can gett. Grate a Little *Nutmeg* on it; and Lay it Warm to the Stomach.

§ Among the Scotch Islanders, M. *Martin* says; For Coughs and Colds, *Water-gruel* with a Little Butter, is the Ordinary Cure.

CAP. XXXVII. The *Breast-beater.*

or,

A <u>Cough</u> quieted.

THE Pores (as we call 'em) of the Body, being duely kept open, they discharge an unknown Quantity of Excrementitous *Lympha* and *Serum,* from the Blood. When those Pores are stop'd, these Liquors are Increased and Stagnated, and become Sharp, and Salt, and full of Acrimony. Yea, and Whether there be such an Occasion for it, or no, the Depraved Blood sometimes is filled with ill-figured Particles, which cannot pass diverse of the *Glands,* where a Percolation is Expected for them. These Humours falling on the Membranes of the Lungs, or the Vessels about the Windpipe, or on some of the Nerves that serve the Respiration, the Irritation causes a *Cough;* which is a Struggle of Nature to dislodge the Enemy.

Tho' some endure a *Cough* many Years, and find it Salutary to them; A Sort of an *Issue,* the Checking and Ceasing whereof would be dangerous unto them; yett it is Easy to tell, when to permitt the Continuance of a *Cough,* will have in it the Danger of breeding an *Ulcer* in the Lungs, or breaking a Vein which will not be Easily Cured.

O *Nightingale,* with a *Thorn* at thy *Breast;*

Under the Trouble of a *Cough,* what can be more proper, than such Thoughts as these?

"My *Irregular Humours,* how Vigorous is *Nature* in me, to cast them up; to throw them off? Will not my Sinful and Faulty *Dispositions,* be as Provoking to the Principle of PIETY in my Soul? O my Soul, Cast them up, and throw them off. Tis the Work of *Repentance* to do so. *Piety* will no more bear an *Ill Frame,* than my Vexed Body will bear a *Sharp Phlegm,* to be Lodged where it should not be. *Repentance* is a Sort of *Expectoration* for Every *Lust* in the Soul. With the *Impatience* of *Repentance* under Every *Lust,* is Every *Inclination to Sin,* and Every misplaced *Love* and *Hope* and *Joy,* to be parted with."

When a Fitt of *Coughing* does come upon thee, my Friend, Lett such a Wish as this, be raised in thy Soul: *O my God, Lett nothing that may hurt my Soul, be left within me!*

And then, as they say, *Tussis ac Amor*,—our *Cough* cannot be any more *Conceled* than our *Love;* Tis a Circumstance, that may lead us to think on the *Infoelicity* of those, who cannot *Conceal* their *Humours* and their *Follies;* The unhappiness of *Ungoverned Passions;* Exalted and Proclamed *Follies.*

May not the Consequences of *Irritations,* be here also agreeably thought upon? What *Violent Motions* People may, if *Irritated* be putt upon! Learn Wisdome, from the Intimation.

Father *Latymer*[1] somewhere in a Sermon speaks of a Terrible *Cough,* which the Justice of Heaven will bring upon them, who have *gotten Riches and not by Right,* compelling 'em to Vomit up their Ill-gotten Goods. Yea, he tells them they shall *Cough in Hell* for it. A *Cough* which Every Wise Man will deprecate.

In certain Memorials of PIETY, I have read such a Passage as This. "I am followed with a Trouble some *Cough.* This *Breast-beater* may be my *Awakener.* It may awaken in me some serviceable *Sentiments.* I propose, that when a *Coughing Fitt* comes upon me, it shall *Raise* in me, [Thus would I *Raise,* when I cough!] Some serious *Thought,* Some Holy *Thought,* and Especially Some *Thought* on a Glorious CHRIST; and on what is to be *Beleeved* of HIM, and what is to be *Expected* from HIM. And this *Thought* I would in a Quick *Prayer* then *Dart up* unto the Heavens. The *Thoughts* of a Soul so disposed for God and His CHRIST, are some of the *Fruits,* wherewith He is to be *Glorified.* How Useful and how Healthful is my *Cough* unto me, if it may have *all Manner of precious Fruits* in this way growing upon it! All that I Suffer from it, will in these Heavenly *Fruits,* have a Sufficient and an Abundant Compensation.

§ A gentle *Vomit,* will be in many *Coughs,* a good Beginning for the Cure.

§ The Balsam of *Copeyba,*[2] is for a Cough, certainly One of the finest Things in the World: The Quantity of a Few Drops taken on a Bitt of Sugar.

§ Some observe; When the Blood and Habit of the Body is foul, and a Load of thick Flegm is to be brought out of the Lungs, your mucilaginous and incrassating Medicines, are very noxiously præscribed; For they further pollute the Blood with an heavy and mucous Chyle, and stuff up the Lungs with a greater Colluvies.[3] And brisk stimulating Things, the Vertue whereof does not reach the Lungs, these only raise a Cough, which tire and spend the Lungs to no Purpose, when a great Mass of tough Phlegm is deposited, and sticks fast in their inner Vesicles.

§ *Mulled Water,* (an Egg beaten in fair Water,) drunk either Cold, or Warm, for a few Nights, does for an ordinary *Cough,* beyond all Imagination.

§ Tis among the *Boylaean* Receits. Boil *Turnips* in Water, and having Expresst the Juice, Mix it with as much finely powdered *Sugar-Candy,* as will bring it into a Kind of a Syrup. From time to time, Swallow slowly a Little of This.

§ Præparations of *Hore-hound;*[4] particularly, the *Syrup* thereof taken in a glass of *Warm Wine;* but especially, shreds of the *Leaves* taken in Milk warm from the Cow; few *Coughs* can stand before them.

§ A Conserve made of *Scabious Flowers,* is a Specific for a *Cough,* hardly to be parallel'd.

§ For a *Cough* attended with a tickling *Rheum,* tis among the *Boylaean* Receits: Take finely powdered *Olibanum,* and *Venice-Treacle,* Equal Parts. Incorporate them, and make Pills. The Dose is half a Dram, at going to Bed; or, if need be, a scruple twice a day.

§ The *Roots* of *Violets,* (which are easily run into a Jelly) made into *Lozenges,* will stop a Cough to Admiration.

§ *Wardens*[5] with a proper Quantity of Honey and Elecampane, baked in a moderate Oven,—afford an Electuary for *Coughs,* famous among the Ladies.

§ For *Coughs,* the shavings of *Castile-sope,* drunk a few Nights, in Wine, or Beer, will do Wonders. Or, you may make Pills of *Castile-sope,* and *Oyl,* and Sugar; which you may take Morning and Evening. This Remedy strikes at the Root.

§ *Liquorice, Liquorice,* in all forms, is a good, safe, marvellous Thing for a *Cough.*

§ From an happy Experience I may recommend this Remedy for a *Cough;* ℞ Conserve of Roses, Two Ounces. Elecampane, Anniseed, Liquorice, powdered; a Dram of Each; Oil of Rosemary, Twenty Drops. Spirit of Lavender, Ten Drops. Mix them with Syrup of Marsh-mallows, q.s. Take the Quantity of a Nutmeg, Morning and Evening. Tis a Matchless Thing!

§ Here's a thing which does Wonders! Take half a Pint of

Rum, and burn it. Add, half a Pound of Honey, and half an Ounce of Liquorice-roots. Boil these well together.

§ Here's another, that can't be Enough Commended; ℞ A Quantity of Barley; Boil it in a Gallon of Water till it be a Sort of a Gelly. Mix with it, half a Spoonful of powdered Elecampane; and a Spoonful or two of Honey. A Spoonful of this, taken several times in a day has cured not only Coughs, but also begun Consumptions.

§ Hearken to me! Ten or Twelve Drops of *Spirit of Turpentine;* taken on a bitt of Sugar, Morning and Evening (or either of them,) Cure a Cough to admiration; and with Safety; It removes the Cause.

§ Some that have had an Obstinate Cough, with a grievous Pain in the Breast, have had a Strange Cure, by drinking for a while Every Day; *Metheglin*[10] in which the Leaves of Sage have been Steeped.

§ There are some *Coughs;* People should have a Care how they Stop 'em. They hold People many Years, and accompany them to their Graves; (they are called, *Church-yard-Coughs!*) and keep them some while out of their Graves. You may make them *Easy,* with *Soothers,* if you please. But if you stop them at once, *All the fat is in the Fire.*

§ Take *Honey* and *Butter* Each a Spoonful; Two Spoonfuls of *Rum,* or *Brandy.* Take it warm, at going to Bed.

§ Here is a Remedy for a *Cough,* (yea, tho' attended with an *Asthma,*) that cannot be too much Commended. *Experto Credite!*[11]

Take Figs half a Pound (Sliced) Raisins, a Quarter of a Pound, (Stoned,) Liquorice an Ounce, (Sliced,) Anniseeds, half an Ounce (bruised,) Ground Ivy, an handful. Stew these in Three Quarts of Water, till they come to two.

Take half a Pint of this hott, at going to Bed.

In the Ensuing Morning, take three or four Small Pills, made of Tar, and Honey, and powdered Liquorice, mixed.

§ Here is a Notable Remedy for a *Cough.* Take Brown Sugar-Candy Powdered; Liquoris also Powdered: Mix these with *Sallet* Oil. [Would not, Oyl of *Sweet Almonds* do better?] Ana, q.s.[6] Use a little of it, four or five times every day.

§ Here is another Infallible. Take powdered *Liquoris,* powdered *Anniseed,* powdered *Mastick,* of Each an Ounce. Mix these with Four Ounces of Conserve of Roses.

§ Some cry up this; Take *Hore-hound* and *Elecampane;* both dried and powdered. *Brimstone* powdered: Mix them in Honey.

§ The famous *Willis,* knows not a better Medicine for a *Cough,* than *Tincture of Sulphur,*[7] from Six to ten drops, Morning and Evening, in a spoonful of Syrup of *Violets.*

Be sure, *Balsame of Sulphur,*[8] a few Drops in Conserve of Roses, or any other agreeable Vehicle, does notable Cures.

§ Old Dr. *Hancock*[9] was cured of an Obstinate Cough, in which it was common for him to throw up Blood and Bloody Matter, With nothing but a few *Stewed Prunes,* taken at going to Bed. He adds, "The taking a Quantity of Stewed Prunes, when you go to Bed, is the Quickest Medicine for Stopping a *Cough,* and taking off a *Cold,* that ever I mett with."

§ *Dolaeus* will tell you, I *highly Commend Medicines of Myrrh.*

§ In some Countreys, for a *Cough* and *Hoarseness,* they Bathe the feet in Warm Water for a Quarter of an Hour; and then rub a little Quantity of Deers-Grease, (the Older the Better) to the Soles of the Feet by the Fire. It must be repeted.

§ *Smith* tells of a young Woman troubled with a desperate *Cough,* who was Cured, by nothing but washing with *Cold Water* Every Morning, behind her Ears, and on her Temples, and on the Mould of her Head.

§ I have known Long and Sad and Obstinate *Coughs,* Wondrously cured with nothing but This. Take only two or three Spoonfuls of *Cold Water;* as often as an hard fitt of *Coughing* returns upon you.

§ Some who find the much Use of *Cold Water* bring a *Diarrhoea* upon them, have putt a Spoonful of *Wheat Flowre* into a Porringer of Water, and setting it by their Bed-sides, have taken a Mouthful of this now and then, as a fitt of *Coughing* afforded Occasion; And the Effect has been very Notable.

§ Some have boiled *Wheat-Bran* in Water, and Strained it; and then drank a little of the Water, every time they Cough'd in the Night; and have drank off the rest in the morning. This Cures a *Cough* to Admiration.

§ What say you, to *Buttered Flip?*[12] With some, tis little Short of the *Grand Elixir.*

§ Some almost worn to Death with a *Cough,* and apprehended far gone in a *Consumption,* have been cured by the Blessing of Heaven upon This. They kept often Chewing a little Malt,[13] with a *Raisin;* Swallowing their Spittle and Spitting Out what remained of the chew'd Substance.

CAP. XXXVIII. *Breath Struggled for.*

or

The Asthma,—
and, *Short-Windedness*, releeved.

PEOPLE sometimes have their *Breathing difficult,* and not without some *Noise* in their *Throats,* and their *Lungs.* Many times, tis no more than what is called a, *Dyspnoea,* and the Difficulty of Breathing is more moderate; But sometimes, it grows into an *Orthopnoea,* and carries with it an hazard of Suffocation.

This *Asthmatic* Indisposition, has been distinguished into, the *Flegmatic* Sort, and the *Flatulent* Sort. Sometimes, it grows into the *Convulsive,* and is very hazardous. *Viscid Flegm* filling the Branches of the *Bronchus,* may cause it. So may, gross Humours filling the *Stomach* to such a Degree as to Lift up the Diaphragm. So may, Fumes of *Metals* imbibed; So may a *Cough,* when it grows tedious, and obstinate, and has long and much disturbed the Breast; And so may, the prevailing of the *Scurvy,* and some other Distempers.

All Diseases of the *Lungs* are dangerous. *This* calls for a *Special Care* in the Patients.

But, the first Thing I would have them Careful about, is, To Entertain the *Sentiments of Wisdome;* which the Malady would more peculiarly call them to.

My Friend, Is it a Trouble some Thing to be so *short-winded,* as thy *Asthma* renders thee? Tis as bad a Disease, to be *Impatient* under the Troubles that are Ordered for thee. *Impatience* under *Afflictions* from the Hand of God; *Impatience* under *Injuries* from the Hand of Man; a Readiness to fall into *Short* and Quick Resentments; An Inability to bear with *Patience, even to Long-suffering;* Tis an *Evil-Disease.* O *Phtisical Soul,* when thy Struggle for Breath, putts thee upon Crying out, *Lord, Help me!* Lett this come into the Cry, *Lord, Save me from all the Short-Winded Impatience, I am subject to!* At the same time, and at all times, *Look unto the* Patient JESUS. He that cannot *Walk,* but is presently *Out of Breath,* by Setting the Exemple of a Lovely JESUS, and of His *Patience* before Him, will come, even to *Run with Patience.*

It is a grievous Thing to *Breathe* with *Difficulty.* Tis *Prayer* that is the *Breath* of the *New Creature.* Man, Dost thou find thyself to *Pray* with *Difficulty?* Not finding a *Freedom of Spirit,* Either in it, or to it? Oh! Lett this be grievous to thee. Find out, and Throw off, the *Faulty Humours,* that may bring this Oppression upon thy Soul. Make thy *Prayer* for the *Spirit of Prayer,* until thou find, that thou canst *Pray With* the *Spirit. Pant* at that rate; *Quicken me, O God, that I may call upon thy Name.*

Think again: "If my *Breath* fail, I feel my *Life* is gone. When my *Breath* Stops, I feel my *Life* goes. What a poor thing is Man, whose *Breath is in his Nostrils!* Man, whose *Breath goes forth, and he returns to his Earth,* and in *that Day his Thoughts perish!*"

Think; "How Criminal am I, if I do not Glorify the God, in *Whose Hand my Breath is, and Whose are all my Ways;* and who can immediately *take away my Breath,* and I *Dy and Return to my Dust!*"

Asthmatic Distempers mightily warn the sufferers, to be, *Always Ready.* A *Sudden Death,* may very probably Sieze upon them. Lett them immediately gett into Such Terms with Heaven, that a *Sudden Death* may be no unhappy Surprize unto them.

Strong Passions of the Mind,[1] have often brought a *Suffocation* at once, upon *Asthmatical People. Anger* has done it. Yea, *Laughter,* has done it. O People under an *Asthma,* keep up a *Constant Calm* of Mind as much as ever you can. Lett nothing *Move* you Inordinately. Tis a thing of great Consequence unto you.

§ A gentle *Vomit,*[2] will do well in Humoral *Asthma's:*—Especially, if the Cause is Lodged in the Stomach. *Bleeding* does well in *Convulsive* ones.

§ *Diureticks* are profitable, and necessary in this, and other Diseases of the Breast.

§ Take *Gum Ammoniacum,*[3] One Dram and an half; having dissolved it Cold in a Mortar, in *Hysop-Water,* four Ounces; and *Rhenish Wine,* Two Ounces; Strain it out for Two Doses. Of this *Lac Ammoniaci,*[4] (for it looks like *Milk*) *Brunner*[5] sais, *In an Asthma, its accounted an Extraordinary and a never-failing Remedy, and putts off the Suffocating Fitt So Effectually, that I have not seen a better.*

§ *Balsame of Sulphur,* is of good Use in *Asthma's.*

§ *Cows Urine,* taken alone (or, Disguis'd and Conceal'd from the Patient, in Beer,) has had an Incredible Success in curing the *Phthisic,* tho' never so Inveterate. But, why must it be a *Red Cow?*

§ *Mustard-Seed,* Unbruised (Some take it in the Pulp of a Roasted Apple,) is a Specific.

§ So is *Elecampane.* It may be made into a Pleasant Syrup. I have known a *Cough* and a *Phtisic,* marvellously releeved, by a Syrup of *Elecampane,* made with *Rum* or *Brandy,* in which it has been infused, and then the Liquor sett on Fire in a Porringer, with, Lumps of Sugar placed on Ranges of Skewers or any such thing, and so melted by the Flame to run into the Liquor. Tis a notable Thing.

§ *Hore-hound,* which does Wonders for the Cure of a *Cough,* will do the same for an *Asthma.*

§ *Eggshels,* (the Inner skin taken off) beaten into a very fine Powder, is a very powerful Specific.

§ In the *Boylaean* Receits, there is, *An Excellent Medicine for a Dry or Convulsive* Asthma.

Take *Saffron;* reduce it (by rubbing it in a Glass or Stone Mortar) to a kind of Powder; and with any Convenient Mixture, give Eight or Ten Grains of it, in form of Pills, at Bed-time.

§ *John Smith* relates, That a very poor Man desperately Ill of an *Asthma,* and in a deep *Consumption,* was advised by a Physician, To Drink nothing but *Water,* and Eat nothing but *Water-gruel* without *Salt* or *Sugar.* He continued this Course of Diet for Three Months, and was perfectly Cured. Continuing it a Month longer, he grew Fatt and Strong upon it. His Rule was, never to Eat, until he was thoroughly Hungry.

§ Monsr. *D'Ube,* sais, The Spirit of *Tobacco,*[6] given from Three Drops to Twelve, in a Glass of Hydromel, is the most Specific Remedy in the World against this Disease.

§ The Breast may be well anointed with Spirituous and Castorine Medicines.

§ *Helmont* sais, whatever will cure an *Epileptic* will cure an *Asthmatic* Person.

Cap. XXXIX. DESECTOR.
the CONSUMPTION;
the Grand <u>Mower</u> felt by the *Grass of the Field:*

A DREADFUL Disease! But so incident unto *Us,* that Foreigners call it, *The English Disease.*

What is the *Spectacle* that we have before us, when we see a Friend, with a *Consumption* upon him; and, *Ossa tegit Macres, nec juvat ora Cibus!*[1] We see the Body Wasting with a Lingring *Fever;* and for the most Part a tedious *Cough,* proceeding from ill-figured Particles in the *Blood,* with which the Lungs are grievously corroded.

How Instructive, how Affecting, a *Spectacle!* How Loudly Preaching to the Spectator, upon the Venom and Mischief which our *Taste* of the *Forbidden Fruit* has brought upon us; and Enforcing that Confession, LORD, *When with Rebukes thou dost Correct / / Man for Iniquity, / / thou makest to waste, Even as a Moth / / that which is his Desire./ /*

But then, Surely the *Patient* himself, is under all possible Obligations, to hear the Voice of his own Malady. *To Day if he will hear the Voice!*

It is a very wholesome Advice, that *Galen* gives for them that are Sick of a *Consumption; Prædict their Danger to them, and forewarn them of their End.* Accordingly, the very first Thing whereto the Languishing are to be advised, is This. *Friend, Suspect thy Danger, Beleeve thy Danger, and putt not off thy Præparation for thy End.* It is a Thing to be observed, That there is hardly any *Distemper,* wherein the Languishing are less aware of their *Danger,* than a *Consumption.* There seems an Unaccountable *Sleep* upon them; a Strange Inadvertency, Stupidity, and Security. Tho' they feel their *Hectic Fever* every day at or near a Certain Hour coming on them; the *Red Spot* in their Cheek proclaiming it unto the Standers-by; Tho' their *Appetite* be gone, their *Midriff* puff'd up with Wind, their *Stomach* Swol'n with a Mass of Ill-humours there; Tho' their *Pulse* grow Slow and Weak; their *Breathing* difficult; their *Cough* so raging, so cruel, so violent, that it can't be long before their *Lungs* are Lacerated and Ulcerated, if they be not so already: Tho' their *Spittle* Stink; and their *Urine* be grown Oily and Fatty; and Colliquative *Sweats* are spending of them; and their *Feet* and *Legs* are tumified; and they are so *Hoarse* they can do little more than Whisper to ye; and, in short, if a *Looking-glass* were called for, they could either not see their *Face* there, or see such an *Hippocratic*[2] one as might astonish them; yett they'l Strangely Flatter themselves. The little *Revivals* they have now and then, they improve into so many *Flatteries; They may gett over yett!* Alas, my Friend; Be not so Vain. Apprehend thyself under an *Arrest,* which there is *Very Little Probability* of thy Escaping from.

Wherefore, the *First Thing* to be done, is to gett out of that *Unregenerate State,* in which if a Man Dy, it will be *Good for that Man that he had never been born.* And in this, if thou *Linger,* I must lay my *Hand* upon thee, as once the Angel upon *Lot,* escaping from Eternal Burnings, and say, *Escape for thy Life; Make Haste, and escape! A Process of Repentance* will now be plainly and briefly sett before thee, and in going through it, it may be hoped, thy *Conversion to God* may be ascertained. Sett apart some Time, without any Delay, and while thy Spirits may be most in Vigour for it. In this Time, first of all, Cry to God, (even to the Holy SPIRIT of God,) with an unspeakable *Agony,* That He would *Quicken* Thee to Turn unto Him; Owning, that thou art of thyself able to do nothing to Purpose without His *Quickening,* and that thou art as unable by any thing to deserve His *Quickening.* Then, with much Contrition of Soul, *Confess* before the Lord, thy Sinful Violations of His Laws, enumerated in some Explanation of the *Ten Commandments,* and lay to Heart above all the *Fountain of Sin* in thy Heart, the *Original,* from which the Vile Streams of thy *Actual Sins* have issued. Now Carefully with Tears Beg it of the Glorious God, that He would pardon all thy Offences, for the Sake of the *Sacrifice* which His Beloved JESUS has offered up to the Divine Justice for thee; The *Sacrifice,* which now plead for thy *Atonement,* with the *Cries* of a Soul in the Jaws of Death; *Cries* that will pierce the very Heavens. Hereupon give thyself up unto God, with *Dispositions* and *Resolutions* for His *Holy Service,* and be restless in thy Petitions to have thy *Heart* Cleansed, Filled, Fired with His *Love;* and say, *What have I any more to do with fools?* Consent unto the *Covenant of Grace,* unto all the *Articles,* unto all the *Proposals* of it; most Heartily, Earnestly, Thankfully Lay hold upon it; and so conclude, *O Lord, I am Thine; Save me. I desire to be Thine, and wait for thy Salvation.* Having thus improved the *Space of Repentance,* which thou dost Enjoy in the *Slow Progress* of thy Distemper, and Repeated this *Action* as often as thou canst, for the better Assuring of it; Now lett the Several *Symptoms* of thy Malady, awaken in thee Such Sentiments of PIETY as may be Suitable and Savoury for One in thy Condition.

Think; "My *Outward Man* is *decaying day by day;* Oh! That my *Inward Man* may be *Renewed!* That as I grow *Weaker* in Body, I may grow *Stronger* in my *Love* to God and my Neighbour; *Stronger* in my *Faith* on my SAVIOUR; Gain more *Strength,* to bear with a

Patient Submission, what it shall please Him to lay upon me, and overcome the Terrors of the *Death* which I am hastening to; Encounter the *King of Terrors* which is now falling on me."

Think; "Tho' my *Blood* be *soured* and full of *Acrimony;* Lett my *Soul* be *Sweetened* with a sense of the Divine Favour to me, and be *full of Goodness.*"

Think; "Tho' I have a Slow *Fever,* burning and melting of me, which at certain Hours rises into more sensible *Paroxysms;* yett, lett the *Passions* with which my Soul is too ready to be fired, be all Extinguished."

Think; "If I *Cough* so vehemently, to *Cast up,* what is *Amiss* within me, Lett me be as Vehement in my *Desires* and *Essays* to *Cast Out* all that is *Amiss* in my Soul; all that is provoking there."

Think; "Have I a Mass of *Ill Humours* gathering in me? Lett not my Spirit have the *Ill Humours* of a Froward, Peevish, or an Envious, Mind, or any *Impatience* misbecoming a Child of God."

Think; "Is my *Appetite* gone? Oh! Lett my *Appetite* unto all the Delights, and Riches, and Honours, of *This World* go with it! Have I the Aspect of a *Dead Man* upon me, *Looking as if I were Laid out* already? Oh! Lett me *Dy* to Creatures as fast as I can; become as Indifferent as a *Dead Man* unto the *Comforts* and unto the *Troubles,* of this World. I must be *Dead,* before I *dy,* or else I am not *Fitt to Dy.* My *Life* lies in such a *Death* as that; Being *Dead with CHRIST,* and feeling myself *Alive* in Conversing with Him alone."

Anon; as the *Cough* begins to Abate, and the *Flux* comes upon thee, which is the *Immediate Harbinger of Death;* NOW, yeeld up thyself, *O Departing Spirit,* unto thy SAVIOUR, with all possible *Resignation.* Walk thro' the dark, *Valley of the Shadow of Death,* keeping a fast Hold on thy SAVIOUR; *Go up out of the Wilderness, Leaning on thy Beloved.*

§ *Borellus* has this Remark, on many Students falling into *Consumptions;* That it often proceeds, *a fumo Candelarum hausto in Musaeis undique Clausis.*[3]—And he quotes the famous *Placaeus,*[4] to confirm the Observation. The Admonition may be of Some Use, by way of prevention: But not as an Encouragement unto Students to throw by their *Lucubrations.*

§ What is the *Hectic Stone,*[5] they tell strange things of? And of the Milk or Water, in which that Stone has been dipped or quenched?

§ Among the *Boylaean* Receits, there is,

A very nourishing Aliment, that has recovered diverse in Consumptions.

Take Eight or Ten *Craw-fishes;* and, after the blackest Gutt or String is taken out, boil them in Barley-water, till they become very Red; Then take them out, and beat them long, Shells and all, in a Stone or Glass Mortar, to a soft Mash; and Strongly Squeeze out the Juice. This may be given, Either Alone, or mixed with an Equal Part of Chicken-Broth, or some such convenient Alimental Liquor.

§ A *Consumptive Cough* has been thus releeved, when other Means have proved Insignificant.

Take a dozen good *Raisins* of the Sun; and having taken out the Kernels, then Stuff them with the Tops, or Small Tender Leaves of the *Rue:* Take 'em in a Morning; and Fast a little after 'em.

§ Tis incredible, how strangely and quickly even far-gone *Consumptions* have been cured, by nothing but this: Lett a Convenient Spott of Earth be opened, and lett the Patient stoup to the Place, and there take the Smell of the Fresh Earth, for a few Minutes together. Why may not a Spadeful of the Fresh-Earth, be brought into the sick Chamber, and there Smelt unto?

§ Our Indians cure Consumptions with a *Mullein*-Tea.

§ Red *Nettle-seeds* taken in *Honey,* a Convenient Quantity, some time together.—This has recovered those, who have been far gone in a *Consumption,* that has been look'd upon, as desperate.

§ Well-præpared *Antimonials,*[6] are of great Efficacy to Sweeten the Blood, and keep off, if not gett off, a *Consumption.*

§ The *Antihecticum* of *Poterius,* in the common Præparation, Often defeats the Expectations of them that use it. But rightly præpared, it often does Wonders, in recovering People out of Desperate *Consumptions.*

§ The Use of *Milk,* is Commended in a *Consumption,* especially, *Womens* Milk. Next unto which, if I præfer that of *Asses,*[7] I should quote an Author for it. It shall be *Avicen.*[8] But then, the *Vicious Acids* in the Stomach must be corrected by *Absorbents;* Else the Benefit of the Milk-Diet will be defeated.

§ *Milk-Thea,* is a pretty Sweetener.

§ The Yolk of an *Egg,* in a Glass of Good Wine, drunk in a Morning, has been sometimes of Good Consequence.

But it is a Just Caution *Dolaeus* gives; *Aqua Vitae* is *Aqua Mortis.*[9]

§ *Pork* boil'd in Milk, and the Broth drunk; This has been cried up as a mighty Analeptic.[10]

§ The Use of *Snails* has done Wonders in the *Speedy Cure* of *Consumptions.*

§ In a recent *Phthisis,* there is often præscribed, *Syrup of Turnips.*

Take *Turnips* sliced, and double refined *Sugar,* of Each half a Pound; putt them in a glaz'd Pott; setting a Lay of *Turnips,* and a Lay of *Sugar,* till it is full. Cover the Pott with Paper, and putt it into an Oven, to bake with Bread. When it is taken out, press out the Liquor, and keep it for use. The Dose is, a Spoonful, Morning and Evening.

§ *Raisins* in Wine, Baked; and a few of these *Raisins* taken every day; have had a marvellous Efficacy.

And so, Dried *Figs.*

§ *Consumptions,* from *Obstructions* within, wherein People sometimes unaccountably Linger and Languish, are Sometimes helped by the Use of *Millepedes.*

§ An *Issue* may be of some Use. Advise about it.

§ *Change of Air;*[11] what may be thought of That?

§ See what may be done, by Sweetening the Blood, with *Thea's,* or Decoctions or Infusions, of *Sassafras,* of *Sarsaparilla,* of *Guajacum,* of *China*-roots,[12] of *Colts*-foot, and the like.

A *Tea* of the Bark of *Sassafras* Roots, has marvellously cured *Coughs,* wherein a *Consumption* has been *Threatned,* if not actually *Entred.*

§ Take *Myrrhe* well powdered; Two Drams; *Saffron,* half a Scruple; *Nutmeg,* half a Dram; *Honey,* two Ounces; Mix. *Th. Fuller* sais, "It is readily admitted into the inmost *Penetralia* of the Lungs; and is a Gallant Medicine for such a *Consumption,* as is not yett gone beyond the *first Stade* of one."

§ Physicians (especially *Spaniards*) tell of Ulcers in the Lungs Cured, with a Decoction of *Guajacum.*

§ Here's a Receipt. ℞ Flowre of Sulphur, Two Ounces; Melt it in a Large Iron Ladle; Then add, by Little and Little the same Quantity of the best *Salt of Tartar;* Stir them together Continually, with an Iron Spatula, till they are well-mixed, and are of a dark Red Colour. Then add, *Olibanum,* and *Myrrh,* of Each in Powder, Two Scruples; and *Saffron,* half a Dram; Stir them together for near a quarter of an Hour more; When tis Cold, Lett this Mass be dissolved in *Canary Wine*, Two Pints; Then add, of Trebly-Refined *Sugar*, Three Pound. Boil this to the Consistency of a Syrup. Of this, give one or two Spoonfuls, four times a day, in a Draught of some pectoral Decoction warmed, or in a Glass of White-Wine.

Woodman sais, "By this only Medicine, I have known People Recovered from this Disease, when they have been thought by others, past Recovery. Tis to be used for a Considerable Time. Tis a Noble Medicine in Hectic *Fevers*, if administred in Time."

§ Several have had the Heate of an *Hectic Fever* not only allayd, but extinguish'd, by the Use of *Succory Tea*.

I knew a young Man recovered from an *Hectic* by using *Whey* as his constant Drink.[13]

§ Here's another, (that is mentioned among Dr. *Lowers*[14] Receits,)—

Take the Yolk of a New-laid Egg; Beat it with Three Spoonfuls of Red-*Rose-Water;* putt to it Half a Pint of the Strokings of *Red-Cows Milk;* Sweetened with a sufficient Quantity of *Sugar of Roses;* Add to it a Little *Nutmeg* scraped. Take this every Morning for a Month, fasting Two Hours after it.

It is added: This alone restored a Gentleman, that was given over by the Physicians.

§ Here's another. Take Two Young *Cocks*, hatched in the Spring, and kill them with Strangling, not shedding any of their Blood; pick 'em, and gutt 'em. Don't wash 'em. While they are warm, now bruise them to a Mash, breaking all their Bones. Putt them into a Clean Earthen Pipkin; adding Two Quarts of Water, and One Pint of Sweet Rich *Wine*, wherein Boil the *Cocks* to Rags. Then Strain it hard thro' a Clean Cloth; and into the Strained Liquor put One Pound and an half of Stoned *Raisins;* Two Drams of *Saffron;* One Ounce of *Harts-horn;* One Ounce of *Ivory;* One handful of *Maiden-hair;*[15] Two Ounces of the Roots of *Colts-foot* sliced; and again lett it be well-boiled. Then Strain it. So, give to the Patient, Half a Pint, or a Gill, or Less, as his Weakness is more or less, and his Stomach will bear it, Every Morning. You may Sweeten it with a Spoonful of Syrup of *Gilly*-flowres,[16] or *Maiden-hair;* until you find the Cough departed. Every full Moon purge a little with *Pill Ruffi.*[17]

The Account added is: "An Excellent Remedy for those that are inclining to a *Consumption*, or any Inward Weaknesses, attended with a *Cough*. Proved by many Experiments."

§ Strong *Wort* boil'd unto the Consistence of a Cataplasm, with a little *Venice-turpentine* added; This laid unto the Breast, will strangely nourish and strengthen the Vitals; and prevent a *Consumption* coming on.

§ Dr. *Morgan* observes, "He who shall go about to Cure an *Hectic,* without a Primary and Chief Regard unto the *Scurvy,* of which it is a Symptom, will find himself unhappily Mistaken." For this he cries up certain *Mercurial* and *Antimonial* Præparations; As, the *Ethiops, Cinnabar,* diaphoretic *Antimony;* and the *Antihecticum Poterii.*

§ Take *Vervain,* a Convenient Quantity. Make a Strong Decoction. Then add unto the Decoction an æqual Quantity of *Honey;* and boil them together into the Consistency of a *Syrup.* Of This, take now and then a Spoonful.

Tis a very *Remarkable,* and often *Experimented,* Cure for *Consumptions.*

Cap. XL.

A Pause made upon,
The Uncertainties of the
PHYSICIANS.

WHEN we are upon a *Consumption,* it may be as proper a *Time* and *Place* as any to make a Remark upon, *The Uncertainties of the Physicians,* on whose Advice the Patients depend so much for their Lives, and the Comfort of them. Their *Uncertainties* appear notoriously and sufficiently in their *Contradictions* to one another; which indeed are very Conspicuous in this Distemper (as Dr. *Marten* in his, *New Theory,* has with a Just Ingenuity observed,) but also to be found in all other Diseases. How rarely does, *A Council of Doctors,* do the Patient so much good, as a Single One *happens* to do! A Famous Physician, Who shall be Nameless, *Died* of a Disease, which at that very Time, he had a Book in the Press, to teach the Cure of. We will single out, *The Consumption,* for our Experiment; because it is One of those *Maladies,* which have the greatest Share in the Deprædations of Mortality; and on which more has been written than upon many others. And here, we will not Concern ourselves with the *Differences* among the *Physicians,* about the *Cause* of this Distemper; (whereupon, who can read the Collection made by *Dolaeus,* and not cry out, *The Diviners* are mad!) but only see, how they *Differ* about the *Cure* of it.

Some Physicans are violent in it, That the Cure of a *Consumption* must be accomplished only by *Alcali's*. Others with as much Violence urge, that it must be only by *Acids*. I will spare the *Names* of the Gentlemen on both Sides.

Many hold, that no Good is to be done in a *Consumption*, without *Opiates*. It is held by others, that they are Pernicious Things, and no better than an Halter. I still spare the *Names* of my Gentlemen.

But, I will do *That* no Longer.

We know, what Shelves of Medicines are prepared with *Sugar*, for a *Consumption*. But *Harvey*[1] Exclaims against Pectorals prepared with *Sugar*. *Helmont* sais, That Syrups and Lohochs[2] have not benefited one in a Thousand. *Heurnius*, and *Wedelius*, and *Capivaccius*,[3] are against all sweet Lambatives.[4] *Dolaeus* affirms, they rather Increase the Disease than Releeve it.

Conserve of Roses, has been in high Esteem for many Ages; And an Army of Advocates, besides the great Names of *Platerus*,[5] and *Forestus*, and *Riverius*, might be mustered for the Defending of it. But *Sylvius*[6] decries it as an useless thing, And *Harvey* asserts the Patients to be rather the Worse than the Better for it.

Balsam of Sulphur is cried up to the Skies: And particularly, by *Sylvius* tis valued above all Medicines. But *Hoffman* and *Walschmid*, as vehemently disrelish it; and say, it rather Increases than Extirpates the Distemper. *Deckers*[7] reports, That some have been brought into the Distemper by using of it. And *Michael*,[8] quoted by *Dolaeus*, will confirm the Report.

The Decoctions of *Guajacum*, and some other such Things, much in Vogue, for a *Consumption;* have had the like Reputation; *Prais'd* by some, and *Scoff'd* by others.

Have not *Snails*,[9] gott as *Early* as any Remedies, into general Esteem and Practice? *Cardan* sais, he has made a Cure of *Desperate Consumptions* with them. Harvey despises them. *Salins*[10] reproaches them.

The *Milk-diet* is recommended by *Dolaeus*, and a Thousand more. *Harvey* sais, Tis useless; and in many Cases, hurtful. And in how Many Cases doe *Morton*[11] forbid it?

Lett *Weikard*[12] and *Harvey* Engage one another upon the *Juice of Turnips;* The former with *Panegyricks*, the Latter with *Invectives*.

Ground-Ivy has mett with the Like Reception.

They warn us against *Aloeticks*[13] in a *Consumption*. And yett, my Friends, how much do you rely on your *Elixir Proprietatis?*[14]— Whereof yett some will tell you, The frequent use of it has brought a *Consumption*.

Helmont, and *Ettmuller*, and *Borellus*, and *Dolaeus*, condemn the Letting of Blood in a *Consumption:* And *Capivaccius* thinks, there will be Seldome, if Ever, any Need of it. Yett *Galen*, and *Mercatus*,[15] and *Spigelius*,[16] and *Sylvius*, and *Willis*, and many others, approve it; especially on the Beginning of the Disease. *Hippocrates* would have us Bleed in Distempers of the Lungs, as most as Long a there is any Blood in the Body. Yea, our *Sydenham* does allow Bleeding on some Invitations; And our *Morton* does advise it, as often as a New Peripneumonick Feaver happens in this Distemper.

For *Emetic* and *Cathartic* Medicines; *Hippocrates* condemns *Vomits;* and *Helmont* as much condemns *Purges*, in this Malady. *Dolaeus* tells us, *Vomits* are Ever Suspected; and *Purges* are Seldom Safe. Whereas *Morton* is not against both gentle *Vomits* and *Purges*, in that which they Call, *The First State of the Distemper*. *Prosper Martianus* is very Zealous for *Vomits*. *Hartman* favours them. *Ettmuller* sais, There is no Remedy that æquals them. *Crato*[17] and *Baglivi* are against *Purges*, in this and all Diseases of the Breast. But *Galen*, and *Avicen*, and most of the Ancients, purged plentifully in this Malady. And *Mercatus* urges it, as almost the only way to Cure a *Phthisis*. *Willis* also, and *Barbette*, and *Deckers*, are for Sleight Purgations.

Morton speaks but Suspiciously of *Diaphoreticks* in this Distemper. But what say others?

Galen Condemns *Diureticks*. But *Montanus*[18] and *Crucius*,[19] and *Willis*, and *Sylvius*, and *Dolaeus* direct them. They are approved by *Morton*, and admired by *Baglivi*.

Authors disagree about all the Methods of *Evacuation*. And there is as much Disagreement among them about *Issues*, and *Blisters*, and External Applications. Alas, what a *Blindmans Buffet* carried on among them!

Of how great Consequence is the Doctrine of *Animal Spirits*, in Physic? And yett, *Morgan* derides it, as an Hypothesis only Serving to Explain those Diseases which the Physicians have been Ignorant of, or Surprised at; Like the common Refuge of *Witchcraft* among the Vulgar!

Oh! the *Darkness* that we find *Sett in our Pathes!* "But from this

Darkness tis *as clean as the Light,* That our *Dependence* must be no longer on our *Physicians* for the Cure of our *Diseases.* T'wil be a very foolish and faulty thing, to fall into the Distemper of him, Concerning whom it is left upon Record: *In his Disease he Sought not unto the Lord, but unto the Physicians.* Relying upon them, We may feel that word fulfilled upon us, *Thou shalt use many Medicines, and thou shalt not be Cured.* Yea, we may be like the Woman, of whom the *Beloved Physician* honestly relates, *she spent all her Living on Physicians, neither could be healed of any.*

O *Thou afflicted,* and under *Distemper,* Go to *Physicians,* in *Obedience* to God, who has Commanded the *Use of Means.* But place thy *Dependence* on God alone to Direct and Prosper them. And know, That they are all *Physicians of no Value,* if *He* do not so. Consult with *Physicians;* But in a full Perswasion, That if God leave them to their own *Counsels,* thou shalt only *Suffer many Things from them;* They will do thee more *Hurt* than *Good.* Be Sensible, *Tis from God, and not from the Physician, that my Cure is to be Looked for."*

Tis a Sad Story told by *Huartus,*[20] That when the *Arabick* Medicine flourished in *Italy,* there was a Physician so celebrated for his Learned Writing, Reasoning, Disputing, Distinguishing, and making of Conclusions, that his Auditors Expected, he would not only Cure Diseases, but Even Raise the Dead. But after all, when he came to Practice, hardly any of his Patients Escaped with their Lives. They did by their Death so generally Expiate the Empty Knowledge of the Professor, that with Confusion he bid adieu to the World, and ended his Days in a Convent.

What an Oracle has *Hippocrates* been to our Physicians, who *Profanely* enough use to put the Title of *Divine* upon him! How extravagantly, is he revered, by those, with whom after *Macrobius*[21] he is Blasphemously Esteemed, as, *Tam fallere quam falli nescius!*[22] How Hyperbolically Extolled by those who like *Heurnius* assert of him, *Cujus tanta fuit Benignitas, ut nihil Sciverit quod nos nescire voluerit; tanta autem Solertia et Sapientia, ut nemo post eum Sciverit, quod ipse ignoravent!*[23] And yett; what are the *Aphorisms* of *Hippocrates;* many of which are *Trivial* Enough, and *known* to our Very *Barbers;* And those that are more Important, many of them found *False* in very many Cases! Many full of *Uncertainty Sanctorius* has done Enough to demonstrate, that they are not so *Infallible* as they have been Commonly taken to be. Even *Celsus* himself, that great Plagiary of *Hippocrates,* is compelled from Experience to make that

Confession upon them, *Vix ulla perpetua praecepta Ars Medicinalis recipit.*[24] There are no *Rules in Physick* to *be relied upon!* What are his *Prognosticks?* Those that are True of them, are Such as fall under the Observation of our poorest *Nurses,* and the meanest who tend upon the Sick! An ingenious Gentleman, who has written a Treatise Entituled *Medela Medicinae,*[25] has made sufficient Remarks upon them. And indeed our Incomparable *Boyl* could not forbear Saying, That he *might venture to say, that some of those rigid Laws of* Draco, *the Severity whereof made Men Say, they were written in Blood, cost fewer Persons their Lives, than* one Passage which he mentions, of *Hippocrates.*

As for *Galen,* the Learned Man who writes, *De Vitandis Erroribus,* hath reckoned up above Thirty of his *Notable Errors.* And whereas *Galen* seems most of all to triumph in his Book, *De Usu Partum;* the acute Anatomist *Vesalius*[26] derides his Ignorance of *Anatomy,* and shows that he never performed one Dissection, and proves him to have Erred in one hundred and sixteen Particulars.

It is a Sad Story, which One of the greatest Physicians that Ever *France* could boast of, has Confess'd unto the World. *Certum est, Numerum Aegrorum a Medicis Curatorum, non attingere, illum Eorum, quos ad Orcum Pomposa cum Latinitate deducunt.*[27] Yea, The Story goes on; *Ars divina Medicinae, metuo ne ad illud deveniat ut juxta Merita Crimina, Obque Perpetua Homicidia, in Exilium, Sicut antiquitus a Romanis, arceatur.*[28]

It was thought, that *Argenterius*[29] far Surpassed *Galen,* in reducing, The *Art of Physic,* to a yett more perfect Method; And yett it is reported of him, That most of his Patients dyed under his hands; or fell into Incureable Distempers: insomuch that his affrighted Countreymen gave over employing of him.

The Result of this Discourse is, To take off our Dependence on an *Arm of Flesh,* and show what Cause we have to Depend on the Glorious God alone, for the *Cure* of our *Diseases.* What should be the Motto on the Curtains of Every Sick Bed, but this; <u>My Help Cometh from the LORD who made Heaven and Earth</u>!

All this, without the least Intention to depreciate the skilful and faithful PHYSICIAN.

The Words in the *Thirty Eighth* Chapter of *Ecclesiasticus,* deserve as good a Reception with us, as the most Oraculous that ever fell from the Pen of an *Hippocrates.*

Honour a PHYSICIAN with the Honour due to him, for the

*Uses you may have of him. Inasmuch as the Lord hath Created him;
—For of the most High Cometh Healing; And the skill of the Physician shall lift up his Head.*

Give Place to the Physician for the Lord hath Created him; Lett him not go from thee for thou hast need of him. There is a Time when in their hands there is good Success.

CAP. XLI. *Icterus* looked upon.
or
The Jaundice Cured.

THERE is a Disease, which has been called, *Morbus Regius,* or, *The Royal Disease;* because it brings with it the Colour of *Gold* unto them that have it. But so poor a Recommendation will not make the *Jaundice* to be wished for. Indeed, if it may bring the Patient into the Sentiments of PIETY, and bring him to be tinged with the *Grace* which is better than *Gold,* it may deserve as high a Title as what the Complement has bestow'd upon it.

In this Disease usually, the Excretion of the *Bile* into the Intestines, meets with some Obstruction, and so it Regurgitates and is Carried with the Blood all over the Body, whereby all the Parts, both the Solid and the Fluid, come to be tinged with a *Yellow.* At the same time a *Viscidity* in the Humour is Evident from the *Stagnation* of it. Perhaps, there may be some other Fault in the *Bile;* it may be too much Exalted, or Abundant; or the Lixivial Salt of it may be too much Weakened; Or an Excess of *Bile* may arise from diverse ill Mixtures in the Blood, so that the Bladder for it shall not receive it. On this, the Mass of Blood, becomes to like that of one bitten with a *Viper.*

The *Bile* growing more *Vitriolic,* and the Malignity of the Distemper increasing, the *Yellow Jaundice,* becomes the *Black;* and is indeed Sufficiently Dangerous and Ominous.

But now, O Man Lying in *Icteritrous Chains,* Why may not thy Malady become a *Chrysostom*[1] unto thee? Hear the Voice of the *Golden Preacher!*

Want of Sleep is One of the unhappy Symptomes, which thy Malady is attended withal. But at this time, and by this thing, Lett thy Mind be *Awakened* unto the Sentiments of PIETY. Particularly,

Bewayl the *Sinful Sleep* which has ever overtaken thee. Hast thou never been *Asleep, When* and *as* thou shouldest not have been so?

In thy Malady thou hast a *Deadly Picture* of that *Corruption,* which since the Days of *Austin,* the Church has Called, *Original Sin,* and under which all Mankind is Languishing. Behold it, and upon the Taste of *the Wormwood and the Gall in it,* be able Sensibly to say, *My Soul is humbled in me!*

The *Jaundice* is usually *first* of all discovered in the *Eye,* which has a *Yellow Tincture* given to it. Our *Original Sin* has this for the *First* of its *Wretched Influences, We see Wrong.* Our *Lust* has tinged our *Sight;* and made us to *Putt False Colours* on what we Look upon.

O *Patient,* Beg it of thy SAVIOUR; *Lord, Save me from a depraved Eye!* And, *Lord, Lett not Prejudices and Prepossessions keep the Eye of my Soul, from a Right View of what I have before me!*

In the *Jaundice;* the Disorder is *Universal:* Every Part is touched with it; All is out of Order. Nor is any Part of us, free from the Taint of *Original Sin.* O Patient, with an Extended Meditation, Employ thy Self-abasing and Self-abhorring Thoughts, upon the Reach of thy *Original Sin,* to Every Part. See and own, how it has Left no Part untainted; and with Anguish Cry out, O *Wretched one that I am!*

A *Listlessness* to Every thing, is one of the Ill Tokens, with which a *Jaundice* is accompanied. Alas, Tis what thy *Original Sin* has brought thee to: To be *Listless unto all that is Good.* Complain of thy *Sloth* unto thy SAVIOUR; Entreat of Him; *Lord, Save me from the Evils, which the Soul of the Sluggard is doom'd unto!*

In the *Jaundice,* a *Bitterness of the Tongue* is One of the Symptoms. And a *Bitter Tongue* is among the Things that grow upon our *Original Sin;* which may truly be called, *A Root of Bitterness.* Repent now of all thy *Bitter Words;* and Resolve; *I will not offend any more.*

There is a *Sadness* with which the *Jaundice* is commonly accompanied. *Patient,* Lett thy *Sadness* run into the Channel of a *Godly Sorrow;* and that *Repentance which is not to be Repented of.* Check the *Worldly Sorrow,* which is *Wrought by* the *Death* now invading thee, and which will *Work Death* by hastening it, if it be indulged. Entertain instead of it, a *Godly Sorrow,* which will be *unto Salvation.* Employ thy *Sad Thoughts* upon thy Departures from God. Then with a Lively Faith *pour out thy Soul* unto thy SAVIOUR, and so be *no more sad.*

§ I am slow to advise the *giving* of *Lice*[2] [I suppose it would not be with much Success if I should advise the *Taking* of them] in the *Jaundice:* Ever since I read the horrid Story in the *Acta Medica* of *Bartholinus;* That the Taking of them has been anon follow'd with a Tragical Death, upon which a Vast Colony of *Lice* has been found in the opened Patient.

§ *Joels*[3] famous Medicine for the *Jaundice.*

Take the Juice of Great *Celandine* sliced, two handfuls; *Juniper-Berries,* one handful. Bruise them, and pour to them, of *Rhenish Wine,* a Pound. Extract the Juice. Give to four Ounces, twice a day.

§ Gently roast a *Sevil Orange,* with a Dram of *Saffron.* Cutt this Orange, and infuse it in a Pint of White-Wine. Take a Spoonful or two, when you feel the Faintness of the Jaundice.

§ The Cure of the *Jaundice* is usually best begun with a gentle Vomit.

§ *Turmerick,*[4] and *Celandine,* and *Gentian,* and *Centaury,*[5] and *Saffron,* and *Rhubarb,* are all of them Famous Vegetables, for the Cure of the *Jaundice,* used in almost any Fashion. Make an Infusion of them.

§ *Dube* sais, That Syrup of *Hore-hound,* with Honey, is a Specific.

§ *Aloeticks* often are good *Anti-Ictericks.*

Hence, *Elixir Proprietatis* is often of noted Efficacy in the Jaundice.

§ The Syrup of *Horehound* is mightily Cried up.

§ Take an Infusion of *Celandine,* in Wine. Or, A Decoction of *Strawberry* Leaves and Roots.

§ Both *Helmont* and *Willis* cry up the use of *Millepedes.*

§ Take Roots of *Turmerick* and *Madder,* an Ounce of Each, *Celandine* Roots and Leaves, of Each, two Handfuls. *Earth-worms* slitt and opened, and washed, Number twenty. Boil in Water, and Rhenish Wine, of Each a Pound and half, to twenty Eight Ounces. To the Strained Liquor, add, Tincture of *Saffron* One Ounce: Syrup of the Five Opening Roots, three ounces. Mix for use. *Quincy* sais, *it Cannot fail of Success, drank four Ounces, two or three times a day in the most obstinate Jaundice.*

§ The *Urine* of an Healthy Lad, Six Ounces, with Six drams of White sugar; drunk fasting, has been very successful in the *Jaundice.*

§ *Sheep-dung* infused in Wine, has had good success, in this distemper.

§ And so has *Castile-Soap,* dissolved in Milk, that is Warm'd and Sweetened. It seldome fails. Or, *Castile-Soap,* in Pills, with a Little Powder of *Turmeric.*

§ Large Blisters raised with *Cantharides* in a Poultis of *Rye,* will soon draw Large Bags of a yellow Gelly and make the Patient faint. But the Success in the *Jaundice,* is to Admiration.

§ *Quincy* sais of, *Soap;* There is not a better Medicine in the World, for the *Jaundice;* Except the Patient *Spitt Blood,* which is a Symptom of a Desperate Case; and such a Detergent as this would rather increase it.

§ The *Boylaean* Receit is, Take an Ounce of *Castile-Soap,* (the Elder the better) Slice it thin, Putt it into a Pint of Small-Beer Cold; Lett it boil gently half away; after boiling Some time, Scum it once; Then Strain it thro' a Small Sieve; warm it; so Drink it all in a Morning, fasting: Take a small Bitt of Sugar after it; and Fast two or three Hours.

§ He adds another. Take two or three Ounces of *Hemp-seed;* Boil them, till some of the Seeds begin to burst; and somewhat longer, in a Sufficient Quantity of New Milk to make a Draught. Lett this be drunk warm; and Renew'd, if need be; for some days together.

§ Here's almost a Specific.

Take some clean Filings of *Steel,* mix them with some Loaf Sugar. Grind them Long, with great Exactness: [*There Lies the Chief-Secret,* as my Author sais!] of this impalpable Powder give about half a Dram for a Dose, twice or thrice a day, in any Convenient Vehicle.

§ Mr. *Ray* Cured himself, with only drinking an Infusion of *Stone-Horse-Dung,* with *Saffron* in *Ale,* for four or five Days.

§ *Shell-Snails,* dried and powdered; a Spoonful of the Powder, in a Little Ale, Morning and Evening; *Woodman* commends this Remedy.

§ *Fuller* has a *Saponaceous Draught* for the *Jaundice.* Take *Venice-Sope* scraped very thin; from two to four Scruples. Boil it in *Cows Milk* from six Ounces to four. Then add *Sugar* three Drams; and strain it. He sais, *Tis reckoned a most prevailing Medicine.*

§ Two Drams of the Powder of *Earth-worms,* taken for a dozen days together; This Cures Even the *Black,* as well as the *Yellow Jaundice.*

§ You will have the Authority of a *Willis* for it, if you mix the Urin of the Patient with sifted Ashes of Ashen-Wood, and make Balls thereof, setting them in a warm Place, near a Fire, or a Stove. He sais; As these Balls grow hard, the *Jaundice* goes away.

§ *Dolaeus* will tell you, *This Experiment will Scarce Ever fail you.* Putt the Patients Urin in a Pott, which you shall cover with a Tile, and boil till it be half consumed; and then Bury it in Horse-Dung.

§ Among the *Boylaean* Receits, there is this *Magnetical Cure.* Take the *Gall-Bladder* of a *Sheep,* and near the Top, without Emptying the Liquor, make a Small Hole; At which putt in Two or Three drops of the Patients Warm Urine. Then ty up the upper Part of the Bladder. Hang it up, to dry.

§ A Dram of the Powder of a *Parrot,* has been Commended. And so has the Heart of a *Wren.*

Yea, so has half a Dram of the *White Part* of *Hens-Dung* dried, and mixed with a Little Sugar, and given in a few Spoonfuls of White Wine.

Cap. XLII. The Main Wheel scoured and oiled.
or, Help for,
The <u>Stomach</u> depraved.
[and, <u>Vomiting</u>.]

THE Grand Wheel in the Machine, being out of Order, how many and how miserable the Consequences!

We will touch upon Two Disorders.

I.   Sometimes a grievous Decay and Failure of *Appetite* is Complained of. A Considerable Quantity of a *Flegmatic* Humour or, of a *Bilious* Humour gathered in the Stomach, may be sufficient alone to produce this *Inappetency.*[1] There may also be other Causes for it.

But be the Causes what they will, the Malady may have Some Suitable *Sentiments of PIETY* raised upon it.

O Man, feeling such an Indisposition to *Eating* or *Drinking* upon thee, that there is a meer Force upon thy *Stomach* in all thy Deglutitions; thy *Stomach* rises against all that is as it were Cramm'd, and Ram'd, down into it; I hope, thou art now Convinced, That thy *Chief Happiness* lies not in *Eating* or *Drinking.* Surely, Thou will gett above the Class of *Brutes;* and none of those *Fools,* who know no *Higher Song* than that, *Soul, Take thine Ease, Eat, Drink, and be Merry.* Thou wilt now look after some *Higher Good,* than what goes down into thy *Stomach:* such is, The *Knowledge* and the *Image* of thy SAVIOUR, and the *Joy* of His *Great Salvation.*

But, thy *Want* of an *Appetite,* for the *Word* of God, the *Necessary Food* of thy Soul, and for the *Spiritual Blessings,* which that Word brings to those who *Desire* them; Lett this be more grievous to thee, than all that *Loathing* of thy *Stomach,* in which thou art Languishing. Alas, what has thy *Stomach* been full of, when thou hast *Loathed this Honey-Comb!*

Lett an *Appetite* for an *Appetite,* be now raised in thy Soul; and Lett the Ferment work in such Wishes as these. *Oh! That I had a Stronger Appetite, for an Acquaintance with my God and SAVIOUR! A Stronger Appetite for Communion with Him, in the Exercises of Godliness. A Stronger Appetite for those Attainments in PIETY, which may qualify me for the Kingdome of Heaven!—*

What? Must the Hand of Heaven at Length give thee some *Affliction,* like a *Glass of Bitter,* to Cure thee?

This is a Maxim, *Ventriculus male affectus, est Origo Omnium fere Morborum.*[2]

Tis another Maxim; He that would have a *Clear Head,* must have a *Clean Stomach.*

Dr. *Morgan* asserts, That of all proper Corroboratives, to Strengthen the Muscular Force and Action of the *Stomach,* the *Peruvian Bark*[3] is the chief, and Stands beyond all Competition against Every thing Else, in Confirming a Good *Digestion.* He sais, In angered Constitutions, where the Appetite is Lost, the Digestion vitiated, and the Natural Heat Exceedingly diminished, from the Weakness of the Stomach, and the Intestines, the *Bark* is *the greatest, and most Efficacious Stomachick in the World.* Consult a wise Physician, (I wish, you could find a *Morgan*) about the Way of using it.

§ A gentle *Vomit,* may be Necessary and Serviceable.

§ *D'Ube* sais, *You can pitch upon*[4] *no better Remedy,* than to infuse *Wormwood Leaves,* in a Glass of proper Wine, with a Little *Sena.* He also Commends, A *Digestive Powder,* of Half an Ounce of *Anniseed,* a Dram of the Powder of *Red-Roses,* and half a dram of *Limon-Peel,* well-bruised in a Mortar. Add a little Sugar, and so take half a Spoonful after Supper.

§ There are *Stomach-Plaisters,* which Every body knows of.

Sir *Kenelm Digby* præscribes a very pretty Plaister, which I have known to be a notable Thing. Upon a Peece of Leather, a Little Broader than your Hand, Spread a good Quantity of *Mithridate,* and grate upon it a good Quantity of *Nutmeg;* then lett a Peece of Thin Leather, So Cover it, that it may not run out at the Bottom. Lett this be hung over the Pitt of the Stomach.

§ *Fuller* mentions a *Testaceous Electuary.* Take fine, Soft, White *Chalk* Washed; *Conserve of* [torn] *Roman* (or *Sea*) *Wormwood;*[5] Each, one Ounce: *Oil of Wormwood,* One Drop; *Oil of Mint,* Two Drops: And *Syrup of Quinces,* Enough to mix it with.

He sais, *This merits a principal Seat among the noblest of the Stomachicks; It causes a comfortable glowing Warmth in the Stomach, and breaks its Acidity. It is prevalent against the Heart-burn, Pain in the Stomach; Belching; Queasiness, Vomiting; Inappetency; Diarrhoea.*

Lett Three Drams be given twice a Day, when the Stomach is most Empty.

§ Here's a Noble *Stomachic Mixture.*

Take Strong *Cinamon-Water,* One Ounce; *Oil of Vitriol,* one Dram; *Oil of Cloves,* twenty four Drops. Mix.

Lett forty Drops more or less, be given in a Glass of generous Wine, on an Empty Stomach.

It strengthens the Stomach, Excites the Appetite, Stays Vomiting, to admiration. So says the Author. But I suppose, that Stomachs disordered with *Biliose Humours,* are they that it will do most Good to.

§ *Lovage-root*[6] infused in Rum, has been mightily cried up, in the Want of *Digestion.*

§ Roots of *Gentian* pulverized; From Twelve or Fifteen Grains to double the Quantity. Taken twice or thrice a day. You may add a little powdered *Sugar* to it, if it be too bitter for you. The famous *Boyl* commends this, not only for Want of Appetite, but for Obstructions; and Vertiginous Affections of the Brain; and Agues.

§ *Wormwood,* and *Mint,* and *Mugwort,*[7] beaten together for a Cataplasm, to be laid, and kept warm at the Stomach has been found a notable Strengthener of it.

§ *Borellus* discovers the Secret, with which a Citizen of *Montpellier* gott a mighty Reputation, for the Restoring of Stomach, and the Strengthening of the Appetite, and killing of *Worms.* Twas a little Purgative. T'was nothing but a *Syrup of Wormwood;* nothing differing from that in the Shops of the Apothecaries, but only the addition of a little pulverized *Rhubarb,* and the gathering of the *Wort* in *May,* before Sun-rise, with the dew upon it.

§ Here's an Excellent Stomach-Plaister.

Take *Storax*[8] in Powder; *Aloes* finely powdered; of each, One Ounce. Boil these together, with half a Pint of *Rose-Water,* till the Rose-water be Consumed. Then lett it Cool. Add as much very good

Honey, as will make it a *Paste*. Spread this upon Leather, and *Lay* it unto the Stomach.

Of this Plaister, Sir *Kenelm Digby* sais; "It will strengthen the Stomach Extremely; and will free it from all Corruption, and give a Natural Heat unto it. It hath Saved the Life of many; Even of those who already had lost their Speech." He adds: "This Paste is very Odoriferous and Incorruptible; it will last forever."

§ Here's a *Stomachic Electuary*.

Take Conserve of *Roman Wormwood*, and of *Sevil Orange* Peele; One Ounce of Each. Powder of Mint, Two Drams; Oil of *Cinamon*, Six Drops. Syrup of *Quinces;* Enough to make it into an Electuary.

The Dose is the Quantity of a Nutmeg, taken about an Hour before Meals: After it Sucking the Juice of half a Lemon.

Tis an admirable Strengthener of a Weak Stomach. It also cures Habitual *Diarrhoea's,* and so fortifies the Solids of the whole Body, as to remove all Kinds of Fluxes.

§ M. *Martin* writing about the Western Islands of *Scotland*, has an Account of a Young Man, who had utterly lost his Appetite; restored unto Health, by boiling the Blade of *Alga Marina*, or *Sea-tangle*,[9] (some call it Sea-wave,) and so drinking an Infusion of it boil'd with a little *Butter*.

§ One that had a Stomach so depraved, that for many, many Long Months together, he Cast up all he Eat, and was thought far gone in a Consumption, was cured with nothing but This. He daily took two (spice) *Cloves;* with a Clove of *Garlick*, and a Couple of *Almonds;* and chew'd them together, and swallowed them.

§ An Eminent Physician writes: "We know that *Warm Water*, will most of any thing Promote and Assist *Digestion* in *Weak Stomachs*, and *tender Nerves*. And by This alone, we have seen several such Persons recover to a Miracle, when Cold *Mineral* Waters, *Bitters, Cordials,* and *Drams*, have done more Hurt than Good."

§ To Persons troubled with *Indigestions*, Dr. *Strother* directs, that a swathing band should be tied round their Middle, so as to compress the Stomach and the Bowels. This is an artificial Supply for the Weakness of the abdominal Muscles; which squeezes the Stomach and Victuals thrown into it. It is an Observation old as *Piso*,[10] that This will [torn] Concoction.

§ The *Amarum Salubre*.[11]

There has been much Noise in the World, about *Bitters* for the

Restoring and Strengthening of the *Stomach;* But here is a Plain and a Short One, which Exceeds all that are cried up in the Common Advertisements, and that have brought no little Gain unto the Publishers.

Take *Gentian Roots,* and *Orange-Peels,* [fine *Sevil* Oranges, clear'd of the white, and carefully dried:] and both cutt very Small: A Pound of Each. Pour upon them in a glass Bottel, a Gallon and half of Spirit of Wine, (or, *Brandy.*) Lett them stand Close Covered in a very Mild Warmth, for Some Days. Then press out the Spirit very Strongly; And lett it fine down for use. An Ounce of *Spirit of Sulphur,* added unto a Pint of this Tincture, makes it every way yett more grateful and useful.

From fifteen to sixty Drops, is a Dose; taken in a glass of Wine, or any other Convenient Liquor. The Irradiations which the *Stomach* receive from it, are wonderful! The good Consequences whereof cannot be numbred.

II. Sometimes a violent, yea, a Dangerous *Vomiting,* siezes upon People. The Enraged *Bile* in their *Stomach,* Setts 'em a *Vomiting,* So that if it be not stop'd, their very Life is a going.

In this Case, Think, O Man; *Have I Cast up the Sins, that are poisoning of my Soul!* The *Confession* of *Sin,* is the *Vomit* of the Soul. This does not *kill,* but *save; Tis a Repentance not to be Repented of.* Tis Time for thee to come unto it. And think; *Has not my Soul, as much amiss in it, as my Stomach?* Add, *O Lord, I am oppressed, undertake for me!*

Reflect poenitently on the Faulty Excess of *Choler,* in which thou mayst at any time have indulged thyself: And now, *Forever Away with it!* How few can have that Stroke in the Elogy on Mr. *Spon*[12] allow'd 'em. *There was no Bile in his Composition. If no People died but of Choler abounding in them, he had been immortal.*

§ For the Cure, an *Hippocrates* would say, *Vomit.*

§ Salt of *Wormwood* a Scruple, in Juice of *Limons,* a Spoonful, is a miraculous thing.

§ *Scalding hott Water,* Stops Vomiting, every body knows it, almost miraculously.

§ A Decoction of *Barberries;*[13] Take a Wine-glass full.

§ The Yolk of an *Egg,* beaten up with a little *Brandy,* does Wonders.

§ Here's a Speedy Remedy. Take a Large *Nutmeg,* and grate off one half of it. Toast the flatt side of the other till the Oily Matter begin to Sweat out. Then clap it unto the Pitt of the Stomach, as hott as the Patient can bear it. Repeat when it Cools, if there be occasion.

§ The Pulp of *Quinces,* in Vinegar, to the Consistency of a Gelly; to which add, a little Powder of Orange Peel. Take a little of This.

Or, An Ounce of the *Juice of Quinces: D'Ube* cries it up as, *A Most Excellent Remedy.* You may at the Same time apply a Bruised *Quince* to the Stomach, outwardly.

§ For Children, taken with the *Vomiting,* (which proves Deadly to Multitudes,) the Oyl of *Sweet Almonds,* mixed with some agreeable Syrup, (e.g. of Marsh-mallows,) has quieted their Stomach, and wrought wonderful Cures.

§ The *Vomiting* and *Looseness,* is a Plague, that annually Visits our Children,[14] and frequently destroys great Numbers of them, in the Months of *August* and *September.* To prevent this Plague, Lett the Children as these Months are coming on, (and in them,) Every day at the Table take a *Spoonful of Wine.* It has been found a Notable Præservative.

§ For the *Vomiting* with a *Looseness,* (the, *Cholera Morbus,*[15]) I have known this Method have almost a Miraculous Efficacy. After the Washing of the Stomach with Scalding hott Water, if there be a Fever, take the Syrup of *Limons,* a Spoonful: Salt of *Wormwood,* Ten grains: powdered *Coral,*[16] two or three grains; mix these with an Ounce of Some *Cordial Water,* (as, *Treacle Water,* or *Aqua Mirabilis.*[17]) Take a Spoonful or two of this; and Repeat it. If the Patient be very Thirsty, mix fair Water with it.

But, if there be no Essential Fever in the Case; Take a Grain of *Opium* well-prepared with Salt of *Tartar.* Mix it with three Ounces of Somesuch *Cordial Water,* as *Aqua Mirabilis.* Take a Spoonful or two.

§ *Woodman* found a Great Success of this Julip, in furious *Vomiting* with a *Looseness.*

Take of *Cinamon* and *Mint* Waters, of Each Two Ounces; Salt of *Wormwood,* Two Scruples; Tincture of *Opium,* Twenty-five Drops; Syrup of *Limons,* an Ounce and half; mix for a Draught. Renew it, if the Vomiting Return.

§ Here's a *Corollate Mixture.* Take *Red Coral* finely Lævigated, Two Drams; *Salt of Wormwood,* Four Scruples; *Juice of Lemons* fresh drawn, Four Ounces; Strong *Cinamon Water,* Two Ounces.

Mix them in an open glass, and lett them Stand Uncorked, Lest their Fermentation break the Bottel.

Dr. T. *Fuller,* sais; "It wonderfully and almost miraculously, (like a *God in a Machin,* as they say,) represseth Subversions of the *Stomach,* and motions to *Vomit.* I have many times observed, That in Continual Fevers, miserably afflicting with anguish at the *Stomach,* and Symptomatic Vomiting, more Good hath been done, with this Medicine alone, than with all that Ever I could find out." There must be Two Spoonfuls given Every Hour, or a Spoonful Every Half-hour, the glass being first well Shaken.

Cap. XLIII. *Edulcorator.*
Helps for
The Heart-burn.
[And, *Stomach-ache.*]

TIS no Rare Thing, for People to have their *Stomach* infested with a *Sharp Humour,* which makes them feel a Sort of *Burning* and *Gnawing* there, that is very painful to them. Tis commonly called, *The Heart-burn;* [A *Cardialgia:*] it being indeed no New Thing for the *Stomach,* to be called, *The Heart.* If it be, as a famous *Helmontian* thinks, *The Seat of the Soul,* tis no wonder, that it is called so. In the Days of *Abraham,* a Repast was, *To Establish the Heart with a Morsel of Bread.* [Compare, Heb. XIII. 5.] Yea, our Blessed SAVIOUR directs Temperance in *Eating* and in *Drinking,* with such Terms, *Take Heed lest at any time your Hearts be overcharged, with Surfeiting and Drunkenness.*

The Patient Vext and Spent with his *Heart-burn,* may do very well, to look *further Inward,* and Enquire, Whether the Passions of *Anger,* and of *Envy,* do not sometimes give him a worse *Heart-burn* there. Those *Passions* alwayes bring *Troubles* with them. Twil be very *Trouble some* unto the Soul of a Good Man, to find them working in him. Friend, gett the *Cure* of these *Passions,* and Watch against their Operations.

The frequent View of the *Goodness* in the *Heart* of thy Lovely SAVIOUR, will cure thy Sinful *Heart-burn,* sooner than any thing in the World.

The *Meditation* of His Grace, will cause another, a better, an Holy *Heart-burn* in thee. Converse with Him, till thou canst say, *Did not my Heart burn within me?* There, *Muse till the Fire burns.*

To take a Glass of *Wine,* will often raise a Fitt of the *Heart-burn,* and sett the *Stomach* a raging, as if a *Live-Coal* were thrown into it. On this Occasion, Think: "How Easily and how Righteously might a Just God, render me incapable of Receiving and Relishing, the most common Refreshments, and Enjoyments."

Think; "How careful should I be, if any *Provocations* are offered me, never to take them in, or lett them go down into my Soul."

Many things are commonly præscribed and practised for the Releef of the *Heart-burn.*

To Swallow Corns of *Pepper.*

To Swallow, *Crabs-Eyes;*—or, *Chalk.*

To Swallow a little *Indian-Meal,* with Water.

To Swallow a few *Pease.*

But the too frequent Use of these Things, (or all but the last,) has a Tendency to Pall and Spoil the Stomach.

§ The best Cure for an *Heart-burn,* is the Continued use of *Conserve of Roses,* dissolved in a warm *Cup of Milk.* I beleeve, it hardly Ever failed.

§ The *Diarrhodon Abbatis,*[1] is of the like Efficacy.

§ Here is an *Emulsio Cretacea.* Take white *Chalk* in fine Powder, Three Ounces. *Barley-water,* three Pints. Boil it unto two. When it is cold, make an Emulsion, with the Four greater Cold Seeds; of Each Two Drams: Eight Sweet Almonds; Then add *Chalk* in fine Powder, three Drams; and *Pearl-Sugar* Enough to make it Palatable.

It is not only a pleasant Remedy in a *Diarrhoea,* but also taken, (but ever shaken when taken,) two or three times a day, about four Ounces at a time, Dr. *Quincy* sais, *It is an infallible in removing the* Heart-burn *almost instantly.*

I have known it Cured, by the *Magnetic Plaister,*[2] worn upon the Stomach.

§ Take *Red Coral* finely powdered; Half a Dram; Every day, in any Convenient Vehicle.

A Mantissa.

The *Stomach-ache,*—a Pain of the *Stomach.*

My Friend, If a *Pain* in thy *Stomach* follow thee, such a *Thorn in the Flesh* may humble thee.

But if thou make out for, and make sure of, *A Spirit reconciled unto the Will of God in all Events,* thou dost forever provide against the worst *Pain within.* All will be easy There.

However, now look after thy *Stomach.*

§ *Orange-peels,* being steep'd in Wine, and given Warm; or, Wine in which you have boil'd *Camomil-Flowres;* have been potent Remedies.

§ *Worm-wood* Wine has been Commended.

§ *Galen* would advise to a Cupping-glass.

§ Here is a *Pulvis Anticardialgicus.*[3]

Take the Purest and Whitest *Chalk,* Six Ounces; *Crabs* Eyes and Claws, of Each, an Ounce and half; Treble Refined *Sugar,* Half an Ounce. Chymical Oyl of *Nutmegs,* Six Drops. Mix and make a Powder, adding thereto fine Bole; six Drams.

The Dose is One Dram, in a Large Draught of Cold Water; Morning and Evening, for about a Fortnight; with a Purge once in Six Days.

Now, hear *Salmon* upon it: "It is a Specific against Pains at the *Stomach,* though never so Extreme; yea, tho' they cause Swooning. It always gives a present Releef; and in a short time, a perfect Cure."

Cap. XLIV. The *Vermine-Killer.*

upon,

Worms.

TERRIBLE Things are done to and in the Children of Men, by *Worms*[1] in their *Bowels,* as well as those found in several other Parts of their *Bodies;* yea, (without a Metaphor!) in their very *Brains.*

Mouffet,[2] and *Tyson,*[3] will Entertain you with the formidable Dimensions, that some of these *Worms* arrive unto. And I can add, That I have seen One in my Neighbourhood, the Head whereof being Siezed in the *Throat* of the Patient by his hand, was pull'd up, until he was found about one hundred and fifty foot long.

How these *Worms* come to be Lodged in Humane *Bodies,* (which way the *Eggs* Convey'd thither?) when tis found, that *Unborn Infants* have had them, has been yett scarce accounted for.

When it is Considered, that Every Joint of these *Worms,* is a Distinct *Worm,* with a *Mouth,* and *Maw,* of its own, and that a vast

Number of these, hanging to one another, do sieze upon the *Chyle,* as soon as it is made, in the Stomach of the Patient, and that it passes thro' these *Little Dragons,* before the Body of the Patient can have the Benefit of it, it is enough to strike One with *Horror* to think on't; and there will be no room left for any *Wonder* at the Dismal Effects which these Devourers have, where they make their Deprædations.

It is one of the Remarkables in History, That faithless and bloody Tyrants, [your *Herods* and *Philips,* and Company] who have been famous *Persecutors,* have died in the Midst of Torments, by *Worms* bred in their Bodies. The Justice and Wisdome of an Holy God, has thus triump'd over the haughty Murderers.

Christian, Beholding the *Worms* at Work upon Thyself, or Others, Think; "*Lord,* What is *Man,* that is a *Worm?* Yea, the *Son of Man,* [the most Excellent Man!] which is but a *Worm?* How little to be accounted of! A *Worm* is a *Match* for him; a *Death* to him. Even a *King,* and when he allows his Flatterers, most of all to make a God of him, finds the *Worms* able to kill his Godship; and to Eat up his Entrails!"

Think, "The greatest Man in the World, is but a *Worm,* and a Peece of *Worms-Meat.* And shall the Favour or the Anger of such a *Worm,* weigh with me any more than the *Light Dust of the Balance,* against that of the Infinite God?"

Think; "The *Worms,* which begin to Sieze and feed upon me, while I am yett above Ground, assure me, [All their *Mouths,* with *one voice* proclaim it!] the Time is at Hand, when *I must ly down in the Dust,* and the *Worms will cover me;* will *feed sweetly* on me. *My God, præpare me for it!*"

Think; "Tho' *Worms destroy this Body,* yett I have an Almighty SAVIOUR, who will Rescue it, and Restore it from them. How Easily can He now Præserve me and Restore me! *O Almighty SAVIOUR, who didst once come into the Humiliations, which did oblige even Thee to say, I am a Worm!*"

Think; "The *Worms* preying on the *Bowels* and the *Vitals,* are formidable Things. But the *Lusts* which prey upon my *Soul,* and *War against it,* are much more formidable. And there is that *Worm* of *Guilt* gnawing on and by the *Conscience,* under Sin unpardoned, which is more to be trembled at than any thing that the *Body* can Encounter with. *O Lord, I Beseech thee, Deliver my Soul!*"

There was a Capital Punishment call'd *Boating;* which the *Jews* borrow'd from the *Persians.* The Criminal was Laid on his Back in a *Boat,* and having his Hands tied fast unto Each side of it, had another *Boat* putt over him; his Head only being left out thro' a Place made fitt for it. In this Posture, they forcibly fed him with Milk and Honey, till the WORMS[4] bred in the Excrements which he voided, Eat out his Bowels, where he Lay, and so killed him. It was usually Twenty Days before the poor man Expired; until which he Lay in horrible Torments. "*Lord,* my Crimes deserve to be punished, with *Worms,* that shall breed in me, and bring a lingring and a dreadful *Death* upon me."

§ *Worms* are so very frequent a Plague, and the Cause of so many Maladies, beyond what is Commonly thought for, that it is not Easy to be too Suspicious of them. When the *Measles* were Epidemical among us, there were few of the Sick, but what voided *Worms.* Especially, When our *Children,* grow Pale, Meagre, Froward, and Feverish: it is not often Enough Enquired, *May there not be Worms in the Case!*

§ Monsr *Andry* assures us, That he has found *Borellus's* Remark to be True: That *Remedies against Worms will Signify Little, Except they be given in the Wane of the Moon.*

§ Others besides Dr. *Leigh*[5] will tell you, Eminent the Vertues of *Coralline,*[6] for the Killing of *Worms.*

§ The famous *Tho. Bartholinus,* in his *Acta Medica,* celebrates the Flowres of St. *Johns Wort,* infused in *Spirit of Wine,* as a *Most Excellent Remedy for the Expelling of Worms. Paracelsus* before him sais, That the External Application of that Plant, makes *Worms* fly before it.

§ Among the *Anthelminticks,* there is reckoned scarce any more Powerful, than *Water* that has had *Quicksilver* boil'd in it. Tho' the Body of the *Quicksilver,* be so dangerous to be taken, yett this *Water* has been thought Innocent Enough, so they say. But,—Several Children have been ruined by it.

§ *Mercurius Dulcis,* given, to Six Grains unto Children, and to Twelve or more unto Men, in Conserve of Roses, or the Pulp of an Apple, is a mighty Worm-killer. But remember, Tis a Remedy commonly adulterated. Tis therefore an Hazardous Remedy. Some have been Poisoned with it. Be Cautious!

§ Purges of *Rhubarb,* and Clysters of Milk and Sugar, are of Use; Especially when joined with other Medicines.

§ J. *Zapatha,*[7] hugely Commends, *Oil of Sulphur,* dropt in Spring-Water.

§ *Weskardus*[8] as much commends a Drink of *Rye*, and *Hop-flowers*, boiled in Milk.

§ *Wittichius*[9] cutts *Onions*, and Steeps them all night in Water, and makes a Drink of the Water.

§ *Garlick* does notable Things.

§ Almost all *Wines*, do quicken and hearten the *Worms*; But *Alicant* Wine,[10] destroys them wonderfully.

§ *Orange-peel*, dried and powdered, has been Commended.

§ A Child miserably perishing with the *Worms*, cried for a very foul *Tobacco-pipe*, with which it saw a Neighbour Smoking. It fell asleep, with the Pipe accidentally lying on the Stomach of it. Anon, it voided a great Knott of *Worms*, and recovered. On the Mention of this I am informed, that a *Tobacco-Leaf* laid unto the Navel of Children, has wonderfully saved them from this Formidable Adversary.[11]

§ *Peach-Leaves* Bruised, with the Gall of an Oxe added unto them; and the Cataplasm laid unto the Navel; has been highly Commended.

So have Earth-Worms wash'd in Wine, and dried, and boil'd, and made up with the Flowers of Saint *Johns* Wort, and Peach-leaves;—Laid unto the Stomach.

§ *D'Ube* sais, There is not a more Excellent Remedy than *Gratiola*;[12] [Hedge-Hyssop,] If you boil the Leaves, and reduce to the Consistency of a Syrup, with Sugar or Honey. A Spoonful is to be given unto Children: Two Spoonfuls to Elder People. Two Hours after, give a Clyster of Milk and Sugar.

§ Sir *Kenelm Digby* writes: Take an Apple of *Coloquintida*: Splitt it: Fry one half with the gall of an *Oxe*, till it be tender. Bind it on the Navel of the Patient, at going to Bed; Remove in the Morning. Renew it for two Nights more. He sais, *This will kill any Worms in the Gutts or Maw, be they never so many or dangerous.*

§ *Pontaeus's* famous Remedy for *Worms*, was, Fifteen Grains of *Mercurius Dulcis*, with Five Grains of *Scammony*, and three times as much Sugar; made up in Lozenges.

§ Take *Rue, Wormwood, Savin*:[13] Boil these with unsalted Butter, till you have brought the Mixture to be very green. Then strain it and pott it up for Use. When you Employ it, Annoint with it, first the Pitt of the Stomach, and Part of the Chest, a little above it. Then, after a little while, rub well upon, and all about the Navel.

§ Oil of *Savin*, on the Navel, kills Worms in Children.

And, so does Ointment of *Sowbread*.[14]

§ If you want a powerful *Worm-killer,* here is a Receipt for you. Take Half a Pint of *Rhum;* a Quarter of an Ounce of *Worm-seed;*[15] A Penn'orth or two of *Aloes;* Lett these gently Simmer together over a Fire, till a quarter be Consumed; Then add a Convenient Quantity of *Molasses,* and boil the Composition to Little. So strain it, and keep it for use.

The Dose is a Spoonful or two, for Children; and thrice as much for a Man. Tis a little Cathartick.

This has been found a most Surprising *Worm-killer.* Tis Incredible what Cures have been wrought by it, on Children troubled with *Worms.* How many Lives have been Saved by this poor, mean, homely Medicine! I am of [the] Opinion, That when Raw Fruits, and Cold Things, have brought the Children into these Maladies, this Electuary may be then most proper for them. In many Cases it may be too Inflammatory.

But then, our Countrey-People make almost a *Panacæa* of it. It strangely releeves *Pains* in the *Stomach;* and restores a ruined Appetite. It helps in *Bloody Fluxes,* and in many other Distempers.

But remember, People troubled with the *Piles* must not be too free with any thing that has *Aloes* in it.

§ The famous *Borellus* has a Notion, that *Worms* may have an Hand in most of the Diseases, which Men are annoy'd withal: *Eorumque Semper Medicus in Curatione rationem habeat.*[16]

He directs the Use of *Wormseed* above, and of Sweet-*Clyster* below, at the same time. Or, a Drop of the Essence of the *Seed,* applied in a Peece of *Cotton,* to the Navel.

He sais, he saw one, *Pro tabida habitum, et quasi Conclamatum,*[17] who was Cured, by drinking thrice a Dram of pulverized *Orange-peels,* in Wine, *Ejectione innumerorum Vermium.*[18]

§ Some say, Drink distilled Water of *Gentian.*

§ The Islanders of *Scotland,* kill *Worms,* with an Infusion of *Tansy,*[19] in *Whey,* or in *Aqua-Vitae;* taken Fasting.

§ Our Countrey People furnish themselves with a Distilled Water of *May-Weed,*[20] in which they find Wonderful Virtues, (for the Releef of *Pains,* but more particularly) for *Worms,* which perish before it.

Cap. XLV. *Intestinal Feuds Composed.*

or, The Disorders of,

A <u>Flux</u>, rectified.

WITHOUT any Puzzle about the Distinction between a *Diarrhoea,* and a *Lienteria,* and a *Coeliaca,*[1] tis enough to say, That Every body now and then feels a Malady, which we Call, *A Looseness.*

A Distemper which they reckon proceeds from a Depraved Acid or Corrupted Ferment in the Stomach, and some Indigestion there; Or from some Obstruction of the Serum, that should have been perspired thro' the Pores of the Skin, and now forces its way thro' the glands into the Intestines.

I have read of one, who propounding that his Life might be filled with *Acts of Repentance,* contrived this among other Points of Conduct, That whenever he went unto, *The House of the Secret Seat,* he would form Some Thought that should carry *Self-abasement* with it, and add unto his *Humiliations.* And certainly One follow'd with a *Diarrhoea* has an *Humbling* Opportunity to Think; "What *from the Belly is Cast out into the Draught,* tho' Lothsome Enough, is not so much to be Loathed, as that which *comes forth from the Heart, wherewith a Man is defiled.* What *Filthiness* is there to be found in my *Body;* which may therefore be very justly called, *A Vile Body;* and may Compel me to Long for the *Body,* wherein this *Corruptible* shall putt on *Incorruption?* But, oh! how much more *Abominable and Filthy is Man,* in regard of the Vile Thoughts and Frames and Lusts, with which my Inner Man is polluted? *Lord, I abhor myself before thee!* I am Lothesome to myself. How much more so to the Holy God, who *knows what is in Man,* and who *cannot look upon Iniquity!"*

The Distempered, finding his *Appetite* gone, in the Progress of his Distemper, and the most pleasant *Food* nauseated, may do well to think, What it would be well for him, to be by *Wasting Afflictions* brought unto. *My Friend,* Evacuated of one Enjoyment after another, Lett thy *Desire fail* for all Creatures, and lose thy Appetite for all that is to be Enjoy'd in this World.

A moderate *Flux,* may be very wholesome; A sort of a *Natural Cathartic;* upon Something Taken in that should be carried off. Don't make too much haste for Stopping of it. It has been particularly noted, That in Diseases of the *Head,* the Supervening of a *Flux,* is often

Useful and Healthful; (in Diseases of the *Breast,* pernicious.) There are other *Inconveniences* too, which may do us good, *if they don't go too far!*

The Malady is for the most Part Easily cured, if it be *taken in Time.* If it be *Neglected,* it may, yea, it will grow *Dangerous.* I pray, *My Friend,* Receive this Instruction, before we go any further; of all the *Ill Things* that are to be Cured, Learn to *Take them in Time.* Don't Neglect *Seasonable,* Early, Speedy Applications for the Cure of them. Delay not proper Methods, *Dum mala per Longas invaluere Moras.*[2]

When one that is in a *Consumption,* finds a *Flux* come upon him, —I hope, he has before now heard the Admonition, *Sett thy house in Order, for!*—Be sure *Now,* the Language of it is, *An End is Come, the End is come, it Watcheth for thee; Behold, it is come!*[3]

§ *Vomits* have done wonders in most obstinate *Fluxes.* Vomit with four or five Grains of *Tartar Emetic;* or, a Scruple or Two of *Salt of Vitriol.* Perhaps it must be Repeated Three or Four times, before the Number of Stools, is very notably abated. Then give Astringents and Opiates.

If in giving a *Vomit* (or a Purge) a Violent Purgation should happen, a Dram of *Venice-Treacle* will presently check it: or, a Plaister of it applied unto the Navel.

§ But *Vomits* are too hard Things for some Nice Constitutions. *Purges* are to be used for them. *Rhubarb,* is ordinarily one of the best Things that can be thought of. Monsr *D'Ube* sais "There is hardly a better and a safer Remedy under the Sun against a *Looseness,* and the *Bloody Flux* itself, than a Ptisan prepared with half an Ounce of *Rhubarb* cutt in Slices, and tied in a Peece of Cloth, while it is boiling."

§ To begin with Astringents and Opiates, in *Fluxes,* is for the most Part very Improper, very Hazardous. Even in weakly Children we must prepare for the Cure, with a *Clyster.* But in due Season for it, this has been mightly cried up; Take an Ounce of the *Juice of Quinces,* thickened with Honey; mix with it a Dram of well-powdered Root of *Tormentil.*[4] Take the Quantity to the bigness of an Hazel-nutt, Every Morning; drinking a Little Wine after it.

§ *Tormentil-Root,* powdered and Infused in Brandy; a few Drops of this on a bitt of Sugar. Tis a most wonderful Remedy in *Fluxes.* How many Childrens Lives have I known saved by it!

§ Unsalted *Butter,* gently boil'd and skim'd. Give a Quantity of this, as the Patient can bear it. It is a potent Remedy.

§ *Clysters,* made of a Decoction of unpeel'd *Barly, Bran,* and *Camomil* Flowers, with a little of the Yolk of an *Egg,* may be of good Consequence. Or, *Mallows.*[5]

§ *Milk* that has had *Mallows* boil'd in it; Sometimes This alone will do. Or, *Mallows-Tea.*

§ For *Fluxes* caus'd by Sharp Humours, Eat a Toast, that is thoroughly drench'd in very well-condition'd *Oil.*

§ To chew a Bit of *Logwood,*[6] and Swallow the Spittle, cures a *Flux,* to Admiration.

§ Tis among the *Boylaean* Receits, Boil a Convenient Quantity of *Cork* in Spring-Water, till the Liquor taste pretty Strong of it. A moderate Draught of this, from time to time.

§ Try *Fennel-Water* with Oyl of *Marsh-Mallows.*

§ *Diaphoreticks* are of great Use in *Fluxes;* And when there is Malignity in them, we must add, *Alexipharmacks.*[7]

§ Mix about a dozen Grains of powdered *Rhubarb,* with half a Dram of *Diascordium.* Take it going to Bed; or Early in the Morning, after the first Sleep.

§ Dr. *Willis* would have you toast a Peece of Bread, Spread it with Treacle, Dip it in some generous Red Wine heated, and apply it unto the Stomach.

§ A Gentleman in my Neighbourhood, cures Fluxes Infallibly, and Immediately, [So *Immediately,* that there is often Occasion to take a little Purge afterwards, to the Inconveniences of too *Quick a Cure!*] with a few Grains of *Ratts-Dung,* dissolved in a Glass of Wine, or any proper Vehicle.

§ *Ireland* suffered a sore Plague of *Diarrhoea's;* and it was never helped, until they litt on the Receit, of *Butter* and *Small Beer.*

§ A Spoonful or Two of the Q[ueen] of *Hungaries* Water, in a glass of Water, will sometimes give a Stop to a Flux.

§ In a *Tenasmus,* or a Continual Inclination to go to Stool, with little or no Evacuation, *Woodman* will tell you, The Fumes of *Turpentine* cast on burning Coals, received by the Fundament, are an Infallible Cure.

Cap. XLVI. *Jehoram Visited.*
or,
The <u>Bloody-Flux</u> remedied.

WHEN we consider the Vast Length of the *Intestines,* their Involution, and their Constitution, how can we do any other than Wonder that they Continue in any tolerable Manner performing their daily and constant Operations for so many Years? Tis no Wonder if *Distempers* do sometimes invade them, and very particularly, That of a *Dystentery,* or *Bloody Flux;* Wherein a Sharp Salt, (perhaps from a *Blood,* or at least a *Stomach,* full of a Venemous Acrimony) corrodes the Gutts, with grievous Vellications; until first the *Exteriour* Coat, thereof, and then the more *Fleshy* One, be wasted; *Ulcers* are produced, and anon *Gangrænes,* that prove mortal to the Patient.

It is marvelous to see, how Diseases of the *Intestines,* do reach, and affect, and weaken the *Mind;* and then, in the Reciprocation, how the Passions of the *Mind,* make Impressions on the *Intestines.* Nothing is of more Consequence in a *Dysentery,* than that the *Mind* be kept Calm, and Quiet and Easy; and if it be possible, Chearful. But that the *Mind* be made *Holy,* and fill'd with proper Sentiments of *Piety,* This I am sure, will be no Prejudice, to any Intention of the Cure to be aimed at.

The Patient often lies *Awake* in this Distemper; *Whole Nights* awake: The Sharp Salts in the Blood, so dilate the Pores of the *Brain.* Lett his *Waking Hours,* have as many *Holy Thoughts* as may be, filling of him. And lett him Consider, whether he has not been sometimes *Asleep* (Either Naturally, or more Spiritually,) when he should not have been so! *Whether no Sinful Sleep have been at any time indulged with him!*

Of a miserable King,[1] who by his *Bloody* Dealings with his Brethren discovered, that whatever *Entrails* he might have, he had no true *Bowels* in him, we read, *The Lord Smote him in his Bowels with an Incureable Disease; in process of time, his Bowels fell out, by reason of his Sickness: so he died of sore diseases.* A *Bloody Flux,* wasting of the *Bowels,* may justly putt the the Patient upon Examining, *What Bowels have I had?* And, *Have I not wanted Bowels toward them, whom I should have been Compassionately Concerned for?*

The Mischiefs of *Intestine Discords* in *Families* as well as *Nations,* are what a *Dysentery,* wherein one has *within his own Bowels* that which destroys him, would very Emblematically lead one to think upon.

The *Bloody Flux,* what a Nasty, Filthy, Lothesome Disease! *Patient,* Cry out, *Lord, what a Loathsome Wretch am I! I Loathe myself before thee. I Abhor myself, and Repent before thee, and thy People also!*

The Malady is *Contagious.* Lett the Wishes of the *Patient* be; That he may receive no *Sinful Infection* from others; (Bewayl it, if he has done so!) But much more That he may never Convey any *Sinful Infection* to any others.

In this Distemper, tis worse to have no Sense at all of Pain, than to be in some sensible *Pain.* When the *Pain* suddenly vanishes, but the Symptoms of the Distemper continue, it may be feared, that a *Gangræne* may have siezed the Bowels. *My God, Lett me Feel what is Amiss within me; Lett it be Painful to me. Lett me not be left unto the Stupidity of an Indolent Soul, under my Corruptions!*

I will add this; The Corrosions of *Envy* in the Soul, are as mischievous as the *Corroding Humours* of a *Dysentery;* and as much to be deprecated.

§ Lett it be well observed, whether the *Dysentery* be attended with Evident *Malignity.* If it be, then Begin the Cure with *Sweating.*

§ *Vomits* are ordinarily of great use and Force, in a *Bloody Flux.* Once *Vomiting* has wrought Sometimes a Cure, when all other Means have been unsuccessful. Twice or Thrice, it may be repeated; with Four or Five Grains of *Tartar Emetic.*[2]

§ *Diaphoreticks* are of great Consequence in this Malady. The Communication between the Bowels and the Skin is admirable.

But the Binding must not be too much or too soon, before the Particles be Evacuated and well-tempered.

§ *Purges* may be Convenient. [Mr. *Boyl* gives Rhubarb with a Grain of *Laudanum;* And then a Milk-Clyster.] *Rhubarb* alone may do.

§ Tis among the *Boylaean* Receits. Take *Pigs-Dung;* Dry it and burn it unto a grey (not white) Ashes. Of these give about half a Dram for a Dose; Drinking after it, about three Spoonfuls of Wine Vinegar.

§ So is This, proposed as, *An Experienced Medicine.* Give about three Ounces of the Juice of *Ground Ivy,* mixed with one Ounce of the Juice of *Plantain;* once or twice a day.

§ *Whey,* plentifully drank; (as also injected by *Clysters,*) is of Considerable Vertue. Several Authors count it, A *great Anti-dysenteric Arcanum.*[3] Now, no longer an *Arcanum.*

§ *Clysters* do wonders in this Distemper. We will not Cry up, One of *Mutton-broath;* so much as One of Entirely Fresh *Butter* melted; (which is also to be drank four or five Spoonfuls of it at a time.)

The most Effectual perhaps of all *Clysters,* is, Fresh Butter wherein the Parings of *Stone-Horse hoofs* has been fried. It prospers wonderfully!

§ A Decoction of *Mallows,* has its Vertues; A fine Soother, and Smoother.

§ An Army in *Ireland,* Sorely afflicted with the *Bloody-flux,* past the Help of Doctors, was almost miraculously releeved, by this Receit of an Irishman. Take the Partition-Pith of a *Walnutt,* and Dry it. So pulverize it, and then drink as much as can be heaped on a Groat, or Sixpence, in Wine, or any Convenient Vehicle.[4]

§ Warm *Cowes-Milk,* taken every morning, with a Red-hott Steel quenched in it. Of this Monsr *D'Ube* sais, *you can't pitch upon a more proper thing.*

§ *Borellus* tells us, Clysters of *Goats-Milk,* have proved the Only Remedy in an *Epidemical Dysentery.*

§ A famous Man sais, There is not a more Specific Remedy, than *Rose-Water* wherein Gold has been quenched several times.

§ A Gentleman of my Acquaintance, wrought very many wonderful Cures of the *Bloody Flux,* (when all other Means failed) with this Easy Remedy. Take *Nutt-Galls,* and (throwing away the Inside) beat the Shells to a Powder. Of this Powder take as much as may ly upon a Sixpence, in a Spoonful of Good French Brandy. Three or Four Doses (in so many mornings) does the Cure.

§ An Infusion of the *Root* of *Tormentil,* in Brandy; a few Drops of this, given in any Convenient Vehicle, or on a Lump of white Sugar. I know a Gentlewoman, who does notable Cures with this, in Bloody, as well as other, *fluxes.* Little Children may take it.

§ *Dolaeus* affirms, That he Cured above an hundred, when this Plague was epidemical; with *Oyl* of *Sweet Almonds* mixed with Juice of *Citron;*[5] Taken often in a day.

§ Here's an *Enema Spirituosum*. Take Spirit of *Wine;* Eight Ounces. Oil of *Turpentine,* and Oil of *Anniseeds,* Ten drops of Each. Broth of a *Sheeps-head,* Eight Ounces. Mix, and Exhibit warm. A Famous Physician affirms, from his own Experience; That it is an admirable Specific against the *Bloody Flux,* and has Cured People that have been at the very Point of Death.

§ *Cataplasms* outwardly applied unto the Region of the Bowels, have their Significancy. *The Crumb of Bread with Tormentil-Root,* boil'd in Wine or Vinegar, is a notable One. So is a Plaister of *Diascordium* and *Venice-treacle.*

§ *Thea,*—(and *Milk-Thea,*) Drink freely of it.

§ *Dolaeus* makes a pious and a discreet Conclusion; *Prayers, the best of Remedies must be frequently used,* on this Occasion. I desire that This Period of *Dolaeus,* may be understood always at the *End of the Chapter,* in Every Article of the Treatise, which is now before us.

CAP. XLVII. *Miserere Mei!*
or, Compassions for
The Cholic,
and, The Dry-Belly-ache.

A MOST grievous Pain, in the Intestines! The *Cholon*[1] particularly so much the Seat of it, as to give a Name unto it.

There is, what they call, *The Humoral Cholic,* which proceeds from a Vitious and Acid Humour, irritating the Fibres of the Intestines. A Viscid Flegm, generating a Wind, which distends the Intestines, is what they call, *The Flatulent Cholic.* There is also, what they call, *The Bilious Cholic,* which may happen to produce *Ulcers* in the Intestines, with the Inflammation which it gives unto them. There is likewise, *The Convulsive Cholic,* which is Exasperated by Catharticks, and such hott Spirituous Medicines as may releeve in other *Cholicks,* but finds a Strange Releef, by Anodynes, and by Bleeding in the Foot. We will here Chiefly Consider the Two first of these; which we will Suppose, they that attend upon the Sick, will know how to distinguish.

Willis will needs find in the *Brain,* the Cause of this Malady in the *Bowels.* The Malady may lead the *Brain* to some Employment in the *Thoughts* of PIETY there to be rais'd and form'd upon it.

The *Passions* of the Mind, must be much Suppress'd and Compos'd in this Malady; Else,—But then, there are *Sentiments* of the Mind, which are seasonably to be Excited in it, and from it.

The Patient is in Exquisite *Pain,* and it is to be hoped, that he will in his Anguish keep crying to a God full of Compassion, in such Terms as these; Psal. XXV. 18. *Lord, Look upon my Affliction and my Pain, and Forgive all my Sin.*

But, my Friend, wilt thou not also confess, *O my God, I deserve all these Pains inflicted on me; yea, Sore Pains and of Long Continuance! What else can he do, who has done like me, and has denied the God that is Above!*

Wilt thou not infer; *If the Effect be so Bad, what is the Cause? Lord, My Sin has exposed me to this Pain. Oh! What an Evil and a Bitter Thing is it, that I have Sinned against my God!*

Wilt thou not infer; *If it be so Sad a Thing to ly Some Hours in this Pain upon Earth; what would it be to ly unknown and endless Ages in the Dolours of Hell, which cause perpetual wailing and gnashing of Teeth?*

Will not these Thoughts quicken thy Flight unto thy SAVIOUR?

But, O *Patient,* wilt thou indeed be *Patient?* Cry to thy God, That He would Strengthen thee with *Patience to Long-suffering;* and that *Patience may have its Perfect Work.* It was with an Allusion to one under the *Cholic,* that the Prophet cries out, *My Loins are filled with Pain; I am bowed down.*

Lett not One *Impatient Word* be heard from thee; Not one Word that shall have in it the least *Complaint,* or *Murmur,* against the Dispensations of a Sovereign and Righteous God; Not a Word but what shall carry in it, a most humble Submission to the *Will* of thy God; with an Hope, That it will at last be found, *God has meant all unto Good.*

If the *Cholic* proceed unto that, which is called, *The Iliac Passion,*[2] (which, because the *Peristaltic Motion* of the Gutts is inverted in it, and the Excrements are vomited at the Mouth, tis called, *The Twisting of the Gutts,*) the Same Sentiments will still be Seasonable.

And as the Name of, *Miserere mei, Deus!* or, *Lord, Be merciful to me!* has been putt upon it, such, *O Miserable,* must be thy Cry to God thy SAVIOUR under it. But, *Hope in His Mercy;* tho' Confessing thyself most *Unworthy* of it. He *takes pleasure in them that hope in His Mercy.*

Methinks, the People who *Speak Wickedly;* profanely, obscenely, or calumniously, (Especially *Profane Swearers,*) have Something like the *Iliac Passion* on them; and what is as much to be deprecated.

Trifling and Endless *Talkers,* also have a Disease that some have called, *The Upward Looseness,* and would have the Guilty affronted, with a Motion for a *Chamber-Pott.*

§ The *Romans,* as *Pliny* assures us, knew nothing of the *Cholic,* before their cursed Monster *Tiberius*[3] had it. Nor had been any thing read of *The Hysteric Cholic,* before our Blessed *Sydenham* wrote about it. Wherefore, in the Cure of the *Cholic,* it must much be considered, whether it be of the *Hysterick* Sort or no.

§ *Vomits* have been known to work Wonderful Cures upon *Cholicks.*

§ *Helmont* cured one that had been long afflicted with violent Pains of the Cholic frequently returning on them, with only perswading them to leave off Drinking of *Beer,* brewed with *Well-Water.* The Clay, it seems, is a Mineral Glebe,[4] which impregnates *Well-Water* with *Metallic Salts,* that some can't Encounter with.

§ An *Humoral Cholic* has been help'd by *Milk* boil'd with *Garlic.*

§ Take four or five Balls of *Stone-horse Dung,* (fresh,) Steep them for about a Quarter of an Hour in a Pint of *White-Wine,* in a Vessel well stopped. Give of it, from a Quarter to Half a Pint. Have a Care of taking any Cold after it. This is good in several other Maladies.

§ *Chamomil-Flowres* infused in Drink of almost any sort. *Woodman* sais, *There is hardly a better Anti-cholic Remedy in the whole Republic of Physick. Baglivi* sais, *Camomil* is the true Antidote of a *Cholic,* from any Cause whatever.

§ Take *Nitre,* One Ounce; rub it well in a clean Mortar. Grind with it a Scruple or more, of *Saffron.* Give half a Dram for a Dose, in three or four Ounces of Cold Spring Water.

§ Laxative and Anodyne *Clysters,* are of good Consequence, if the Body be costive.

§ Smoke of *Tobacco,* so administred:—has been a frequent Experiment.

But *Ettmuller,* as well as *Bartholin,* decries, glisters from a Decoction of *Tobacco,* as extremely dangerous. However, The Smoke of a lighted Pipe of *Tobacco,* blown into Water, and the Water drunk, has been a notable Remedy.

§ Take a Quart of *Clarett,* with Two Ounces of *Nettleseeds,* in a Bottel well stop'd. Keep it in boiling Water, till the Water has made three or four Warms, to assist the Wines Inprægnation with the Seeds. Of this Liquor take a Draught once or twice a day.

§ *Sperma Ceti* taken with Oyl of Sweet *Almonds,* in hott Brothe. *Crato,* a famous Physician to Three Emperours, reckon'd that among *Arcana,* for the *Cholic.*

§ Tis among the *Boylaean* Receits. Take about half a Dram of *Mastick,*[5] and mix it with the Yolk of a *New-laid Egg.* Lett it be given once or twice a day.

§ *Dolaeus* cured a Student given over for Dead, with nothing but a Decoction of *Tamarinds.*[6] He highly Commends also *Sperma Ceti* (fresh and not grown rancid;) in a glass of generous Wine.

§ In a Fitt of the *Cholic,* Scarce any thing like Half a Dram of Express'd Oil of *Nutmegs,* dissolved in some Spoonfuls of Good Wine. Take it hott.

§ *Whey,* and all Testaceous Powders and things which will imbibe the turbulent Acid, are Commended in a *Cholic* which is of a *Melancholic Original.*

§ A *Flatulent Cholic* has been cured, only by taking a dozen drops of the *Oyl of Juniper;* four times a day, for three days together.

§ Here is, *An Excellent Remedy for Fitts of the Cholic, and some Kinds of Convulsions.* [Among the *Boylaean* Receits.]

Take Flowre of *Sulphur,* and *Sugar-Candy,* of Each, an Ounce; grind them; On this drop Thirty drops of Oil of *Caraway-seeds;* as much of Oil of *Orange;* and as much of Oil of *Anniseeds.* Incorporate these well, and of the Mixture give Twenty or Thirty grains for a Dose.

§ I have often helped the *Cholic,* with a few Spoonfuls of the Queen of *Hungaries Water,* thrown into a Porringer of *Beer;* taken very hott.

While others will tell you, that a little *Hott Flip,*[7] with Butter in it, is the most potent of all Remedies, for this Distemper.

§ A Decoction of *Burdock seeds,* often cures a *Cholic.*

§ A few Cloves of *Garlick,* infused in White Wine; (to which add a Little Juice of *Horse-dung;*—and *say nothing:*) A Little Draught of this; for Two or Three days; does Wonders in the *Cholic;*

yea, in that which they call, the *Stone-Cholic;* and the *Strangury;* and the *Stone* itself.

§ The yellow Peel of *Oranges,* powdered; Half a Dram. The *Boylaean* Receits call this, *An Incomparable Medicine.*

§ *Black Rhadishes,* pared and dried and powdered; as much as may ly on an half-crown, drank with a little warm Ale. This has been a great *Secret* for the *Cholic.* Tis now *divulged.*

§ Here is, *an approved Remedy for inveterate Scorbutic Cholicks, and Pains of the Bowels.* [Among the *Boylaean* Receits.] Take *English Barley,* and having well washed it, boil it in a sufficient Quantity of Spring Water, till it be ready to burst. Then pour off the clear upon the yellow Part of the Rinds of *Lemons,* freshly cutt off from the thick Part. Keep it well stopt in a Bottel. Make a common drink of it.

§ Obstinate *Bilious Cholicks* have been cured by *Riding.*

§ Some that have been used unto frequent Returns of the Cholic, have had a wondrous Cure, by a Spoonful of *Carduus Benedictus* pulverised, which you may take in Sugar, or any Convenient Syrup, for some little while.

§ Be not over free with *Topicals.* If you use any, they should be Nervine ones. Spirit of *Sal-Armoniac,* with Ointment of *Marsh-mallows,* may do very well.

§ *Manlius* tells us, he commonly cured the Scholars of their *Cholicks, Hoc Levissimo Remedio;*[8] applying a little Bag of *Oats,* warm to the Place.

§ A *Consulsive Cholic* usually retreats before a *Tea* of *Anniseeds, Fennel-seeds,* and *Caraway-seeds,* plentifully taken.

§ In the *Iliac Passion,* all possible Endeavours must be used, both Inwardly and Outwardly, to make the Belly Soluble. *Opiates* are hurtful.

Loos'ning and Cooling of *Clysters* are of great Consequence. (Made of Mutton borth [sic.] and Butter; with a Decoction of Marsh-mallows.)

§ *Whey,* with a little *Sèna* infused;—Or, *Sena* in the Juice of *Sweet-Prunes;*—These are good Things in Constipations of the Bowels.

An Appendix; of the
Dry-Belly-ache.

A Grievous and Fearful Disease, an Appendix to the *Cholic,* is now broke in upon a miserable World; called, *The Dry-Belly-Ache.*

Of this, there are indeed several Sorts; There is the *Scorbutic;* and the *Rheumatic;* and the *Nervous.* The *Fibres* of the Nerves in the Intestines, are usually affected in this Malady. And the Malignity, which does Corrode them, or Inflate them, not being wisely Carried off, it is dispersed all over the Body, and a Loss of the Limbs Ensues. There is oftentimes a *Splenetic* and *Hysteric* Addition to the Malady, which not being duely Observed and Managed, it frequently issues in the Death of the Patient, by terminating in a *Consumption.*

Under the Torments of this horrible Disease, we may recommend unto the Patient, such Sentiments of PIETY as we found the *Cholic* leading to.

And be sure, a *Perfect Work of Patience,* is to be Endeavoured. My Friend, Lett thy Cry at the worst be that; *Why should a Living Man Complain? a Man for the Punishment of his Sin!* Yeeld so profound a Submission to the Will of God, as may afford an agreeable Spectacle to the *Angels,* as well as the *Neighbours,* who are the Spectators of thy Sufferings, and of thy Patience under them. *If any Man lack this Wisdome, Lett him ask it of God.* And if thou find Him, *the God of Patience,* thou wilt anon find Him, *The God of Consolation.*

If *Bad Courses* have brought this Malady upon thee, then lett *Repentance* also have its *Perfect Work.* Poenitently own, *I have sinned, and I have done very foolishly.* Poenitently beg, *Lord, Look on my Pain, and forgive all my Sin!*

§ In so Difficult a Case, and where so nice a Conduct is required, I dare not offer any Præscription, but, *A Wise Physician.* Consult such an One; and follow his Directions, relying wholly on the Blessing of God. He will præscribe *Opening Apozems;*[9] and then—he knows what.

§ And yett I will venture to report; That I have known some good People gett a Living by præparing the following Drink, for this obstinate Malady. It may be, Reader, Thou knowest, how little it may differ from *Daffy*'s famous *Elixir Salutis.*[10]

℞ Senna, or Rhubarb; Liquorice; Anniseed, Coriander[11]-seed, Elecampane; of Each Four Ounces; *Lignum Vitae*[12] dust; Eight Ounces; Raisins of the Sun, Two Pounds, Brandy or Rum, Six Quarts. Infuse it, Nine Days in a Vessel, stop't close; and Stir it once a Day. Strain the Infusion thro' a Cloth, and bottel it.

The Dose is an Ounce or Two at a Time:—and so continued as to keep the Body Soluble with it.—

§ The Plant called *Cajacia*[13] in *Piso,*[14] and by the Spaniards called *Erudos Cobres;* that is to say, a *Snakeweed;*[15] I find the Physicians in the *West-Indies* use it as a Specific for the *Dry-Belly-ache.* They give a Dram of it powdered, in any Convenient Liquor; and Repeat once in three or four Hours, till the Symptoms abate. Sometimes they give one, two, three Ounces of it, in Syrups: They give it also in Decoctions and Clysters.

§ Yea, I will venture to report, that there has been an astonishing Success of this Method and Medicine upon this terrible Malady. First give an *Emetic:* (but of that Sort, which is also *Cathartic,*) And then, Three or four Grains of *Paracelsus's Laudanum.*[16]

Tho' *Opiates* are so dreaded and so forbid in this Distemper, *Virginia* will show you multitudes Cured by the aforesaid *Laudanum.*[17]

CAP. XLVIII. *Ashdodes.*[1]

or,

The Piles.

TIS no rare thing, for the *Hæmorrhoidal Veins,* to be distended, and Even Corroded, by the Resort of a *Blood* full of Acrimony thither. A grievous Pain accompanies it; with an Inflammation. And oftentimes a Flux of pure *Blood* follows; even in such a Quantity as greatly to weaken the Patient, and bring on the Hazards of a *Dropsy.*

The Patient ought certainly to *humble* himself before God and Man, and *walk softly* under the *Humiliations* of such a Malady.

The *Seat* of it, in the *Parts of Dishonour,* which can't be mentioned among people of any Breeding without a sort of Blush, seems to oblige the Sufferer unto *Self-Abasement.*

It was, by the infliction of this Malady, upon a Wicked People whose *Cry went up to Heaven* upon it, that there was that thing accomplished; *He smote His Enemies in the Hinder Parts; He putt them unto a Perpetual Reproach.*

O Child of Man, thus under the *Corrections* of Heaven, make these Reflections.

"*My God,* am I Chastised like One of thy *Enemies.* I mourn, that I have been so much among them. I fly, I fly, from *the Tents of those Wicked Men.*

My God putts me to *Shame. Lord,* I ly down *in my shame.* I own that all possible confusion belongs unto me.

I am not more concerned, that my Blood should be *Sweetened,* and kept from all painful Ebullitions, than I should be, that I may obtain a Sweetness of Spirit, and become *Full of Goodness.*"

§ When the Flux of the *Hæmorrhoids* is moderate, and season-able, it purges the Body of its fæculent Blood, and Prevents and Re-moves Diseases, that cannot be Numbred. But if it grow too much, behold, a Secret for it. Take the Juice of *Yarrow*,[2] depurated,[3] One Pint; White *Sugar* Two Ounces; Mix. The Dose is Three or Four Ounces, twice a day.

Riverius tells you, the Decoction of *Yarrow* taken as an usual Drink, for three days together, takes off the Pain of the *Piles.*

§ Our common People have a common Medicine for the *Piles.* Take the *Inside Leather* on the *Sole of a Shoe,* which has been Long Worn, and had the Sweat of the Foot Sufficiently tingeing of it. Pul-verize This; and lett the *Powder* be taken Inwardly.

§ To appease the Pains of the *Hæmorrhoids,* there is a good use of *Blood-Letting,* both in the Arm and the Foot. And an Application of a Fomentation made of *Linseed* boil'd in *Milk,* unto the Part affected.

§ *Fresh Butter* beaten in a *Leaden Mortar,* or with a *Leaden Pestle,* or well-tinged by being wrought with any *Leaden* Instrument, has been applied with good Success.

§ Some take an *Onion* bruised, (and the Root of a *Lilly,* some add) made up with *Linseed* Oil.

§ *D'Ube* sais, Among all Remedies, the *Oil of Box*[4] deserves the preference; Apply only a Drop at a time, with a little Cotton-wool.

§ If the *Hæmorrhoids* are gone so far as Exulceration, Take a Dram of *Frankincense*[5] well-powdered; the Yolk of an Egg; Two Grains of Opium; and a Little Linseed Oil. Mix it well, and apply to the Part affected.

§ A most excessive *Bleeding* of the *Hæmorrhoids,* has been cured with nothing but the Syrup of dried *Roses.*

§ When the Blood falls with a violent Motion towards the *Hæm-orrhoidal* Veins, there may be occasion for Blood-Letting in the Su-perior Parts; for Violent Frictions; and Strong Ligatures on the Arms; perhaps, for *Cupping* on the Breast, and other Parts that may be proper for it.

§ For Fomentations there may be used, the Decoction of the Root of the great *Comfry*.

§ Rags dipt in the Gelly of *Quince seed,* made with *Plantain-water,* Stop the violent agitation of the Blood in those Parts.

§ Tis among the *Boylaean* Receits, Take powdered *Earth-Worms;* with as much *Hens-grease,* as will serve to make it up into an Ointment. Apply to the Part affected; it commonly, safely, quickly mitigates the Pains of the *Piles.*

And This; A Suppository of *Hogs Lard.*

And this; The Sole of an *Old Shoe* burnt unto a tender Coal, and powdered; and mixed with unsalted Lard.

§ Here's an Internal. Take two Scruples of good *Sulphur Vive;*[6] mix it with a Little Sugar. Give this Dose once or twice a day.

§ Or, Take *Yarrow-posset.*[7]

§ After all, if the Violent Bleeding so continue that the Strength of the Patient is likely to be quite Exhausted, Monsr *D'Ube* sais, Take some of the same Blood, which issues from the *Hæmorrhoidal Veins,* and mix it with a little powdered Mud; make it up into a Thin Paste; and being applied unto the affected Part, it will infallibly stop the Bleeding.

§ For Dolours and Tumors of the *Hæmorrhoids;* Fresh *Leeks,*[8] being shred and fried with fresh Butter, make a Poultis, which is in the *Boylaean* Receits called, *A Choice Medicine.*

And so is, *Album Graecum*[9] well-powdered, and mixed with Goose-Grease.

§ Or, Take the Fume of Boiled *Milk.*

CAP. XLIX. *Scabiosus.*

or,

The Itch, safely and quickly chas'd away.

A FREQUENT, but a Grievous, Malady. A Salt, a Sharp, a Biting *Humor,* gott in between the Skin, and the Scarfe-skin; first breaking out in lesser, and Itching Pimples; and anon in more Troublesome Scabs, especially about the Joints, and between the Fingers.

Too well known, to need any Description.

Under this Calamity, the afflicted have the *Love of their Neighbour* wanting in them, if they do not think, that it would be a sad

Addition unto their Calamity, to be the unhappy Instruments of Conveying it unto *Others,* and if they do not use all possible Caution and Faithfulness, that *Others* may not be infected from them.

At the same time, O *Scabby Creature,* Be humbled in a Sense of thy *Lothsomeness;* and if thy *Itch* has made thee *Lothsome,* think, that thy *Sin,* has much more made thee so.

Think; "Twas a culpable *Itch,* to *know Good and Evil,* that is, to know Every thing, that was a Sad Ingredient of our First Fall from God. Lett my *Itch* putt me in mind, of that woful *Fall;* and Quicken my *Repentance* for it, and my Flight, unto thee, O my SAVIOUR, who art the *Second Adam,* and the Restorer of the Fallen."

Think; "A much worse *Itch* than that upon my *Body,* would be, a Criminal *Itch* in my Spirit for to know the *Secret Things* which *belong unto the Lord. Lord, Save me from a Sinful Curiosity.*"

Think; "An *Itch* in my *Soul,* after *Novelties,* may betray me into worse mischiefs, than that which my *skin,* is infested withal, if it be not limited by the Rules of Wisdome. *Itching Ears* have betrayed many unwary People, into the *Error of the Wicked. My God, Keep thou thy Servant from them!*"

Think; "I am a *Mangy* Creature; And shall I not be an *Humble* One! The Best Friends I have, *Shun* me, are afraid of *Touching* me. Did I know myself, I should Even wish that I could gett away from myself. What an Abhorrence am I, to the Holy *Angels* of God! I am advised unto *Brimstone* for my Remedy; how much do I deserve to be thrown in the *Lake that burns with Fire and Brimstone, for my Punishment!*"

A famous Man, was ambitious to have his Fame established on his being the Author of that Sentence, *Disputandi pruritus est Ecclesiae Scabies.*[1]

§ Tis wonderful that after so many Exemples of the Horrid and Fatal Effects, which *Quicksilver Girdles*[2] have had, when worn for the *Itch,* any People will still be so hardy as to venture upon them. Dr. *Fuller,* in his *Medicina Gymnastica,* from his own Experience, when he had *catched a certain cutaneous Infection, more Troublesome than Dangerous,* and would needs *apply a Substance well-charged with a dangerous Mineral,* gives a Just Warning to you all.

§ And yett this Remedy is Commended by Mr. *Boyl.*

Take Strong *Quicklime* one Pound, with a Gallon of Spring-water, and lett them lie together for Some Hours, and then warily pour off the clear, and filter the rest. Then take Two Ounces of *Quick-*

silver tied up in a Linen-Bag. Hang in the Liquor; and Boil it for half an hour or more. Then pour off the clear Water once more; And wash the Hands only therewith, twice or thrice a day.

However, I can tell you, That Even this Remedy, as Innocently as it Looks, has thrown Some into a *Salivation.* I therefore entreat, that such an Edged Tool as *Quicksilver,* may in this Case, be no more plaid withal.

§ A little of the *Flowre of Brimstone*[3] (as much as may ly upon a six-pence) must be taken inwardly, in Milk, or Sugar, or Mollasses, at going to Bed, while the Cure is going on.

When one is but *suspiciously guilty* of the *Itch,* This will presently so drive it out, as to discover the *Thief.*

§ Then, an Ointment of *Brimstone* with *Hogs-fatt,* is the Grand unsavoury Remedy. If while this operation is carrying on, you keep the Patient sweating in a warm Bed *Eight and Forty hours,* a total Cure is usually wrought in a *Minute,* that is to say, in *Eight and Forty Hours.*

§ But some find, a Lotion, of *Brimstone* with *Elecampane* boild in *Vinegar,* to be as Effectual, and less unsavoury.

§ Some chuse to mix their *Brimstone,* with *Soft Sope,*[4] rather than *Hogs-fatt;* and find it, more Penetrating and Efficacious, and less offensive.

To those who are so nice that they cannot endure Hogs Fat or any Unguent outwardly applied; *Borellus* would have a Decoction of *Mallows* with *Allum* applied: He says, that thrice washing with This Warm is exceeding good to cure the Itch.[5]

§ An Unction with Oil of *Bays,*[6] is a sovereign Remedy.

§ Some that have an Horror of *Brimstone,* think they have a Sufficient Remedy, in *Dock-root*[7] and *Elecampane,* sliced, and mixed with Hogs-fatt. Lett the Patient anoint himself a Week, and then have the Patience to forbear Changing his Cloaths for another Week; and the Business is done.

Or, Boil them in Water, and wash the Parts with the strained Liquor.

§ *Borellus* would have *Souldiers,* and *Beggars,* use only to wash themselves with *Black Sope;*[8] which indeed should quickly be wash'd off again, to prevent Excoriation.

Cap. L. *Singultus finitus.*
or,
A Stop to the <u>Hiccough</u>.

THE Stomach Elaborating a certain Volatil *Salt,* of great Use to all the Body, Sometimes this degenerates into an Acid and Viscid Filth, which sticking fast unto the upper Orifice of the Stomach, the *Diaphragm* to which it is Connected, is thrown into a convulsive Contraction, accompanied with the Noise, which we call, *The Hiccough.*

The *Hiccough,* [or, the *Hicket* rather, for tis a *Teutonic* Word, that signifies, To *Sob,*] appears a Lively Emblem, of the Struggle between the *Flesh* and the *Spirit,* in the Life of PIETY.

The Conflict, O pious Mind, gives all the Troublesome Uneasiness of an *Hicket* unto thee. The *Remainders of Indwelling Sin,* which give so many and endless Vellications to thee, I know, trouble thee, more than all the Calamities in the World.

But, Never give over the *Throws* of the Good Principle in thee, to Cast off this *Filth:* Never lett the Battle Cease, till thou art *a Conqueror and more than a Conqueror.*

Faint not; But almost ready to faint, when thy *Hicket* gives thee an Agony, turn thine Eyes *Inward* upon the Corruption whereof thou dost feel the Daily Irritations; and so turn thine Eyes *Upward,* crying out, *O wretched one that I am, Who shall deliver me?*

Lett it Reconcile thee to the Thoughts of *Dying;* That thy Death will putt an End unto the Conflict.—

§ For an ordinary *Hicket,* which People every day fall into, there are abundance of Remedies known to Every One; Besides, that of a little *Fright,* or some Intense *Thought,* into which, we pleasantly Betray our Friends. e.g. chew *Anniseeds.* Or Take powdered *Nutmeg.*

There are *Magical Superstitions* practised Sometimes on this Occasion, which a *Good Christian* must have an Abhorrence for.

§ Two or three preserved *Damsons* at a Time, Sometimes will do.

§ *Sneezing* has been found a powerful Remedy, when the *Hicket,* has not been otherwise quickly Conquered.

§ A Carminative Clyster, has been a Cure, for a long *Hicket,* otherwise Invincible.

§ Of *Opiates* joined with appropriate Præcipitaters, *Dolaeus* will tell you, *They never can be sufficiently Commended.*

§ When things have come to the Last Extremity, and the *Hicket* has continued very many Days, I have known a *Vomit* bring an Effectual Cure.

Cap. LI. EPHPHATHA.

or,

Some Advice to STAMMERERS.[1]

How to *gett Good* by, and how to *gett rid* of their
grievous Infirmity.

THERE is a great Number of Mankind, that have the unhappy and uneasy Infirmity of STAMMERING, to lay Curbs upon them.

Sometimes a Weakness, upon that Pair of *Nerves,* which give Motion and Vigour to the Organs of *Speech,* may be the Original of this Infirmity. And hence I have known such a Thing as the *Spirit* of *Lavender,* or the Q[ueen] of *Hungaries* Water, (used both outwardly and inwardly) still presently and sensibly unfetter one that spoke with Difficulty; when the Drinking of *Coffee* would increase the Fetters. But with Some, there may be a silly *Trick* of *Stuttering,* which a Little Discretion might reform and releeve to admiration.

My Bretheren: Tis a very grievous *Humiliation,* under which the Glorious God has Laid you in this Infirmity. Our most merciful SAVIOUR beholding *One that had an Impediment in his Speech,* it is remarkable, *He Sighed upon it:* It grieved his Merciful Soul, to See Such a *Sad Case,* among the miserable Children of Men. Indeed All that hear the *Stammerer,* if they have any Goodness in them, employ a *Sigh* upon the Sufferer. And they that have no Goodness nor Honour nor Breeding in them, are too ready to make him the Object of an *Inhumane Derision:* whose *Mocking* has indeed been so *Catching,* that we have seen many of these Uncivil Creatures, who have in this way *Reproached their Maker,* by a Conspicuous Vengeance of Heaven rendred Incureable and Contemptible *Stutterers* all their days. Be sure then, the *Stammerer* himself cannot but fetch many a *Sigh,* when he feels God continually *Binding* of him: and when Every *Business* and Every *Company,* wherewith he is concerned, putts him in *Pain,* how to gett thro' the *Speaking Part* which he has before him. Certainly, such a *Misery* should not be Endured, without many Essays to *fetch Good out of Evil:* And a *Prudent Conduct* under it, should be mightily Laboured for.

It will not be amiss for me here to transcribe, what Mr. *Hezekiah Woodward*[2] relates of his own Experience.

"I disquieted myself about my *Imperfection in Speech* very much: So much, as more cannot well be imagined: And all that, *But a Disquieting in Vain.* But yett, this Good was in it: The *Sowre* yielded the *Sweet;* it kept me close *Within,* when others were *Without,* perhaps merrier, but not so well Employ'd. It made me Look up the oftner unto *Him,* (for I saw, I had need of Him) *who made Mans Mouth.* The very Thought of my infirmity kept me *Low;* Every way *Low;* in my Thoughts also; it kept me from *Aspiring;* and it was well so; Else I had been perking too high. Assuredly, I could not have wanted this *Defect.* But it was Long before I thought so; *Long* before I could Cast Anchor upwards. *After all,*—God crossed my Friends Designs, and dashed all our Projects, and placed me in such a *Calling,* and that Place, *which was least thought of!*—I would conclude from hence; *Whatever is wanting to the Child, Lett not Education be wanting,*—What know we, *what the great God intends them for?" Thus that godly Minister.*

I proceed with saying; Your *First Care* must be to make a very *Pious Improvement* of your very *humbling Chastisement* which a Sovereign God has Laid upon you. It calls for such a *Self-Abhorring* and *Self-Abasing* Frame of Mind in you, and such a *Lowly Carriage* towards all about you, as may become one who apprehends himself *marked of God,* and Exposed for the Compassion of all that he has to deal withal; being deprived of a *Faculty* and a *Liberty,* wherein every *Prating Fool* thinks himself Superiour to him.

Yea, how Sollicitously ought you in the Methods of PIETY, to make sure of it, that tho' you here carry about with you, a perpetual *Mark* of one whom God will have to be *Laid Low* in this World, yett you may hereafter be found among them whom God has chosen for *Vessels of Honour,* and such as He has (even in this way) *prepared for Glory!*

And the more you are Chased out of Conversation, and *Unfitt* for, and perhaps grown *Averse* to, the Delights of *Humane Society,* the more you will do well to Converse with your SAVIOUR in the *Religion of the Closett.* You *Sitt alone and keep Silence, because you have born* what you have *upon* you: yea, you *putt your Mouth in the Dust* and speak little more than the Dead: But you will make the Experiment, how far, *the Lord is good unto the Soul that seeks Him.*

One would imagine, That there should be Little Need of advising you, to avoid *Loquacity*. And yett such is the Senseless Folly of them who should *Shew themselves Men,* that there is nothing more frequent, than for *Stammerers* to speak Ten times more than they need to do it. One would think, that there were Danger of their growing like some of the Mahometan *Dervises,*[3] that will not speak *One Word,* Lett the Provocation be what it will, for *Six* or *Seven* years together. But they are not so on the *Reserve.* No, they are on the *Reverse.* It Seems as if thro' the Joy and Pride of their being able to speak *Some Words* freely, they must ostentate This unto all People, at the Expence of showing their *Foible* also to them. Certainly they are not aware, how ungrateful a *Jar,* their broken and blundering way of Speaking, which has intermixed so many *Inanes sine mente*[4] *Sonor* in it, makes in the Ears of those that hear them. Did they *Design* to *afflict* and *affront* the Company, they could not act much otherwise than they do. Or, They act as if thro' a *Judgment* of Heaven upon them, they had a Design to *Expose themselves* unto Pitty wherever they come. There can be nothing more *Advisable* for *Stammerers,* than the *Wisdome,* of being very *Silent People,* and not forward at all, to run into a way wherein Every Step will be a *Troublesome Stumble.* In some *Religious Houses,* a Sentence of Imposed *Silence* for such or such a Term of Time, has been a considerable Article of their *Discipline.* An Imposition of much *Silence* is a *Discipline* of God, which the *Stammerer* ought prudently to submitt unto. The ancient Gentleman, known by the Syrname of, *Silentiarius,*[5] was not the most Imprudent Man in the World. We read of, *A Fool that holdest his Peace,* and is counted *Wise* for doing so. *Friend,* If thou wouldest not proclame thyself, *A Fool,* then Learn to *hold thy Peace.* Never Speak, but upon very just Occasions; and then, lett it be as *Laconically,* Properly, Concisely, and in as *Few Words* as may be.

Stammerers are often of too *Choleric* a Disposition; and *Sooner Angry* than they should be: whereas they of all People, should always maintain the *Meekness of Wisdome.* For Anger will cause them to *Stammer* with *unspeakably* more of observable, and Even Ridiculous Titubation,[6] than they do at other times. Indeed there was one *Slow of Speech,* and *of a Slow Tongue,* of whom we read, That *he was very meek, above all the men which were upon the face of the Earth.* It were well, if all the Tribe of *Stammerers,* would Seek and Strive to be so.

Be sure, For *Stammerers* to *Speak Wickedly,* what can there be more Abominable, more Intolerable? For a *Stammerer* to be a

Swearer; for *Lying,* or *Obscene,* or *Profane* words to come out of a *Stammering* Mouth: what can be so Odious, what so Hideous? A *Thief* on a *Cross,* blaspheming the Son of God was a Sad Spectacle. *Wretch,* Thou art as bad and horrid and shocking a Spectacle! *Boring thro' the Tongue* has been Sometimes a Punishment for *Blasphemies.* Thy *Tongue* is in some sort already *bored;* and shall it *now* give an hissing Articulation unto *Blasphemies?* How worthy such a *Tongue,* to be thrown into a Torment, where a *Drop of Water* to cool it, will be in Vain wished for!

But for the *Little Talk* of *Stammerers,* if they must have any, I would propose, that they Endeavour a *Compensation* for their inconvenience, by as Exquisite Contrivance as may be, *To Speak Usefully.* May they be awakened by their *grievous Exercise,* To Study a very *Fruitful Conversation,* and forever to project, that what little they say, may be what the Hearers may be the Wiser and the Better for; and what may *Minister some Grace* unto them.

One that was very much a *Stammerer,* found a Strange Consolation and Encouragement, in a Speech of *Romanus,* a celebrated Person among the primitive Martyrs, who, when they were going to cutt out his Tongue, said, *He that speaks CHRIST shall never want a Tongue.* And the Story of its Literal Fulfilment, would be very marvellous; hardly credible. Nor has it been altogether unworthy of Observation; That there have been *Preachers* of CHRIST, (like Mr. *Gellibrand,*)[7] who in their *Ordinary Talk* were *Stammerers,* but in their public Ministrations had a *Fluency* which their Auditors have wondered at.

Who can tell, what a Release from the Extremity of your *Infirmity* may be obtained, by your ardent and constant Prayers, to a SAVIOUR, who by one Touch of His Almighty Hand can *open a Door of Utterance* for you; and who has promised it among the Glories of His Kingdome; Isa. XXXII. 4. *The Tongue of the Stammerers shall be ready to speak plainly.*

I know not what well to make of what is related by *Marcellinus Comes,*[8] who was an *Eye*-and-*Ear* Witness, of a Man that was born *Dumb,* and however had also his *Tongue* afterwards cutt out; but yett, when he had Occasion to refute the *Arian*[9] Impiety, *veras voces emisit,*[10] and could speak very Articulately and Intelligibly. One would have been the more *slow to beleeve* it, if it had not been affirmed by no less a Person than the Roman Emperour himself; who in such an Incontestible Instrument as a *Rescript* of his own, [Col.

Lib. I. Tit. XXVII. *de offi praefect. praetor. Africae,*[11]] positively
sais, *Vidimus venerabiles viros, qui abscissis radicitus Linguis,*—It
seems, there were more than one of those *Venerable* Men, who when
their *Tongues* were cutt out at the very *Roots,* yett continued plainly
speaking the Truth of Christianity, against the *Arians.* The Emperour *Justinian*[12] himself had seen them. *Æneas Gazaeus*[13] declares himself also to be a Witness of the Matter affirmed by *Justinian,* and by
Marcellinus; And so does *Procopius.*[14] Nor are these all the Witnesses, which you shall find Subpoena'd for the Relation, by *Cujacius*[15]
and by *Witsius.*[16]

If this History will animate your Zeal, to employ your *Tongue*
as much as you can for the *Glory* of your SAVIOUR, you will make
no ill use of it; I am sure, you will take the Best Course that can be,
for your *Tongue,* tho' a *Stammering* One, to become your *Glory.*

But for the Cure of your *Infirmity,* I will præscribe no more than
One Remedy; which I will introduce with a Story of something that
was an Introduction to the Experiment. It is a Passage in our Sacred
Oracles, *The Heart of the Rash shall understand Knowledge, and the
Tongue of the Stammerers shall be ready to Speak Plainly.*[17] Truly,
if *Stammerers* had less of the *Rash* in them, and would not so hastily
and suddenly and with so much *Præcipitation* rush upon their Words,
nor, as we say, lett their *Tongue* try to *run before their Witt,* but use
a wise *deliberation,* They would *Speak* more *Plainly* than they do.

I know one,[18] who had been very much a *Stammerer;* and no
words can tell, how much his Infirmity did Encumber and Embitter
the first years of his Pilgrimage. The Thousands of *Supplications* for
a *Free Speech* which he poured out unto the Glorious JESUS on this
Occasion, were at last accompanied with *Vows,* That the Grant of
such a Remarkable Favour, would oblige him to Beleeve and assert
this Blessed One, to be very God, even the Almighty God. Having
been One Day Extraordinarily thus Engaged, there came an Aged
Schole-Master, to visit him at his Chamber in the Colledge where he
then resided; and addressed him with a Discourse to this Effect. *"My
Friend,* I now Visit you for nothing, but only to Talk with you about
the *Infirmity* in your *Speech,* and offer you my Advice about it; Because I Suppose tis a Thing that greatly Trouble you. What I advise
you to, is, To seek a Cure for it, in the Method of *Deliberation.* Did
you ever know any one *Stammer* in Singing of the *Psalms?"* [*He then
Exemplified, the Pronunciation of the first Verse in Homer with a
long Prolation of Every Syllable, which a Stammerer might without*

any Interruption conform unto.] "While you go to *Snatch* at words, and are too *quick* at bringing of them out, you'l be *Stop'd* a thousand times in a day. But first use yourself to a very *Deliberate* way of *Speaking;* a *Drawling* that shall be little short of *Singing.* Even this *Drawling* will be better than *Stammering;* Especially if what you Speak, be well worth our waiting for. This *Deliberate* way of Speaking will also give you a great Command of pertinent *Thoughts;* yea, and if you find a word likely to be too hard for you, there will be time for you to think of Substituting another that won't be so. By this *Deliberation* you will be accustomed anon to Speak so much without the *Indecent Hæsitations,* that you'l always be in the way of it; yea, the *Organs* of your *Speech* will be so Habituated unto *Right-Speaking,* that you will by Degrees, and Sooner than you imagine, grow Able to *Speak as fast again,* as you did, when the Law of *Deliberation* first of all began to govern you. Tho' my Advice is, Beware of *Speaking too fast,* as Long as you Live."

This Advice was follow'd. The young Man soon became a *Preacher* in Great Congregations; which was a Thing as much despaired of, as anything in the World. He continued more than Forty years in the Service of the Churches; wherein his *Delivery* was generally accounted far from any Ill Circumstance of his Ministry; and he was Employed in making of Speeches on the most public Occasions, (whereof some have been published unto the whole World,) more than any Person that ever was in the Countrey. *Deliberation;* I say it again, *Deliberation;* I say it once more; *Deliberation,* was the Thing that Heaven gave this Happy Success unto.

But, if after all, your *Infirmity* must, like *Moses's* continue upon you, and you must all your days make those Lamentations, *God hath made my Chain heavy, and I am a Derision to all the* Baser *People;* Now, lett *Patience have its perfect Work,* and Submit patiently to the *Thing Appointed for you;* waiting for the *Blessed Hope* of the Cure, which you shall receive at the *Resurrection of the Dead,* when God *Redeeming your Life from Destruction,* will *Heal your Infirmities,* and particularly *Satisfy* your *Mouth,* with all the *Good* it can wish for.

And if this may be, *Solamen Miseris,*[19] you may take the *Comfort* of the *Company* whereof you have the *Honour* under your Calamity.

Moses I have told you of: A man that was an *Angel* of a Man. I will say nothing of *Aristotle,* whose *Futilities,* have Tyrannized over humane Understanding, in so many Nations for so many Ages.

Nor will I say any thing of *Virgil,* a Gentleman who has done less hurt in the World, and whose Poems no Man reads Intelligently, without finding himself disposed unto *Vertue,* as well as to *Wonder,* from them. These were both of them *Stammerers.* Nor will I enlarge upon the Character of *Michael* the *Stammerer,*[20] who was cried up as a *David,* and as a *Josias,* as long as a Wicked Clergy, had hopes of his doing the Part of a *Persecutor* for maintaining the *Worship of Images;* but anon his more Equal *Toleration* of different Sects, made them Revile him, as *A Common-shore of all Religions.* It seems, *Emperours* have been *Stammerers;* and they that have worn *Crowns* upon their *Heads,* have yett had *Chains* upon their *Tongues.* But I could with Delight call in one of the most Honourable and most Valuable and most Religious *Philosophers* that ever were in the World, and a *Stammerer.* Or, if here be not *Fellow-Sufferers* Enough to keep you a little in Heart, wee'l presume to reckon the great Apostle PAUL among them. He had, *A Contemptible Speech.* This could not mean that he wanted Eloquence of *Style:* His Writings declare him a Master of That. It seems an *Infirmity* in his *Utterance;* and what gave a *Disadvantage,* perhaps, a *Derision,* to his *Discourses:* an ιχνοφωνια, or a *Stammering Speech,* for which the Seducers disparaged him. Some of the Learned think, *This* was the *Thorn in the Flesh,* and that for which the Ministers of Satan buffeted him, and Laughed at him. *Friend,* if thy *Thorn in the Flesh* do thee as much Good as *his* did unto *him,* thou mayst well count the *Grace of God* in other Points favouring of thee *Sufficient for thee* and be *content* with thy Condition.

§ Dr. *Fuller* speaks of *Stammering* in Children, Cured with a Certain Application, whereby the *Organs of Speech* were Strengthened. It is a *Cephalic Lotion.* Take *Bay-leaves, Betony, Vervain, Marjoram,*[21] *Rosemary, Lavender,* Each Two handfuls; Boil them in a *Lixivium*[22] of Wood-Ashes, Three Quarts to two; Adding at last, powdered *Cloves,* and *Nutmeg,* Each Two Drams. Mix.

Lett the Head be shaved, and fomented in the Mornings (a quarter of an Hour at a time,) with a Spunge dipt in this Liquor hott, and Squeezed out again. But have a special care of catching any Cold upon it.

Rulandus[23] cured the *Loss of Speech,* with an Infusion of *Lavender-flowres* in *Wine.*

CAP. LII. *Muliebria.*

or,

Foeminine Diseases.

THE Sex that is called, *The Weaker Vessel,* has not only a share with us, in the most of our Distempers, but also is liable to many that may be called, Its *Peculiar Weaknesses.* Many others besides *Varandaeus,*[1] have written Large Treatises *of Womens Diseases.* I have readd (in *Graunts* Observations,) That Physicians have *Two Women-Patients* to *One Man:* And it is only likely to be True. But inasmuch as both Sexes Dy in a more Equal Proportion, This is very much for the Honour of the Physicians, who cure them, or for the Dishonour of us *Men,* who Dy as much by our *Extravagancies* as *Women* do by their *Infirmities.*

Poor Daughters of *Eve,* Languishing under your *Special Maladies, Look back* on your *Mother,* the *Woman,* who *being Deceived,* was first *in the Transgression,* that has brought in upon us, *all our Maladies.* Beholding your *Affliction* and your *Misery,* in the midst of your *Lamentations* under it, *Remember that Wormwood and Gall* of the Forbidden Fruit; Lett your *Soul have them still in Remembrance,* and *be humbled in you.* Under all your Ails, think, *The Sin of my Mother, which is also my Sin, has brought all this upon me!*

But then, *Look up* to your SAVIOUR, who will one Day sett you free from all these *Maladies:* And in the mean time will make *all things work together for good unto you.*

And oh! That this Good may come out of these *Maladies,* That you Shall be distinguished by the *Blessings of an Healed Soul;* and that you shall be the more *full of goodness;* the more Exemplary for *Whatsoever Things are Lovely, and Whatsoever Things are of good Report!*

Lett your *Patience* also, bear a proportion to your Humbling and Grievous Exercises.

And the more obnoxious your Tender and Feeble Constitutions are unto a Variety of *Distempers,* the more lett your Temperance and Caution be, that you may not bring *Distempers* on yourselves.

Fitts of the Mother.[2]

§ A Plaister of *Taccamahach,*[3] out of the Shell, covering the Navel, and Belly, has been counted an Infallible.

§ *Willis* mentions, *A Medicine by some accounted Infallible in Fitts of the Mother.*

Take the Seeds of *Parsnips*[4] [or, of *Columbines,*][5] in Wine, or in a proper Water.

§ He sais, Take twelve Drops of the *Spirit of Soot;* (or, of *Blood,*[6] or of *Harts-horn,*) twice a day in an Appropriate Vehicle. He adds, *I have seen this more Beneficial than all other Medicines.*

§ This also proposed as, *An Excellent Tincture for Hysteric Convulsions.*

Take of *Assa-foetida,* or *Galbanum,*[7] two Ounces; Dissolve them in Spirit of Wine, till a Red Tincture is Extracted. A Scruple of this, is to be taken in two or three Spoonfuls of *Mugwort-Water.*

The Green Sickness.[8]

There is a Malady which is called, *The White Jaundice,* as well as, The *Green Sickness;* An Enquiry into the *Causes* and *Symptoms* whereof, we will not here Look upon as Necessary.

It will be well, that they who are under the pernicious Obstructions, which their Viscid Blood suffers in this Distemper; feeling all their Powers Unactive, and Languishing; their Appetite impaired, and perhaps very Depraved and Vitious; their Breathing Difficult; especially upon any Motion; and their Bowels rumbling with Wind filling of them; would consider their Distemper as a Lively Picture, of, *A Mind listless to all that is good.* Even such is the *Carnal Mind,* which is a continual Matter of Complaint, with such as *know themselves.*

Yea, *Hearken, O Daughter, and Consider!* And *beholding thy Natural Face in a glass;* beholding how pale, how wan, how like a ghost it looks; consider, the worse, and more ghastly Aspect of thy Soul in thy Sins.

But then, Lett the Terror of thy Condition drive thee to thy SAVIOUR, and make thee Cry out unto Him, *O Lord, Say unto my Soul, I am thy Salvation!*

§ The most famous and potent Remedies, in this Distemper, are Præparations of *Steel.* Consult a Skilful and Faithful Physician, about the best Way of giving them.

§ Take a convenient Quantity of *Sheeps-Dung;* Make an Infusion of it in White Wine, or, Cyder; Standing a Night in the Embers. Drink a Glassful of this, Twice a Day.

§ *Elixir Proprietatis,*[9] taken in agreeable *Wine,* every morning, has been found a considerable Remedy.

§ For three Mornings together, about the Time of Expectation, give a Dram, of the Galls and Livers of *Eels* dried and powdered.

§ The Tops of white *Hore-hound* infused in *White-Wine,* drunk for a few Days, has been found a Remarkable Remedy:—and a mighty Strengthener of the *Stomach,* and what will recover out of an *Ill Habit* of Body.

❡ But then, there is a Distemper very Contrary unto this; Exemplified in the *Eighth* of *Luke* and the *Forty-third.*[10]

In this Case, the first Thing to be done, is what was done by the Good Woman, who could have no Help from the *Physicians;* and who took a Course, to commemorate which, there has been in a Tradition of Antiquity, a *Statue* Erected for her. *Touch the Fringe of thy* SAVIOURS *Garment; Begging and Hoping for Healing Vertue to proceed from the SON of God cloathed in our Flesh.*

§ Now, try a Decoction, (or a *Tea*) of the Inner Rind of a White *Oak Bark.*

§ Two Ounces of an Infusion of *Hogs-dung* mixt with one Spoonful of *Nettle-Juice,* and given Morning and Evening, is a famous Remedy. Some add, wearing a Shift, which has been wett with a Strong Decoction of *Hogs-dung.*

§ A yett pleasanter Medicine, rarely fails. A Mixture of *Claret* Wine, and Old Conserve of *Roses;* and Old Marmalade of *Quinces.*

Cap. LIII. Retired *Elizabeth.*
A Long, tho' no very *Hard, Chapter*
for, A WOMAN whose *Travail* approaches.
with Remedies to Abate the *Sorrows of Child-bearing.*

FROM a Short ESSAY [Entituled Elizabeth in her Holy Retirement,[1]] formerly given to the Publick, Some Advice is now to be offered, unto a *Daughter* of *Eve,* [Lett her also give me Leave to call her, *An Handmaid of the Lord!*] who Expects anon the Arrival of a Time, when her *Loins will be filled with Pain, Pangs will take hold on her, the Pangs of a Woman which travaileth.* Tis *Now,* Sure, if ever, a Time wherein it may be Expected, that she will hearken to the

Counsils of God; *This,* if any, is the Time, wherein the Methods and Motions of Divine Grace, will *find her.* Certainly, she will be concerned, that a *Sudden Destruction,* and a fearful and endless One, may not *come as Travail upon a Woman with Child,* when the *Time of Travail* shall come upon her. The Truth is, That tho' the Hazards and Hardships undergone by *Travailing Women,* be a considerable Article of the *Curse,* which the *Transgression* whereinto our *Mother* was *Deceived* has brought upon a Miserable World, yett our Great REDEEMER has procured this *Grace* from God unto the *Daughters of Zion,* that the *Curse* is turned into a *Blessing.* The Approach of their *Travails,* putts them upon those Exercises of PIETY, which render them truly *Blessed* ones; *Blessed* because their *Transgression is forgiven; Blessed* because they are *Turned from their Iniquities.* And hence in Part it may come to pass, that tho' thro' the Evident Providence of God, watching over Humane Affairs, there is pretty near an Equal Number of *Males* and *Females* that are Born into the World, the Number of the *Males* who are apparently *Pious,* and partakers of a *New Birth,* is not so great as that of the *Females.* Be sure, twil argue a wonderful Stupidity of Soul, and Obstinacy in Sin, if the View of an *Approaching Travail,* do not make the poor Women Serious, and Cause them seriously to Consider their Condition, and bring them into a Considerate, Sollicitous, Effectual Preparation for Eternity.

Ye Daughters of Marah,[2] it is to be proposed unto you in the *first* place; That you do not indulge any indecent *Impatience* or *Discontent,* at the State, which you find ordered for you. Finding yourselves in a State of *Pregnancy,* Froward Pangs of *Dissatisfaction,* harboured and humoured in you, because you see that *in Sorrow you bring forth Children,* may displease Heaven, and bring yett more *Sorrow* upon you. How *Unnatural* will it look in you, to Complain of a State, whereinto the *Laws of Nature* Established by God, have brought you! The *Will* of the Great God has been declared in those Terms; *I will that the younger Women Marry, and bear Children.* When you find that a Conception has brought you into *Child-bearing* Circumstances, Lett your Submission to the *Will* of God cause you with all possible Resignation to say, *Great God, I am Thine; And I am willing to be all that thou wilt have me to be!* One principal End of *Marriage,* is thus far in an *Honourable Way* of being answered with you. Tis what was acknowledged a *Mercy* in *the old Time,* among the *Women who trusted in God,* and who counted themselves *mercifully visited of God,* when they had Conceived. An *Offspring* was promised as a *Blessing:* How frequently, how fervently *Pray'd* for! It was Esteemed, The *taking away of a Reproach. Barrenness* was Threatened and Bewayled, as a *Calamity;* A Punishment for a *Michal.*[3] I shall speak but in the Language which *your Sex* of old would have allow'd of, if I now tell you, *That God has look'd upon His Handmaid, and Remembred her, and not forgotten her, but given her to Conceive.* Yea, I may go on to tell you, That upon your giving up yourselves unto the Lord, your Children become the *Children of God. They are my Children,* Saith your God. It is a *Child of God,* which you now have within you. Tis a *Subject* and a *Servant* of a Glorious CHRIST, whose *Bones* are now *growing in the Womb of her that is with Child.* It is a *Member* of His mystical Body, which is now *Shaping in Secret,* and *Curiously to be Wrought.* I add, you are to bring forth a Creature of Excellent Faculties; God will have Eternal Glory from it. And you know not what an *Instrument of Good* this Child may prove in the World. Who can foresee, how far, *This same shall comfort you,* or Honour you.

But now, The *Next* Thing to be proposed unto you, is, That you hasten into a *State of Safety for Eternity.* For ought you know, your *Death* has Entred into you; and your *Præparation for Death,* as it will not *hasten* it at all, So it will but fitt you to *Live* as well as to *Dy.*

Wherefore, you must, in the First Place, be very sensible of This; That Except you are *Born again,* it had been *good for you that you never had been born* at all: The *Sorrows of Child-birth,* will be to you, but the *Beginning of Sorrows,* and of such as know no *End:* your portion must be in a *Place of Dragons,* and of *Torments:* you are Falling into *Hands,* which it is *a Fearful Thing to fall into.* The Sense of This, must then mightily Quicken and Hasten your *Flight from the Wrath to Come.* In this Flight, you must first Acknowledge; *O Holy Lord, I am neither Able to Turn and Live unto Thee, nor Worthy that Thou shouldest Enable me.* Without this *Humiliation,* how can it be imagined, that you should ever *Turn?* With Humble Acknowledgments of *Sovereign Grace* go on to beg of the most Gracious Lord, *O glorious One, Turn thou me, and I shall be Turned.* Proceed now, and ponder on your Sinful and Woful Circumstances before the Lord: and Confess, *O great God, I have Sinned and have perverted that which is Right: I have Sinned, and have done very Foolishly.* Examine your Past Life; On Every Violation of the *Ten Commandments* that you can call to Mind, make a Bitter Pause. Be as much afraid of leaving any Sin unconfessed, as you would be of having the

After-birth Left in you, after your Travail. With Astonishment cry out; *O my God, Innumerable Evils compass me about; my Heart fails me when I go to Think upon them!* At the same time, go up as far as the *Original Sin,* which is the *Fountain* of all your *Sins.* The Terrors of *Child-bearing,* which are now upon you, do very properly lead you to Bewayl your Share in the *Sin of your first Parents;* and to Bewayl as with a *Fountain of Tears,* that *Corrupt Nature* which by a Derivation from your *Next Parents* you brought into the World with you. Think, *Lord, I was Conceived in Sin; I was born a Leper; and my poor Child will be so too.* Deeply affect yourself with the horrid and heinous *Evil* in all the *Sin,* wherein you have *Denied the God that is Above.* Go on to an amazing View of the *Deplorable State* into which you are fallen by your *Sin;* and with Amazement Think, *Wo is unto me, that I have Sinned! The Almighty God is Angry with me; And who knows the Power of His Anger? The Devil demands me as his Captive; I am a prey to the Terrible One. Sin Tyrannizes over me: I am held in the Chains of Darkness. If I dy as I am, what will become of me? Who can dwell in those Everlasting Burnings, which the Unpardoned must be doom'd unto! O Wretched One that I am! Who shall deliver me?* Being brought into the *Contrition* of this Distress, NOW behold the admirable SAVIOUR provided for you: The JESUS who is *God manifest in Flesh:* God and MAN in one Person: The SAVIOUR who is *Able to save you unto the uttermost;* the SAVIOUR who has Invited you to *Look unto Him and be saved;* the SAVIOUR who has Assured you, that if you *Come* unto Him He *will not cast you out.* Cry to Him, *O my dear SAVIOUR, Draw me to thee: Oh! make me Thine and Save me.* Lett no Apprehension of your own *Vileness* make you despair to find Acceptance with Him. Come to Him under no Recommendation, but that of your own dreadful *Necessity,* and *Confusion,* and the *Triumphs of Grace* which will arise from the Salvation of such a *Lothesome Sinner.* NOW Behold the *Sacrifice* of your SAVIOUR, and plead; *O Great God, Lett the Blood of thy Son cleanse me from all my Sin. Be Reconciled unto me, because thy JESUS has been my Sacrifice.* Behold the *Righteousness* of your SAVIOUR, and plead, *O Great God, Thy Son has answered thy Law as a Surety for me. My Advocate shews His Righteousness for me; therefore deliver me from going down to the Pitt.* That this your *Precious Faith* in the *Sacrifice* and *Righteousness* of your SAVIOUR may be *Justified* with a Good *Evidence* to the Sincerity of it, Resign yourself up to the *Holy Spirit* of your SAVIOUR, desiring and expecting that from and thro' your SAVIOUR as the *Head* of His People, the Influences of His *Holy Spirit* may flow down into you. Yea, Consent that the *Spirit of Holiness* take possession of you. Yield the Consent of a Conquered Soul; *O my SAVIOUR, I am willing: Do thou make me willing; and given Thou thy Order for it; That thy Holy SPIRIT should Renew me in the Spirit of my Mind; make me a New Creature; produce the Lovely Image of God upon me; Render all Sin odious to me; Wean me [from] this World; Restore the Throne of God unto Him in my Soul; Dwell in me as a Temple of Thine, an Eternal Habitation for thee.* So in the promised *Strength* of your SAVIOUR, take up the *Resolutions* of universal and perpetual PIETY. Thus the *New Birth* is carried on. Thus you have gone thro' the Work, which will disarm *Death* of all its *Terrors;* and whereupon you may Sing, *O Death, where is thy Sting?* If you should now be *Teeming* with your *Death,* yett you may keep *Rejoicing in the Hope of the Glory of God.* When the Handmaid of the Lord had the Proposals of Heaven made unto her, She Complied, *Behold The Handmaid of the Lord; Be it unto me according to thy Word:* And she became in a *Transcendent Sense* owner of a CHRIST immediately. O Handmaid of the Lord, The Great SAVIOUR, who condescended once to make a Virgin, *The Tabernacle of God,* proposes this to you; *Shall I be thy SAVIOUR, and Heal thee, and Lead thee, and Rule thee forevermore?* Lett your Answer be: *Behold the Handmaid of the Lord; Be it unto me according to thy Word.* In an *Agreeable Sense* you become owner of a CHRIST immediately. Now, if you *Dy,* to *dy will be a Gain unto you!*

Having thus managed your *Grand Concern,* Lett the Words of an Apostle now come into Consideration with you; 1 Tim. II. 15. *She shall be Saved in Childbearing if they continue in Faith, and Charity, and Holiness, with Sobriety.*

HOLINESS; It lies in a *Dedication unto God.* Now may God assist you to Study and Contrive *How you may be the Lords;* and in what Methods you may Employ all your *Powers* to Glorify God. If the Breach of the *Old Covenant,* be that which has brought the Difficulty of your *Travail,* with all other Mischiefs upon you, what can you do better, than gett as far as you can under the *Wings* of the *New Covenant?* Kneeling before the Great God, most heartily Say unto Him; *O Great God, Thou shalt be my God. I Resolve to be thy Servant. I depend on thy JESUS to make me Righteous and Holy before thee; and Quicken me for thy Eternal Service.* But when you bring yourselves under this *Consecration* unto God, you must bring your *Children,* even the unborn Child, into it with you. When you are Sensible, that you have Conceived, without any Delay Carry Even this *Embryo* unto the Lord; and Say, *O God of the Spirits of all Flesh, I bring to thee, even my Hoped Offspring; Oh, Lett thy Holy Spirit now take an Early Possession of it; Form it; Fill it; make it an Everlasting Instrument of thy Praises.*

But *Holiness* is that which *cannot look upon Iniquity. Loathing* is One of your frequent Indispositions; But may a greater *Loathing of Sin* than ever, be now raised in you. Have in you a growing *Detestation* for that Vile Thing; *When Lust hath Conceived, it brings forth Sin, and Sin when it is finished brings forth Death.*

After all; you will find, that *Meditations* on a Glorious CHRIST, are both *Instances* and *Incentives* of *True Holiness,* beyond any that you can be advis'd unto. It is the *Strange Work* of God, and the most astonishing that Ever was done in the World; Gal. IV. 4. *God Sent forth His SON, made of a Woman.* Oh! Meditate much on this; and with much Astonishment. "My Great SAVIOUR; my Glorious *Immanuel!* How Gloriously didst thou *Humble thyself!* Was there a *Sinless Man* conceived in a *Virgin!* Did the SON of God, vouch safe to Assume this Man into His *own Person!* Is there now lying in the Bosom of the Eternal SON of God, a Man who was once an *Infant* in the Womb of a *Virgin!* A Man *born of a Woman,* who is *more than a Man:* Even *God manifest in Flesh.* A Man Bred and Born, and Nurs'd by a *Woman;* But this *Man-child caught up unto God and His Throne;* and become the Lord of all the Angels, and of whole Worlds, and the *Judge* to whom all must be Accountable. We are *Saved through* that illustrious *Child-bearing.* O the *Dignity* putt upon our poor Sex, in the Birth of such a Redeemer! O the *Assurance* which the Distressed Ones have to find Help with such a Redeemer when there comes a Time of Need upon them!" Yea, you may improve this Contemplation, in your Supplications for a *Safe Deliverance,* in the Hour that is coming upon you. Plead; *O my Good God; The Humiliation of my SAVIOUR in the Circumstances of His Nativity, has purchased this for me, that I should be Sav'd in Child-bearing: O Save me graciously! O my SAVIOUR, Since thou wast born of a Woman, certainly Child-bearing Women, may Cry to thee for thy Protection, thy Assistence, I hope in thee for it. Such Salvation belongs unto Thee, O Lord: Thou, Thou art the God of my Salvation.*

You may be pointed unto another Description of *Holiness.* Tis

that, *A CHRIST formed in you.* You have a *Child formed in you.*
But, may you have, *A CHRIST formed in you.* Now, if you take
up the *Right Thoughts of the Righteous* concerning a Glorious
CHRIST: If you have such a *Mind* in you, as in a CHRIST you see
a Pattern of; If your *Walk* be such as a CHRIST has left you a Pat-
tern of; or, If you *Love* what a CHRIST Loves, and *Hate* what a
CHRIST hates, and bear Afflictions and Abasements with a
CHRIST-Like Patience, and are *Crucified* unto a World in which a
CHRIST was Crucified; Then you have a *CHRIST formed in you.*
A CHRIST will be gloriously concerned for the Welfare of such
Holy Women.

SOBRIETY must accompany this *Holiness.* The *Passions* or
the *Surfeits* of the Mother make a Strange Impression on the Infant;
yea, on the very *Soul* of the Infant. Be *Temperate in all things.* If
such Counsil had not been of some Consequence to the *unborn Infant,*
the Angel would not have counselled the Wife of *Manoah,*[4] as you
may remember he did.

But Prayers must accompany all you do. Certainly your *Præg-
nant Time* should be a *Praying Time.* If you have never yett *Prayed
Earnestly,* tis now a Time to do it: and Lament it poenitently before
the Lord, that you have been so hardly and so lately brought unto it.
Your *Prayers* must be *Cries;* and of that Importance; *For thy Names-
Sake, O Lord, Pardon my Iniquity, for it is Great!* And, *O Lord,
Order my Steps in thy Word, and Lett not any Iniquity have Do-
minion over me.* And, *Oh! Shew me thy Marvellous Kindness in thy
Strong City, and the great Goodness thou hast Laid up for them that
Fear thee.* With the *Pangs* and *Throws* of a Distressed Soul in your
Prayers, you will *Cry* for such Things, and *Lift up your Voice* for
these things. But then, you will more particularly Employ your *Pray-
ers,* for an Happy and an easy *Delivery* in your Approaching *Travail.*
In your *Prayers* for this *Mercy,* (a *Mercy* which is *Big* with a thou-
sand Mercies!) you will plead the *Power* of God. Think on the Word
Spoken to an Hand-maid of the Lord; Luk. I. 37. *With God nothing
shall be Impossible.* The God who made the *Hebrew Women* so
Lively, that they were ordinarily *delivered* before a *Midwife* could
come to them, What may He do for *you,* if Suitably Pray'd unto?
Plead the *Mercy of* God. Think on the Word wherewith she of old
Comforted her Soul; Lam. III. 25. *The Lord is good unto them that
wait for Him; to the Soul that Seeks Him.* Remember, That the Name
of our God, is, *O Thou that hearest Prayer.* You know how to turn
these things into *Prayers;* how to make them the *Plea's* of your *Pray-*

ers. But, in all, Don't forgett now to plead the Mediation of the SAVIOUR, who was pleased for to be, and sometimes for to call Himself, *The Son of the Handmaid of the Lord.* Lett Such as these be your *Groans* before the Lord. "O most *Powerful* God; *I know thou canst do Every thing.* There is nothing that can Stand before the *Power* of thy *Almighty Arm. Lord, if thou wilt, thou canst,* give me a *Good Time,* in the *Time of Trouble* that is now before me. *According to the Greatness of thy Power* preserve one that is *Appointed to dy,* if thou dost not powerfully step in to uphold and strengthen her. *O Father of Mercies, Deal* mercifully with thy Distressed Handmaid; *Look Mercifully,* and with Pitty, on the Miseries, which the Sin of the World had entail'd upon me. *God be merciful to me a Sinner.* But, oh! What a *Joy have I sett before me!* The God whom I now pray unto, is He, who in His own *Second Person,* took a *Man,* into a *Personal Union* with Himself; and was *Born of a Woman.* Oh! Behold thy Beloved JESUS; The *Blessed* One, who was *made a Curse,* that so we might either *not feel* the *Curse,* or Else *gett good* from the *Curse.* For the sake of thy JESUS, the *Son of Man,* who is the SON of God, and whom thou Lovest, above all the Works of thy Hands, and for the Sake of whom thou Lovest all that fly unto Him, oh! Be Favourable to me!" Lett your *Prayers* be those; Psal. XXXVIII. 21, 22. *Forsake me not, O Lord; O my God, be not far from me. Make Haste to help me, O Lord my Salvation.* Or those: Psal. XXII. II. *Be not far from me, for Trouble is near; and there is none to help.* In these your *Prayers,* it would be of admirable Advantage, for you, to search and find out, the *Precious Promises* of God, that may most of all Suit your Condition. Present these *Promises* before the Lord, as Containing and Engaging of Blessings, which the *Blood* of the *Lamb of God,* has bought for you. And say, "Therefore has thy Handmaid *found in her heart to pray this Prayer unto thee. O Lord GOD, Thou art that* God, and these be *thy Words,* and thy *Words be True,* and thou hast *promised this Goodness* unto thy Handmaid. *Therefore now lett it please Thee to Bless the House* of thy Handmaid; For Thou, O LORD God, *hast Spoken it.* Behold, Some of the *Promises* and *Cordials* you have to live upon! Take that; Psal. XXXIV. 22. *None of them who Trust in the Lord shall be desolate.* And that; Psal. LV. 22. *Cast thy Burden on the Lord, and He shall Sustain thee.* And that; Psal. LVI. 3. *At what time I am afraid, I will Trust in thee.* And that; Isa. XLI. 10. *Fear thou not, for I am with thee: Be not dismayed for I am thy God: I will Strengthen thee: yea, I will uphold thee, by the Right Hand of my Righteousness.* And that; Heb. XIII.

5,6. He hath Said, I will never Leave thee, nor forsake thee. So that we may boldly Say, The Lord is my Helper. And that; Isa. LXVI. 9. *Shall I bring to the Birth, and not cause to bring forth, Saith the Lord!* And that; Job. V. 19. *He shall deliver thee in Six Troubles; yea, in Seven there shall no Evil touch thee.* And now, *Having these Promises,* go plead them with God: And lett your Experience be, that which is related, Concerning an *Handmaid of the Lord,* praying for a Child. 1 Sam. I. 15, 18. *She said, I am a Woman of a Sorrowful Spirit, but I have poured out my Soul before the Lord.—So the Woman went away, and her uneasiness continued no Longer.*

That you may be the better furnished and quickened for your *Prayers,* you will *Read the Scriptures.* In the *Scriptures* you may Especially single out, *The Book of PSALMS,* for your Companion and Counsellour and Comforter. Yea, The Pious Author of the Book Entituled, *A Present for Teeming Women,* propounds this to you; That you would *Sing* the PSALMS Considerately alone by yourself; and he adds, *It will be most unquæstionably pleasant, unto those good ANGELS, who are Ministring Spirits to attend you for Good.* Accordingly then, for the *Songs,* by which you *Harmonize* with Heaven, and call in the Help thereof, I commend unto you, multitudes of passages, which ly scattered all over the PSALTER. Especially in the III PSALM; the IV; the XVIII; the XXIII; the XXV; the XXVII; the XXXI; the XXXIX; the XLIII; the LI; the LXXI; the LXXXVI; the XCI; the CXVI; the CXVIII; the CXIX; the CXXVII; the CXXX; the CXXXVIII; the CXLII. To which you may add, The Prayer of *Jonah;* The Song of *Hannah;* and, The Song of *Mary.*

Nor are *Psalms* only, but *Alms* also, to accompany your *Prayers.* The XLI Psalm will tell you, what you are to Think of them. Our SAVIOUR, how frequently, how Earnestly, does He insist upon them! Say, *Thy Merits, O my SAVIOUR, are my Only Ones; I shall never imagine my Alms to have any. But thy Commands, O my SAVIOUR, have directed them; Therefore by my Alms, I will prepare for thy Mercies.* This is *Pure Religion.* The *Prayers* have a Distinguishing Efficacy, when it may be Said, *Thy Prayers and thy Alms are come up as a Memorial before God.* You are taught: That *the Merciful shall obtain Mercy.* Especially, when you sett apart your *whole Dayes for Prayers* (which you will Sometimes do, as you shall be able to bear it) you will on these *Days* dispense your *Alms* with a particular *Liberality. Is not this the Fast that I have Chosen,* Saith the Lord? And what if in the Dispensation of your *Alms,* you should have a Special Eye, to *poor Child-bearing Women,* if you can hear of any Such, in Wants, and Straits, and grievous Necessities? You will have yett a more Special Eye, to such *Poor* as can *Pray* for you; and you will Engage them to do it, with a *Daily Remembrance* of you.

And now, your FAITH! You Read, *Thro' Faith* Sarah[5] *was delivered of a Child.* By *Faith* keep continually committing yourself into the Glorious Hands of a SAVIOUR, who said unto a Godly Woman, when her *Faith* began to fail her: *Said I not unto thee, That if thou wouldest Beleeve, thou shouldest See the Glory of God?* Were your *Husband* able to give you an Happy *Travail,* how willing would he be to do it! Yea (were there any Goodness in him,) tho' it were to be by bearing your Trouble for you, as a rare *Sympathy* has caused Some to do! But by *Faith* you make Sure of your SAVIOUR to be your *Husband.* The Voice of your *Faith* is, *O my SAVIOUR, I am Thine; Do thou possess me; And by Thee lett me bring forth Fruit unto God.* And now, by *Faith* depend on your most mighty and most gracious *Husband.* Say to Him, Cry to Him, Weep to Him; *O my SAVIOUR, How canst thou cast me off!* Hope in Him, to see the Fulfilment of a Word that once dropped from Him: [Joh. XVI. 21.] *A Woman When she is in Travail, hath Sorrow, because her Hour is Come; But as soon as she is delivered of the Child, she remembers no more the Anguish; for Joy that a Man is born into the World.* Yett by *Faith* submitt unto His Holy Will. We read of a *Rachel; She Travailed, and She had Hard Labour; Her Soul departed, and She died.* And of another: *She was with Child, near to cry out; She Travailed, her Pains came upon her; It was the Time of her Death.* Suppose this may, by the Sovereign *Lord of Life* be the Portion appointed for you, yett by *Faith* triumph over the *Fear of Death:* By *Faith* Resign yourself into the Hands of the Glorious Lord; *Lord JESUS, Receive my Spirit!* And so, *Rejoice in the Hope of the Glory of God.*

When your Time arrives, meet it with an Honourable *Courage,* bear it with an Honourable *Patience.* But in the Minutes of your Anguish, Lett your Cry be like That; Psal. XXVI.11. *Oh! Redeem me, and be merciful unto me.* Or That; Psal. XXX. 10. *Hear me, O Lord; Have Mercy upon me; Lord, Be thou my Helper.* Your Omnipotent REDEEMER is One who *Commands Deliverances* for them who *weep and make Supplication;* That is, He *Commands* His Good *Angels* to bring and work *Deliverances: Deliverances* come as Effects of His *Commands* unto His *Ministers.* No *Midwives* can do, what the *Angels* can!

While you are in a Doubtful Expectation of your *Travail*, you will do well to avoid all *Rash Vows*, which usually prove the *Snares of Souls*. But yett Entertain some Holy *Resolutions* of a more Exact, a more Watchful, a more Fruitful *Walk with God*, when He shall have *Delivered* you.

And being *Delivered*, your *Next Work* will be, To Consider, *What you shall Render to the Lord*. Think, *Seeing thou, O my God, hast given me Such a Deliverance as this, Should I again break thy Commandments, wouldest thou not be Angry with me, till thou hast Consumed me?* But then, go on to Think, *What* you will do, that you may maintain more Communion with God in the *Religion of the Closett*. Think, *What* you will do, that you may be a greater Blessing in your *Family*, and unto your Several *Relatives*. Think, *What* you will do in Abating of your *Superfluities*, that you may Employ the more upon *Pious Uses:* perhaps, to cloathe poor Widows, Like another *Dorcas*. Beg the Help of the Divine Grace, that you may do such Things; and Glorify your SAVIOUR with a *Reasonable Service*.

One of the First Things to be now done, is to give up your *Newborn Child*, unto the Lord, in His *Holy Baptism*. Thus rescue the Child from the *Great Red Dragon*, which is watching to devour it. Lett the Child be either *Male* or *Female*, this is a Matter to be Entirely Left unto the Wisdome of the Glorious God. Either of them, if it be a *Perfect Child*, brings Ten Thousand Mercies with it. And, if it may be a *Child* of God the FATHER, a *Subject* of God the SON, a *Temple* of God the HOLY SPIRIT, think, *This Enough; Lord, I have brought one of thy Children into the World*. As a Declaration of this Intention in you, Lett the Child be *Washed* and *Blessed* in the Name of the Glorious One, and in a Congregation of His Faithful People; and be Laid under Everlasting *Bonds* to be the Lords. But at the same time, Look on yourself as laid under *Bonds*, to bring up the Child for Him; and *in the Nurture and Admonition of the Lord*.

§ Doubtless, the poor Women think, there is as little Sense in speaking of, *An Easy Travail*, as the Frenchmen think there is, in speaking of, *An Easy Prison*.

But, the Illustrious *Boyl* tells us, The *Livers* and *Galls* of *Eeles*, dried slowly in an Oven, and powdered, and given to the Quantity of a Walnut in White Wine, have kept Multitudes of Women, from dying in Hard Labour.

The Admonition of Dr. *Morgan* must not be forgotten, "most pernicious is the Practice of those, who at the Supposed Time of Delivery, give what they call, *Forcers*,[6] to hasten on the Work."

§ The *Labour-powder* is thus made.

Take *Date-Stones, Amber, Saffron,* and *Cummin-seeds*.[7] Beat and Scrape them all Severally, into very fine Powder. Take of Each, as much as may Ly on a Groat. Only Double the Quantity of the Cummin-seeds. Mingle them. And when the poor Woman is in her Extremity, give her a Spoonful of it in Mace-Ale.

§ Here's a *Digbaean* Projection, to facilitate a *Travail.*

Take a Large White *Onion,* (or two small ones,) and slice it, and fry it with three Spoonfuls of the best *Sallet-Oyl,* till it be tender. Then putt all into a Little Pipkin,[8] till it be Tender, with half a glass-full of Water. Boil it well together. Strain it out. And so drink it in the Morning. Continue this for a fortnight or three weeks before the End of the Reckoning.

§ Agreeably to this, the Great *Borellus* has an Observation; *Saepius Compertum est;*[9] It is often found, that by Drinking of (good, clear, sweet) *Sallet Oyl,* before the Travail, Women obtain an easy Travail:—*nec tormina ulla*[10] *patiuntur puerpetae.*

The same Gentleman brought on an *Hopeless Travail,* with Six Ounces of the *Essence of Amber,* in a glass of Wine.

§ Our *Boyl* writes; *Betony-Roots* wonderfully prevail against the Distemper of the *Womb;* and *Hysterical Affections.*

§ Here's an *Hysteric Mixture.*

Take *Assa foetida,* (Extracted with *Spirit of Wine*) Tincture of *Galbanum,* of *Castor,* and Spirit of *Sal Armoniac* (or, *Harts-horn,*) Each one Dram; Oil of *Amber,* Thirty two Drops. Mix.—Shake the glass, when you give it.

Dr. T. *Fuller* sais, "Its an Extraordinary Medicine for *Hysteric People;* and singularly to be noted for *Women in Labour,* whensoever the Spirits being Hysterically Confused, flow not in plentifully and powerfully Enough to the Muscles of the *Abdomen,* and other Parts promoting the Birth, and so the necessary Pangs fail, and the Womb itself riseth not up to make strong Effort of Expulsion. In this Case, I say, this uses to bring, as t'were *Divine Help,* beyond almost anything Else, if Twenty or Thirty Drops be ministred in an appropriate Vehicle, and at due Times repeted."

§ Among the *Boylaean* Receits, there is This; *For Women in Labour, to bring away the Child.*

Take one Dram of Choice *Myrrh,* and having reduced it unto a

Fine Powder, Drink it in a Draught of Sack; or, if you would have the Liquor less active, take it in a Posset, or any more temperate Vehicle.

§ To *bring away Every thing* that may be left, tho' it were a part of a Dead Child:

With the Juice of *Sheeps Sorrel,* and some of the Strong Infusion of the Same Herb (unpress'd) in Water, and a Sufficient Quantity of Sugar, make a Syrup. Of this, the Patient is to take about a Spoonful, twice or thrice in a day.

§ In *Child-bed Fevers,* tis by *Willis* Commended as a *Good Medicine.* Take of *Laudanum,* a Grain; and of the Powder of *Saffron* half a Scruple: Mix, and give it in a Spoonful of *Treacle-Water.*

§ In *Childbed* the Piles are often very troublesome. The usual Releef, is, *Mullein-leaves* beaten and stewed in *Hogs-fat,* cool'd and applied.

§ To prevent *Miscarrying,*

Wear a *Load-Stone,*[11] about, or above, the Navel. When any Danger of this appears, the Common Practice is, Only to *Keep Quiet,* and take a Tea of *Double Tansey.*

Hear the Words of Dr. *Cheyne* upon it. "The most Effectual Method I have Ever found, to prevent such Misfortunes, is, To drink plentifully *Bristol-Water,*[12] with a very little *Red Wine,* for their Constant Drink: To lay the Plaister *Ad Herniam,*[13] with *Oil of Cinamon* and *London Laudanum,*[14] in a due Proportion, to their Reins: To keep them to a *Low, Light, Easily digested Diet,* Especially of the *Farinaceous Vegetables,* and *Milk-meats;* to strengthen their Bowels with *Diascordium* and *Toasted Rhubarb,* if they become too Slippery; To air them once or twice a day, in a Coach or Chair; and to keep them *Cheerful* and in *Good Humour* as much as may be. This Method, will Scarce Ever fail, unless a latent *Scrofula,*[15] or some other *Hæreditary Sharpnesses* in their Juices, destroy the *Birth.*"

§ For an *Ague in the Breast.*[16]

Take *Aqua Vitae,* and *Linseed Oyl:* Warm them together on a Chafing-dish of Coals: Dip a proper Clothe in it, and Lay it on as hott as may be.

§ For the *Hard Swellings* in Womens *Breasts.*

Use *Turnips* boil'd, and made unctuous with a little fresh *Hogs-Lard.*

The Old Medicine of the *London-midwives* to break and heal Sore Breasts, was this.

Take *Red Sage* and *Oatmeal;* Boil them in Spring-Water to a

Consistency. Then add a fitt Proportion of *Honey*. Boil it a while. Take it off. A While boiling hott, thicken it with *Venice-Turpentine*. Make a Plaister of.

§ To increase *Milk*, with Nurses.

Potage made with *Lentiles*, or *Vetches*, does it. So does Powder of *Earth-worms*, well-cleans'd and dried. A Dram in any Proper Vehicle. So does, *Milk* turn'd with *Beer*.

Here's an *Infallible*, and I hope, not an *Unacceptable*.

Take *Chickens;* make a Brothe of 'em. Add thereto *Fennel* and *Parsly*-Roots: and butter the Roots with New Butter. Having so done, Eat all the Mess.

But above all, Try this. Drink for a few Days, twice or thrice a Day, the Water wherein *Fresh Fish* has been boiled. This will fetch back the Nurses *Milk,* when it is gone: and will so supply her *Breasts* that they shall be better to the *Infant* than the richest *Clusters of the Vine.* The Infant may *suck and be satisfied with the Comfortable Breasts: Milk out and be delighted with the Abundance* which it finds there provided for it. *Hoc mea me Conjux Experta docere Volebat.*[17]

However, the Nurse won't Expect from the Use of these Things, to become like the French Nurse, whereof *Borellus* relates, that she not only Suckled at once a Couple of Boys, but also from her *Milk* supplied an Apothecary with *Butter,* which he found the Noblest Remedy in the World for a *Consumption*.

CAP. LIV.

Great Things done by Small Means, with Some REMARKS, On a Spring of Medicinal Waters, which Every Body is at home, an owner of.

Rebus in Exiguis Vis bona Saepe Latet.[1]

WHAT *Great Effects* a Small and a Mean Thing may have; tis what cannot be without some Wonder thought upon.

§ There is a certain Water called, *All-Flower-Water;* The process whereof is this: Take Fresh *Cow-dung*, that is gathered in the Morning, Twelve Pound; *Spring Water,* Thirty Pound; Mix them, and Lett them Stand for Digestion Twenty four Hours; And then Decant the Brown Tincture.

Such a Water as this, the *Pharmacopaeia Bateana*,[2] commends as good against the *Gout, Rheumatism, Stone,* Stoppage of *Urine;* An Excellent thing against the *scurvy:* as also against the *Palsey,* and other Diseases of the *Nerves.*

But now hear Dr. *Salmons* Report about it. "There was a Certain Woman, who from the most obscure Condition, sett up for a Doctoress; and undertook the Cure of all Diseases with this only Remedy; and from the State of a Beggar became a Mistress of more than Twenty Thousand Pounds.[3] This she gave in all Distempers and against all Diseases; and so happy and successful she was, that she cured almost all such who were given over by others for Incurable: and it was rare that any thing came under her hands that miscarried. This was her *Catholicon.* It is without doubt, a good Thing, and so much the better because of its general Tendency, and being constantly used with such an approved Success. Her usual way of giving it was thus, she ordered the Patient to take about five or six Ounces in the Morning, fasting; and Last at night going to Bed; and if the Disease were stubborn, as much an hour before Dinner. And if there was any External Effect, to Bathe the Part two or three times a day therewith, for a quarter of an Hour at a time. By this only thing and method (said Dr. *Salmon*) She did even almost Incredible Things. Tis true (*he adds*) the Medicine is but a mean thing; but it is not to be despised."

§ What *Miraculous Things* have been done, with *Fasting Spittle!*—Especially, in *Pains,* and *Sores* and *Swellings.* The Eyes moistened with it every Morning, præserve their *Sight* unto Admiration. Yea, it has done *Incredible Things.*

And, Christian, won't *Fasting Prayer* do so too?

Every Body knows, that *Sheeps-Dung* is a Medicine, which has done many notable Cures. One might write almost an *Elephantine Book* upon the Virtues of it!

Yea, How many Lives have been saved by *Stone-horse Dung,* [with which *Manlius* tells us, that his Brother, who was *Luther's* Physician cured *Pleuresies.*]

How many Lives have been saved by *Pigeons Dung!*

Even a *Dogs,* has its Vertues.

And for what Cases has an *Hogs* been Celebrated!

Concerning the *Excrements* of *Animals,* it is reported, That Old *Xenocrates,*[4] fetch'd his Remedies for all Diseases from them.

It seems, there is *Rime* as well as *Reason* for it. *Stercus et Urina Medicorum fercula prima.*[5]

But of all *Dung,* One would think a Præscription of *Humane Dung,* should be the Least Agreeable. I know the Name of a *Prophet,* who would have thought so. And yett, even while this *Foetid Sulphur* has not undergone a Change (as it may into a Real *Civet,* but Ironically been called, *Zibetha Occidentalis,*[6] it has been used as a Remedy in many Cases.) It won't be wondered at, for *Becherus*[7] to say, *Internus usus non adeo Delicatus;*[8] And yett this *Foetid Balsam* used so, has made a Speedy Cure of the *Jaundice.* And *Joannes Anglicus,*[9] pulverising it, and giving it in Wine and Honey, cured *Agues* with it! Yea, a *Tavernier*[10] will tell us, That in the Isle of *Java,* the Darts which they shoot in their Fights, are poisoned with so strong a Poison that whoever are struck with them Dy Suddenly. But whoever has any of his own Exrements about him dried unto a Powder, and presently takes a Little of this Powder in a glass of Water, Shall feel no Effect of the Venom; the *Fiery Darts* will not prove so mortal. But the *External Use* of it, was known in *Galens* Time, for a grievous Tumour in the *Throat. Mundererus*[11] asserts, that the Stench of it, next the Heart, in a Morning, præserves from the *Plague. Weickardus* præscribes an Application of it, for *Cancers. Rocheius*[12] and *Corbeius,*[13] have a notable Preparation of it, for that formidable Malady. The Learned make a *Water* of it, and an *Oyl* of it, whereto they ascribe very many Vertues; which I don't insert, because I suppose no body will take them indeed; the Powers that *Salmon* ascribes to this *Dung* used as a *Plaister* for Dangerous and Obstinate *Ulcers,* are very Surprising. Slowly dried and pulverised, the Powder blown into the Eyes twice or thrice a Day, wondrously clears the Eyes, Even takes away Films growing there. But Enough of This. Tis hardly *Good Manners* to write so much about it.

And yett there is another *Excrement* of *Humane Bodies,* wherein there is found a *Remedy* for *Humane Bodies* that is hardly to be parallel'd! *Medicinal Springs* have been of great Esteem in the World, and much Resorted to. People Expect much from *Going to the Waters.* But, my Friend, thou hast one within thee, that Exceeds them all. The *Uses* and *Vertues* of Humane URINE, St. *Barnaby's* Day were Scarce Long Enough to Enumerate them. The People, who take a Daily Draught of it, (Either their own, or some young healthy Persons,) have Hundreds of Thousands of them, found it a *Præservative of Health,* (even to Old Age) hardly to be æqualled.

It is true, Very much of the Skill to Judge of the *Health,* by the *Inspection of the Urine,* pretended unto, has been meer Fallacy and

Imposture: And the *Piss-Prophets*[14] commonly carry on their Trade, with Juggles, wherein People are strangely imposed upon.

But the *Urine* is doubtless capable of being used as a *Medicine,* to procure *Health,* whereof the Benefits cannot be Numbred.

Urine mixed as an Ingredient with other Things, is used in so many Remedies, that it would require a Volume to exhibit them. I cannot Omitt One Experiment. Ones own *Urin,* mixed with the Yolk of an Egg, and sweetened with a Little Sugar, Taken for a While, has cured the *Coughs* and other Ails, of those that have been thought far gone in a *Consumption.* But, It is *Crude Urine* alone, that we will now make some Remarks upon.

If *Pliny* tell us, That the Barbarians used *Urine* that was Five Years Old, as a notable Cathartic, I can sooner find an Author that will call it, *Barbarum Remedium,*[15] than I can direct any Reader where to find it immediately, to make the Experiment.

Mundererus[16] will tell you, What the Drinking of *Urine* will do in *Obstructions* of the Bowels. Now Remove *Obstructions,* and you help any thing!

Mizaldus will tell you, of strange things it will do in the *Dropsy* and *Jaundice;* And *Hildanus* will confirm it with Some Rare Stories upon it: And *Pausa*[17] will add unto the Number of them.

A Considerable Number of Eminent Physicians, besides *Weckerus,*[18] will tell you, That in a Time of *Pestilence,* they who drink a Mornings-Draught of *Urine,* find it a Marvellous Præservative.

It has done Wonders in *Intermitting Fevers.*

Platerus præscribes it against *Worms.*

And the same Gentleman commends it against the Stoppage of *Urine.*

People troubled with what we call, *A Cold,* find it the most Suitable Drink for it in the World.

Suckerus[19] admires it for Children troubled with the *Falling-Sickness:* when used for diverse Months together.

Crato cries up a Lotion with it for Suffusion in the *Eyes;* And *Stockerus,*[19] for all Watry, and Feeble *Eyes.*

Weickardus applauds it for Pains in the *Ears,* and for Worms lodged there.

Mundererus recovers *Lost Hearing,* with a Lotion of it.

Reusner[20] makes it a mighty Cleanser of the *Teeth.* Joined with Bran, it makes a *Dentifrice.*

When Limbs have a *Tremor* or *Shaking* on them, *Forestus* and

Rondeletius[21] will inform you, what a Bathing with *Urine* will do for them.

Hippocrates commands a Fomentation with it, for the Bearing down of the *Womb*. And *Rodericus a Castro*[22] will suppress *Hysteric Fitts,* with the Smell of a Chamber-pott.

Besides what *Urine* will do for the *Itch, Bacmeister*[23] does with it help the Swelling of the *Piles.*

Weickardus does great Things in the *Gout,* with a Lotion of it.

And *Reusner* assures you, That in the same way, you may find Releef against *Weariness,* when your Feet are weary with Walking.

Quincy mentions *Urine* as commended in *Rheumatic* Pains, when boil'd into the Consistence of *Honey.*

In *Ulcers,* yea, in *Cancers,* and in *Bruises,* it has been found of admirable Efficacy.

In *Wounds,* yea, very desperate ones, it has been Very efficacious. *Becherus* tells of a Fellow who cutt his own Throat, that was cured with it.

But if I go on so far as I might, I should stay as long upon it, as the Man in the Pitt that *Schenkius*[24] tells of; but yett not want a *Cordial* and a *Strengthener.* For, *Sustentario Virium,*[25] is one of its Excellencies. He relates a Pleasant Story, of a Man who fell into a Pitt, the depth of near Forty feet, where the Earth fell upon him; however a Board falling with it, he enjoy'd some hollow Shelter there for *Seven Days* together. At the End of *Seven Days* they dug him up, and found him in such an Hearty and Jolly Condition, that he came out boasting and bant'ring of his Cheap Living so long, where his *Diet had cost him Nothing:* For, *he had all this Time lived upon his own Urine.* The Story was thought worthy to be dressed in a Poem; wherein the Writer having affirmed that the Man

> *Viribus integris, Sensu et Sermone Valenti,*
> *Sanus ad Extremos Vixit et inde Dies;*[26]

He at last so Confirms it;

> *Porro ne quis et hoc fictum putet esse; Ego vidi*
> *Scriptor! Quid visu certius esse Potest?*[27]

But now, *what shall we say to the Præserver of Men?* Certainly, We cannot but admire His Bounty to miserable Man, in Surrounding us and Befriending us, with so *many Releefs* of our Calamities, and So *Easy to be Come at.* Certainly, we cannot but Confess our Dependence on *Him* alone, for the *Cure* of our Maladies, when we find it may be convey'd by such Improbable and such Despicable Instruments.

Cap. LV. *Mirabilia* et *Parabilia*.

or,

More, great Friends to *Health,*

very <u>Easy</u> to come at.

WE are Enumerating Some Very *Small Means,* very Plain, and Cheap, and Scarce probable Ones, wherewith *Great Things* have been done, to Restore and Præserve the HEALTH, for which *Dissolved Pearl,* and *Potable Gold,* would not be too precious. But they so grow upon our hands, that we may furnish out *Another Chapter* of them.

§ A Physician wrote a whole Book, about, *The Vertues of Warm Beer.*[1] And indeed, many Invalids, by the Constant Use of *That,* have grown Healthy, and Strong, and Fatt, and thought it almost a *Cure of all Diseases.*

But the same Physician, afterwards finding Some Constitutions, which his *Grand Remedy* had not the Expected Effects upon, he very Conscienciously wrote Another Book, to prevent Peoples *Relying too much,* on what he had formerly published.

Be sure, *Strong Beer,* if it be much used, is Poison to *Weakly* and *Studious* People. Instead of what may be called a *Malt-Soupe,* Lett *Small Beer* be the Drink. *Strong Beer* sufficiently diluted with *Water,* cannot be too much Commended.

§ *Beer* having a Glass of *Wine* incorporated with it, and invigorating of it, is for the most part as wholesome a Drink, as any that can be commonly taken. It will mightily Suit the *Stomach;* and Correct and Prevent *Flatulencies.* And Such a *Sheathed Wine,* will do the *Stomach* much less Damage, than the *Naked Wine* constantly used at the Table.

Quincy has an Observation: "They who intermix *Wine* with their Common Drink, are not so Subject unto *Coughs,* with other Distempers of the Breast, and *Dropsies;* Yett they are more afflicted with both *Nephritic* and *Arthritic* Pains."

§ Were the Vertues of *Hott Water* known, very much of the *Physick* used in the World, would be Laid aside, and the *Physicians* would find unknown Abatements of their Employments. It fluxes the Salt of that *Viscid Flegm,* which depraves the *Stomach,* and produces very many of our Diseases. We have known Some Languishing under a Complication of Distempers, very Strangely Recover *Health,* and

Flesh, by nothing else but a Draught of *Hott Water* taken Every Morning.

§ It is a Custome with some, to *boil Water in an Iron Vessel* over night, Letting it stand there, until the next Morning; then take a Draught of it. A long Summers-day, would be much of it spent, in hearing them, tell the Vertues and Praises of this *Universal Medicine.* It will Recover People out of Numberless Disorders; and Establish them in a Vigorous Condition; and perhaps do them as much Good, as many *Mineral Springs* that are with much Cost repair'd unto.

§ Issues[2] have been of such wonderful Service in a vast Variety of Cases: [*One might write a Large Volumn on them!*] Especially on the *Prophylactic* Account; and for the Prevention of a Thousand Mischiefs; Above all, to prevent *Convulsions* in little Children, and *Consumptions* in Elder People; that I can't forbear the *Mentioning,* yea, and the *Commending* of them. Tis true, Some do needlessly run into the *Troubles* of them. Wherefore, *My Ailing Friend,* Advise with thy *Physician,* whether an *Issue* will be proper and useful for Thee.

And, perhaps, if he know not well what otherwise to do for thy Ails, THIS had best be the *Issue* of it.

But, when we see how much we abound with *Bad Humours,* methinks, It should *Humble* us; And it should also make us afraid of *Worse.* Those of an *Ill Temper,* and an *Ill Carriage,* are so.

§ If People would gett and use the Skill, of Managing the Muscles, wherewith *Ructation* is carried on; and Rasp up the *Wind,* as much and as long as they have any Occasion for it, and until they find rising the very bottom of the Vapour that has offended them with the Sensible Relish of it, they might free themselves from a World of *Sick Fitts,* and Qualms, and Pains, which would else arise from those *Flatulencies* not well discharged, and would putt them to the Trouble and Expence of *Many Medicines.*

§ The Effects of *Cupping,* are more Numerous and Marvellous, than has been commonly thought for; and the Operation is applicable to more Cases than tis easily imagined. I have known a Colonel, who always carried a *Cupping-Glass* with him, wherever he went, and wrought Strange Cures with it; and would almost have beaten any Man, that should have quæstioned, whether he could not with it have much releeved, almost any Malady that could be mentioned. Since we have now gott the Way of *Cupping without Fire,*[3] t'wil doubtless be the more easily and more frequently ventured on.

§ Who would imagine that a Diet of poor, mean, plain *Water-gruel* should be such an Effectual Remedy for so many Distempers? But I can tell of Countreys, where they Cure not only *Colds* and *Coughs* but Even *Consumptions* with it.

Suppose the Vertue of this Diet may ly only in This, that while People confine themselves unto it, they Suspend the Actions of *Self-Destruction:* yett even this is far from Contemptible.

§ Some of my Neighbours apprehend a mighty Benefit unto their Health, from a *Lye* commonly used with them. They throw a Spoonful or Two of hott *Ashes* into a Porringer of Water, and letting it Subside a few Minutes, they drink the Water. Tis a great Cleanser and Strengthener of the Stomach; And that *Grand Wheel* doing its Duty well, the whole Engine fares the better. Yea, tis a sort of a *Panacæa* to them.

§ A *Milk-Diet* has had wonderful Effects, in Curing many, and grievous, and such as have been thought Incureable, Diseases. Dr. *Ziegler*,[4] who was cured of the *Black Jaundice* by it, when his Case was grown desperate unto all Physicians and Medicines, wrote a Book upon *Milk*. But he observed, That Milk will do hurt, with other meats; but being used *alone* it has Vertues that may be wondred at! He releeved Hæreditary Maladies, by Living Entirely upon *Milk,* Sometimes for fourteen days together.

Wepferus[5] mentions a Matron, who had been for many years afflicted with terrible Convulsions, and Hysterical Suffocations, miraculously releeved by Drinking of nothing but *Milk* for a long while together.

Reader; Canst thou Reflect on such Things as these, without celebrating the Compassion of the Glorious One, who *Remembers us in our Low Estate, because His Mercy Endures forever;* and who conveys His *Healing Mercy* to us, in Ways that are so Easy to be practised, but so unlikely, without His Blessing, to do *much good* unto us?

§ For the Scattering of *Wens,* and of many and grievous *Tumours,* which being lett alone, (or, imprudently irritated) would prove not only beyond all Expression Troublesome to People, but also anon bring their very Lives in hazard, the Efficacy of a *Dead Hand,*[6] has been out of measure wonderful. It must be kept on, till the Patient feel the *Damp* sensibly Strike into him; and sometimes there may be Occasion for the Repetition of it.

The famous *Greatreats,*[7] the *Stroker,* never did Such Cures with his *Living Hand,* as a *Dead Hand* has done upon the living.

But, My Friend, The Repeted *Contemplation of Death,* and of the *State* which it brings Mankind into, will be as profitable to thy *Soul,* as the Application of a *Dead Hand,* Can be unto thy *Body.* Continue the *Contemplation,* till thou feel it Strike to thy very Heart within thee. All the *Tumors* of a *Carnal Mind,* will be notably discussed and suppressed by such a Method of PIETY.

Methinks, The lifeless, pallid and squalid *Object* which thou hast before thee, when thou hast the *Dead Hand* upon thee, gives thee a very particular Opportunity and Invitation, to form such Thoughts, with a most lively Impression from them; *Lord, How soon may I come into the Condition of this Breathless Carcase!* And, *Lord Where will my Spirit be Lodg'd, when it has left the Carcase!*

CAP. LVI. The Eyes of poor *Hagar*[1] opened.
or,
A Discovery of Unknown Stores for Cures,
which every Body is Master of.

THE Vertues of *Bread,* are what every Child, that can but manage a peece of *Bread and Butter,* can declaim upon.

But then, Who would have thought that a Peece of *Chewed Bread,* should be recommended as, *An Universal Medicine?* And yett, among the, *Annotations upon* Mr. Hartlibs[2] *Legacy,* a Gentleman Employs a Whole Chapter on this Intention. *White-Bread,* Chewed in the Mouth, to a Kind of a Pap or Paste, has cured Sores, that no Salves did any good upon; yea, Sores that seemed as having something of the *Kings Evil* in them.

Green Wounds; Yea, the Bites of *Mad Dogs,* have been Cured with it.

It has releeved *Pains* of an uncommon Obstinacy.

It has mollified *Corns* at such a rate, that they have been Easily rooted out, and never grown any more.

It stops *Bleeding:* Draws out *Poison;* does a Thousand Things, that would not have been Easily imagined.

But lett us leave *Bread,* and go to *Water.*

We shall quickly find greater Authors than *Darby Dawn,* to tell us,

The greatest Part o' th' World's Content

With Adams Ale, *pure Element.*
And when the Stomach's out of Order,
No Cordial, like a Glass of Water.
This, This has baffled all the Slops,
Of Ladies Closetts, and the Shops.
Its Uses are too manifold,
And marv'lous great e'er to be told.

Dr. *Morgan* observes, "Of all Liquors, *Water* is beyond Controversy the most Excellent and Effectual, to Cool, and dilute the *Blood,* and wash off the Viscidities and Obstructing Cohæsions of the Glands, and keep the animal Fluids in a due State of Fluxility and Motion. And therefore, this had doubtless been still retain'd as the Common Drink of Mankind, had not the Abuse of Reason in Artificial Intemperance prevailed so far, as to sett aside one of the main Principles and greatest Præservatives of Health."

Dr. *Cheyne* observes, That all *Malt-Liquors* (except only clear, *Small Beer,* of a due Age,) are Extremely hurtful to *Weakly* and *Studious* Persons.

But, for *Strong Waters,*—They cannot be Enough decried: When People have come to a State wherein these become Necessary, they may justly be reckoned among, *The Dead;* Both as to the *Little Time* they have to *Live,* and the *Little Use* there is like to be of them while they *Live.*

As for that famous *Diapente,*[3] which we call PUNCH [The *Indoustan* Term for for the Number *Five,* which, you know, is the Number of its Ingredients,][4] however a little of it may be of use in some Cases, and particularly, under the Excessive Heats, of our hotter Days in the Summer, it is yett *ordinarily taken* a Dangerous and a Venemous Composition: and will anon prove a Sort of *Arsenic* to them who *tarry long* at the *Bowl.* A Learned Foreigner has informed the World, *est Anglicus quidam Potus quem Vocant,* Bola Puncha;[5] and has Reported the *Virtues* of it. The True Report would be, Its *Virtues* are to Poison, and Besot, and Enrage the Children of Men, and to *Destroy them wonderfully.* The *Drinkers* won't beleeve me; but will *run Violently down into the* Bowl, and will *perish in the* Liquor.

A Learned and Acute Physician, whose Name I have lately mentioned, makes this Observation:

"To releeve a Surfeit of *Meat,* with a Surfeit of *Wine,* is to *Light the Candle at both Ends.* Both Weak and Strong, who drink only *Water* (or *Small Beer,*) will digest as much again, as if they drank *Stronger Liquors.*"

As for the Richer, Stronger, Heavier *Wines,* the Rule is, *Ad Summum Tria Pocula Sume,* or, *Stop at the Third.* My Physician adds, *Whatsoever is more, cometh of Evil:* and must be diluted with the Tears of *Repentance.*

But, for WATER! WATER!—

Hyrodopota Encouraged.

Rustici—qui nil bibunt praeter Aquam frigidam, gentium Sanissimi sunt, et attigunt grandaevam aetatem.[6] Bartholin.

No longer tell me of *Wine,* in any other Terms, than *Hector* in *Homer* treats it withal.

> *Inflaming Wine, pernicious to Mankind,*
> *Unnerves the Limbs, and dulls the noble Mind.*

His Commentator *Pope* observes, That the best Physicians agree with *Homer* in this Point. *Sampson* drank as little *Wine,* as *Hector.* We will now celebrate a *Liquor that was made before it!*

We were Speaking of Significant, and almost Universal *Remedies,* which are *Easy to Come at.* But if I mention *Common* Water, Certainly none can mention a thing more *Easy to Come at!* And I Entreat, that the *Compassion* of our most Gracious God unto a Miserable World, may be celebrated with proper *Praises* and *Wonders,* when I have demonstrated, that among the *Remedies* that will answer and releeve a World of uneasy Cases, *Common* Water has often had Effects, that few can pretend unto; yea, that would Surpass all Imagination.

Festus[7] fancies, That the Temple of *Esculapius* was built in the middle of the *Water,* to Signify the Custome of the Physicians, who cure their Patients by obliging them to drink *Water.* Verily, it would be well for us, if they more obliged us unto it than they do.

It is not enough to say, That a *Sweat* from a Draught of *Cold Water,* taken in the Beginning of any *Fever,* is the most powerful Fever-killer, that has ever yett been known among the dying Children of Men. This One Thing alone, were Enough to render it more precious to us, than the most Costly Liquors and Cordials, that have ever yett been known in the World.

We will pass on to a few more of the many Observations, that have been made upon the Matter.

Dr *Curtis*[8] will assure us, that the use of *Water,* for a Common Drink *Preserves the Native Ferment of the Stomach in due Order, keeps the Blood Temperate, and helps to Spin out the Thread of Life to the Longest Extent of Nature. It makes the Rest at Night more quiet and refreshing, the Reason and Understanding more Clear, the Passions less disorderly,—Cold Water exceeds any other Cordial, to cause digestion. Water* is not so Cold and Lifeless, *he says,* as many imagine.

Vander Heiden, in his Book, *De Sero Lactis, Aqua frigida, et Aceto,*[9] observes;

That *Cold Water* not only præserves from the *Gout,* but also Conquers it, Quiets it, Cures it: And that the Immersion of the Hands and Feet in *Cold Water,* does not Repel the Humours, but cool them, and Soften the Skin, and so draw out the Vapours.

That the *Sciatica,* or, *Hip-Gout,* if taken at the Beginning, is cured in four or five Days, only by the Drinking of *Cold Water.*

That the Pain of the *Stomach* from Crudities or, what we call the *Heart-burn,* is Cured by Drinking of *Cold Water.*

Yea, That a Strange Ease is procured in Fitts of the *Stone,* by drinking of *Cold Water.*

Sir *Theodore Mayherne* in his *Medical Counsils,* affirms, That for most of the Diseases that afflict the *Head,* there is nothing better than to Bathe it with *Cold Water.*

And *Smith* cured a desperate *Pain of the Ears,* upon taking of Cold, by keeping on a Towel often doubled, and wett with *Cold Water,* for about half an hour; and upon a Return of the Pains repeating it.

Every Body knows, what is done for *frozen Limbs,* by an Immersion in *Cold Water.* And how the Dipping of the Head in *Cold Water* cures the *Headache.*

Dr. *Cockburn*[10] in his Treatise of *Sea-Diseases,* observes, Under *Want of Sleep* in *Fevers,* there is a Wonderful Success of dipping a Towel four times doubled, in *Oxyorat,* [which is, six Parts Water and one Part Vinegar,] and binding it about the Head and Temples. *John Smith* says, He often found *Cold Water* alone, to have the Same Effect.

But, who would have imagined, what *Vander Heiden* sais, That *Paralytic* Members may be in a little time Cured, by a frequent Washing of them with *Cold Water?* Yes, *Pitcairn* advises it.

Or, who would have imagined, That where any *Pains* are vexatious, the washing of the Parts often with *Cold Water,* will Sooner and Surer take them away, than the more *Spirituous Embrocations,* which are commonly used on such Occasions? Yea, that holding the Hands and Feet and Legs in *Cold-Water*, will disperse the Winds that cause the *Cholic?* But so *Vander Heiden* sais. Be sure, The Internal Use of *Cold Water*, has in the *Cholic* been found of most happy Consequence.

Dr. *Wainright*[11] says, That *Water-drinkers* are never troubled with the *Cholic*.

The Candid Gentleman, who has recommended *Cold Water* to the World, as the, *Febrifugum Magnum*, adds, That from Experience he knows *Cold Water* to be good in all kinds of *Asthma's;* And that Water gives twice as Good Breath for *Easy Walking*, as Wine or Ale can do.

He affirms, he has by long Experience found, that *Water* is the best Thing that can be, to cure a *Surfet*.

When our *Food Corrupts* by lying too long in the Stomach, or, when we are vapoured into *Præternatural Heats*, by Meats and Drinks taken at a Full Table, in too much Variety, a Draught of *Cold Water*, will *do good like a Medicine*.

Vander Heyden cures *Hoarseness*, with a little Supper of a *Raw Apple*, and a Draught of *Cold Water*.

Excessive *Bleeding* at the Nose, is cured by the Drinking of *Cold Water*. [*Heiden* tells you, the most Speedy, and Certain Remedy for *Bleeding at the Nose*, is, To putt the Feet of the Patient into *Warm Water*. He may stand up to the Knees in it, if the Bleeding be violent.]

Galen sais, The Drinking of *Cold Water* will cure *Hecticks*.

The *Rheumatism* is cured by drinking of *Cold Water*.

Clysters of Water, yea, of *Cold Water*, have done Strange Cures; even in *Bloody Fluxes*.

Yea, we will again Speak of the *Gout*, from others besides *Heyden*. We have Authentic Stories of a Regular, and Obstinate *Gout*, utterly taken away, so as never to return any more, only by taking to the Drinking of *Cold Water*. Be sure, it would so imbibe the *Gouty Salts*, that the Distemper would have Longer Intermissions, and be Less Painful in the Returns of it. It is affirmed, the using of *Cold Water* for some Days together in *Spring* and *Fall*, or, a little before the certain Times, when the *Gout* usually siezes the Party; tis a wonderful Præservative.

Old *Piso* sais, a Morning-Draught of *Cold Water*, Continued a few Days, marvellously helps the *Stone* in the Kidneys.

Borhoeve[12] will tell you; Nothing is a greater *Diluter of Thick Blood,* than *Warm Water* drank in great Quantities. But then, how much is *Health* and *Life* befriended by it!

The daily washing of the *Mouth,* is an useful Practice. But if with it, we wash the Joints of the *Jaws,* and behind and below the *Ears,* with *Cold Water,* we præserve ourselves, from the Weary and Grievous Hours, with which the *Toothache* afflicts millions of People.

Strainings, Bruises, Tumours, are strangely relieved by *Cold Water* used upon them.

Tis amazing, how much the Cure of *Wounds* is forwarded by wetting them with *Cold Water,* for a few Minutes together. *Vander Heyden* will tell you enough of This.

Memorandum. If your *Water* be not Such as will make a Good Lather with Soap; You must *Boil* it before you use it.

But after all these Remarks, *Wisdome will be profitable to Direct.* People may sometimes be in Hazard, of *Over-Cooling* their *Stomacks.* As soon as ever they perceive this (and it will be Easily perceiv'd,) Lett them stop a Little; and recruit the necessary Heat of that important Bowel. *Drink no longer Water, but use a Little Wine, for thy Stomachs Sake.*

But then, tis an Everlasting Maxim, That when People are *over-heated* by *Labour* and *Fatigue,* they must beware of drinking any thing that is *Cold;* as they would of taking *Poison.* An Experienced Old Gentleman writes, *The Want of due Care in this Case, has kill'd more than the Plague ever did, or ever will do.*

I will take this Occasion, to offer one of the best *Refreshments for a weary Man,* (I beleeve, and I have often tried it) that ever was known in the World.

Cutt a Large and Thin Slice of *Bread.* Let it be (Without Burning) thoroughly toasted. Putt it hott into a Pint of Cold Water. Lett it Stand a While; And then Sett it on the Fire, till it come to the Heat in which we Ordinarily drink our *Tea.* Drink as many Dishes, as you please of it; my first Adviser said, *Without Sugar.* But our *Philosophical Transactions* tell us of a Gentleman coming to be an Hundred Years Old, whose great Age was ascribed unto his great Use of *Sugar.* A bitt of *Sugar* in it will do it no Harm. Nor will the Mixture of a little *Milk* with the *Bread-Tea* be a *Milk-Tea.* The World can hardly shew another so Refreshing a Liquor.

Our *Ministers* coming home from their public and heating and spending Services, cannot be advised unto a better Thing than This!

Tis impossible to come out of this *Capsula,* without thinking on The COLD BATH. Do but read Sir *John Floyer* and Dr. *Bainard,*[13] and say whether the *Psychrolusia,*[14] be not one of the most Salutiferous Operations that ever was heard of! In abundance of *Deplorable Cases,* and the Sorrows of *Chronical Ails,* the Cold-Bath is most certainly One of the most Seasonable and Profitable Resorts, that can be imagined. People under *Innumerable,* and such as have been thought *Incureable* Infirmities, repeating their Immersion into the Cold Bath, have often seen such an astonishing Success of it, that it has look'd almost, as if the *Angel of Bethesda* had led them to it.

Patients, I Exhort you, Consult your *Physicians* about it. *Physicians,* I Entreat you, Direct your *Patients* unto it, *Oftener than you do!* And yett nicely consider their State. Remember Dr. *Quincy's* Caution: *Corpulency,* and any Unsoundness, or Corruption, in the *Bowels,* forbid the Use of the *Cold Bath.* Be Sure, the Vessels had need be Sound, that they may bear the Sudden Changes in the Vibrations here given to them.

Cap. LVII. A *Physick-Garden.*

or,

A Consideration of the admirable Vertues,

in certain Plants which every *Common Garden* is furnished with.

THE celebrated *Helmont,* tho' he understood and Asserted *Chymistry* as much almost as any of them that *Labour in the Fire,* yett makes this Ingenuous Confession: *I beleeve that Simples in their Simplicity, are Sufficient for the Curing of all Diseases.*

While the *Spagyrical*[1] Gentlemen sometimes too much *Neglect* the *Simple Vegetable,* the *Galenical* do too much *Confound* it, by mixing a needless Heap of Plants together in their Medicines, among which it would be Strange if the *Single Vegetable* should Exert its proper Vertues.

I must indeed allow the Censure of Dr. *Fuller;* That *our Herbals give such poor, sorry, deficient, false and undistinguishing Accounts, of the Vertues of Simples, that we must not Venture to practice upon their Authority.*

Nevertheless, we will proceed.

One Vegetable sometimes has Vertues Enough to Supply an Ingenious Physician with matter Enough to write a *Whole Treatise* upon it. The *Naturae-Curiosi*[2] in *Germany* have produced a meer Library of Examples; [indeed a *German* can hardly write of a Plant but he cures all Diseases with it!] and *Mallows,* does no longer monopolize the Title of, *Omnimorbia.*[3] The famous *Moly*[4] of *Homer,* we can't come at; or indeed know what it was, or, whether it ever Existed any where but in the *Iliad,* but Among the Ancients, there were Several *Plants* which bore the Name of *Hercules.* In *Theophrastus*[5] and in *Dioscorides,* and in other Botanists, there is a *Poppy,* called, *Hercules's.* There was another Plant called *Heracleum.* The *Nymphaea* was, as *Pliny* tells us, called *Heraclea.* There is a Sort of *Panax* also, and there are Some other Plants named from *Hercules.* Tis probable, the Name was given, to denote the *Extraordinary Force* of these Plants; which they compared unto the Strength of *Hercules.* (As the *Epilepsy* is called, *The Herculean Distemper.*) I will now sett some *Herculean Plants* before you.

Among the Plants of our Soyl, Sir *William Temple* Singles out *Five,* as being *of the greatest Vertue and most Friendly to Health:* and his *Favourite-Plants* are, *Sage, Rue, Saffron, Alehoof, Garlick,* and *Eldar.*

The Wonders of <u>Sage</u> can't be reckoned up.—*Cur moriatur homo?*[6]

Sage-Tea, would be of more use to you, *Gentlemen,* than what you give a *Guinea* a Pound for.

<u>Rue</u>. The Juice of it made up, with Sugar into Small Pills, and Swallowed, when there is Occasion;—Tis Excellent for all Illness of the *Stomach,* proceeding from Cold or Moist Humours. Tis a notable *Digester;* and a Restorer of the *Appetite.*

<u>Saffron</u>. Tis a matchless *Cordial;* a mighty Comforter of the Spirits. It cannot be of too Common Use in *Diet,* any more than in *Medicine.*

Your *Tea* would be worth taking, if there were a Pinch of *Saffron* in the Pott. There would be *Life in the Pott.* Sir *William* sais, "I have known the Spirit of *Saffron* restore a Man out of the very Agonies of *Death,* when Left by all Physicians, as desperate."

But he observes, the frequent Use of *Spirits,* does destroy the Natural Heat of the Stomach; and the *Common Drinking of Wine* at Meals, has a Degree of such a Tendency.

It is given in almost all Disorders of the *Lungs;* And for its great

Efficacy in promoting Expectoration, and relieving the Breath, it is by some called, *Anima Pulmonum.*[7]

Alehoof.[8] Tis a Sovereign Thing for the *Eyes.*

In *Frenzies,* Outwardly or Inwardly Used, it will do Wonders.

This is the Plant, with which our Ancestors made their Common Drink, when the Inhabitants of *England* were Esteemed the Longest Livers in the World. In Old English, the Name Signifies, *What was necessary to the making of Ale.* Tis a mighty Cleanser.

Hear what Sir *Kenelm Digby* sais.

"A good Handful of Leaves of *Ground-Ivy,* boil'd in a Draught of Ale, drunk morning and evening; it is admirable to Cure all *Headakes,* Pains, Inflammations, Defluxions in the *Eyes; Jaundices; Coughs, Consumptions, Spleen, Stone* and *Gravel,* and all Obstructions. The Herb stamped, and applied like a Plaister to a *Felon,*[9] cures it marvellously and speedily. It is admirable for old Sores."

Sir *William* sais, "If there be a Specific Remedy or prevention of the *Stone,* I take it to be, the Constant Use of *Ale-hoof-*Ale."

Etmuller mentions one cured of a *Scorbutic Consumption,* with nothing else but a Strong Decoction of *Ground-Ivy,* after a Vomit had been first given for it.

Quincy sais, The Herb when pick'd clear from the Stalks, and carefully dried, is much better than when it is green, and will make the Infusion stronger and finer.

Garlick. It affords much Nourishment unto them who Eat little Flesh.

It is of great Vertue in *Cholicks.*

It is a mighty Strengthener of the *Stomach,* upon Decays of Appetite, and Indigestion.

Sir *William* sais, Tis a Specific for the *Gout.*

In *France,* tis usual to fall into a Diet of *Garlick,* for a fortnight or three weeks, upon the first fresh Butter of the Spring: And the Common People esteem it a Præservative against the Diseases of the Ensuing year. A Broth of *Garlick* is used by them, the day after a Debauch. They who procure the *Occasion,* deserve not the *Benefit!*

Tis called, *The Poor Mans Treacle.*

It is a wondrously Penerating Thing. Dr. *Lower* observes, that if it be laid unto the *Feet,* the *Breath* will Smell of it.

Eldar. The *Anatomia Sambuci,*[10] published by a German Physician, and since Translated into English, would almost perswade one to attempt the Cure of almost all Diseases with it. Be sure, The *Eldar-*

berry Wine, is as fine a Drink, as almost any that we can treat our Friends withal.

But these *Five Plants* may admitt of Some Competition.

The Quinquina.[11] How Celebrated; Immoderately, Hyperbolically Celebrated!

In the Use of this Powder, what Violent Commotions of the Blood, Humours, and Spirits,

Pulveris Exigui Jactu Compressa quiescunt![12]

Colts-foot, has been found a most potent Analeptic, as *Rensueras*[13] assures us: And *Hillerus*[14] cured Atrophies, in Children with it; making them out of the Herb fried, after the manner of *Clary.*[15] A Strong Decoction of it until the Liquor was grown glutinous, has done Miraculous Cures for the *Kings-Evil;* as well as Restored People from desperate *Consumptions.*

Liquorice, was of old called *Adipson,* for being a great Quencher of Thirst, and therefore præscribed by *Galen* in *Dropsies. Theophrastus* calls it, *Scythica:* and *Pliny* sais, because the *Scythians* would live a dozen days together upon it, with a little *Mare-Milk Cheese.* It was esteemed then a great *Sustainer of Nature.* It strangely helps Pains in the *Stomach* and the *Bladder.* It is One of the greatest Correctors of *Acrimonies.* But then take it alone; mix nothing with it. There is hardly a greater Analeptic to be found in the World. It is as Dr. *Fuller* sais, A Kind of *Balsam in Fieri,* and the most likely to be wrought up to Perfection in the Blood. Lett the *Fresh Juice* be taken, Every Day.

I have heard Celandine Tea cried up at such a rate, that if *Half be true,* tis One of the best Things in the World.

The *Oil of Sweet Almonds:*[16] if the Vertues of it were known, how many Tuns of *Almonds* would be brought under the Torture for it! *Rivers of the Oil* would hardly serve the Occasions of the Physicians for it. It is incredible, how much this *Oil* does Temper, and Correct and Govern the *Bilious Salts* in the *Stomach,* when they grow Disorderly; And how finely they sheathe Such *Salts* (or what else you'l call them) that fire the Blood in most of our Fevers. I have known *Epidemical Fevers,* that generally killed all but those, who were saved by Remedies, whereof *Oil of Sweet Almonds* was the principal Ingredient.

In the Want of this *Oil,* there may be great Things done for the Health of People, in abundance of Cases, by the use of, what has been ignorantly called, *Sperma-Ceti,* but is nothing but the Oil of the

Whale finely and fully digested, and what in Opposition to the Ignorance of the old Appellation, I will call, *Parmisitty.*[17]

Christian; The *Vertues* of Every *Plant,* call for thy *Praises* to the Glorious God, who has made the *Plant,* and has taught us the *Vertues* of it.

And, if thou art a *Plant of Righteousness,* thou wilt Study to be One, upon other Accounts, of greater *Vertues,* than any that are to be found, *from the Cedar that is in Lebanon, Even unto the Hyssop that Springs out of the Wall.*

§ But while We are thus Contemplating the Emblems and Pictures of, *An Useful Man,* in the Vegetable World, and admiring the Goodness of our GOD and SAVIOUR unto us, in making Sometimes *One Single Plant,* a Subject of so many Vertues, I must ask, that One Instance may be more Considered, which has hitherto had very little Notice taken of it.

It is, The *Balsam* of *Copayba.* [or, *Capivy.*] The Words of Dr. *Tho. Fuller,* in his *Pharmcopoeia Extemporanea,* shall Express all that I shall offer on this Occasion.

"*Copayba* I know, by great Experience, to be a most noble Medicament, and had I the placing of it, it should stand in the *Fore-front of the very best of Balsams.* But because its not commonly known so well as it deserves, I shall not grudge a little Pains in setting forth, and briefly Explaining some of its Properties.

Tho' it seems to be of the *Turpentine* Class, yett it gives not the Violet Smell to Urine, but imbues it with a Manifest Bitter Taste, and wonderfully takes off the *Muriatic Saltness* of it, and of the *Serum* of the Blood, and of the *Saliva.*

It impresseth a *Balsamic* Character on the Mass of *Blood;* Cures its Scorbutic, rancid, and putridinous *Cachexy:* is prevalent (both Externally and Internally) against Ulcers, the *Palsey, Gout,* Weakness and Pains of the *Back.* It in a wonderful Manner deterges the *Reins, Ureters,* and *Bladder,* when obstructed with Sand, *Mucus* or *Pus;* strengthens them when relaxed, and heals them when ulcerated. It provokes *Urine,* Extinguishes its *Heat,* and cleanses off its Bloody, foul, and purulent Contents, more Effectually than any thing I ever yett mett with.

It may very justly be accounted the Best of all *Thoracicks;* deterges the *Bronchia,* and Vesicles; recovers the Tone of the *Lungs,* heals their *Breaches;* and (as I have thought) Even dissolves the *Tubercula Cruda.* For I have seen where this *Balsam* alone hath (beyond all Expectation) perfectly cured dry, deep *Coughs,* that ap-pear'd horribly dangerous, and manifestly threatened a *Consumption.* And I have more than once cured with it, coughing up of *Blood* and *Pus* in frightful Quantities.

And notwithstanding it is intensely Bitter, and manifestly *hott,* yett (which is an admirable advantage of it,) I have found it mighty agreeable to *Hectic Persons;* it rather abates than augments their *Heats,* as one might fear it would: The Reason of which is, I suppose, because it so powerfully subdues Saltness and Acrimony, and obliter-ates Putredinous Inquinations."

I will add this; That some of my Neighbours, who have been for many months followed with wasting *Fluxes,* till they have thought their Bowels all Excoriated, have by the Use of this *Balsam* alone, been perfectly and wondrously cured.

The Way of using it is, To take the Quantity of Eight or Ten Drops, with a little Sugar. It may be taken at any time: the best is at going to Bed.

I suspect, the too large Use of it, may be too hott, for some Con-stitutions.

§ Allow me to add a Word of <u>Apples</u>.

Dr. *Thomas Fuller* sais, "Of all Juices, I count that of <u>Apples,</u> beyond Compare, the Best; Because Nature has wrought it up to an high Degree of Generosity and Maturity. They are not fitt for Use, until they have been gathered a While, and sweat in an Heap. The best Way, is not to drink their Juice, but Eat them raw, or scoop out and Eat the Pulp, for a long Course of Time, Every Morning.

Thus they have given more Help, to *Scorbutic* and *splenetic* Persons, (Especially such as were of an hott dry Constitution and apt to be Costive,) than any thing Else, the Shops or Fields could furnish out. Dr. *Baynard* highly cries them up, as a most Noble Pectoral, and cured himself twice of a Confirmed *Consumption,* by the Use of them."

Dr. *Morgan* says, "*Apples,* Especially the gratefully Acid and Oily Sort, Such as the Kentish Pippin, Pearmain, Pomroy Non-pareills—under all hott, flatulent, and rarefactive Disorders of the *Chyle, Lymph,* and *Blood,* they are an Excellent Stomachick, Pec-toral, and Diuretic."

§ Allow me also to annex a Short Quotation, from Dr. *Daniel Coxes* Discourse on, *The Interest of the Patient.*[18]

He sais; "An Eminent Physician assured me, that most Ill Habits of Body, Occasioned by feeding much on Salt-meats, are soon cured, by Eating daily for a few Weeks, almost any Edible *Green Herbs*. And another no less considerable, who hath great Dealing with Sea-men, protested to me, that he cures all those among them that are Scorbutically affected, only with *young pease,* ordered all manner of Ways; Eaten crude, or boil'd, with, or without their Shells; the Juice whereof is to be plentifully mixed with their Broth; This Remedy never failed him nor the Sea-men, of Cure; and this Sometimes after the Disease had eluded many very promising Methods and Medicines.

I shall only mention that Method, which is of general Use, in order to the Extricating the Vertues of the Simples; which is This. The Ingredients are to be hung in Fermenting Liquors, whether Wine, Ale, Beer, or Cider, etc. and that their Medicating Properties are Extracted by this Method, daily Experience doth attest:—As for what refers to Cures Effected by these Means, I dare boldly affirm, *That there is Scarcely any Chronical Disease, that is cured by the Shop-medicines, which may not be cured with more Certainty, Ease, and Pleasure, by Drinks thus ordered, joined with a Regular Diet."*

The Brasen Statue of our SAVIOUR, (with her own) which they tell us, Mrs. *Veronica,*[19] the Person who was cured on her touching the Border of our SAVIOURS Garment, Sett up at *Paaneas,* they also tell us had at the Foot of it a certain *unknown plant,* which growing up to the Border of the Garment, was a *Cure of all Distempers.* Perhaps, we have mentioned Several Plants, the Virtues whereof may be as Considerable as those of that *Unknown* One. Whether it be so or no; The Course taken by that Good Woman, the Story whereof is more certain than the Fable of the Statue, is the *best Cure of all Distempers.*

Mr. S. Bowdens[20] Remark.

§ Plain Remedies, at first, were valu'd most,
   The Drugs were few, and moderate the Cost:
   The Sick were cured without a gilded Pill,
   A Sovereign *Bolus,* or a pompous *Bill.*
   As *Vice* increas'd, So *Physic* by degrees
   Increas'd its *Empire,* and increas'd its *Fees.*

§ I conclude with a true observation of *Rob. Godfrey's,*[21] That commonly, the *Simpler* a Medicine is, the *Better* it is.

And I will transcribe the Words of Dr. *Morgan.* "There cannot perhaps be a surer Mark of a Novice or *Ignoramus* in his Profession, if he be not Something Worse, than the Affectation of a *Multiplicity of Ingredients,*[22] in almost Every thing that is given; by which the Doctor seems to præscribe more for the *Apothecary* than for the Patient.

When any particular Morbid Constitution, Exists distinctly, and is not mixed or complicated with any other, Some *Primary Simple Medicine,* of peculiar Efficacy under that Constitution, Such as *Nature* has præpared, will suffice for the Cure; and any further Artificial Pomp or Apparatus would be needless."

My *Angel of Bethesda,* has therefore Exhibited very few, that are Tedious and Laboured Compositions.

CAP. LVIII. *Thaumatographia Insectorum.*[1]

or,

Some Despicable *Insects* of Admirable *Vertues.*

SOME Animals that at first appear *Despicable* to us, how *Serviceable* has a Good God anon made them to us! The Spectacle calls for our *Praises* of His Goodness.

I will not mention the *Sheep;* that Noble Quadruped, which for *Usefulness* has not its Equal among all the Things that go upon Four. Besides the Supplies of our other Wants, how many Succours for our *Distempers,* does it afford unto us! Its very *Dung* is a most Sovereign Remedy in how many of our most grievous Distempers!

But I will only call in Two or Three Insects, to Illustrate the Matter, from whence I would invite my Reader to join with me in praising the Glorious God, who does us Good in Ways and by Means, which we could have so little imagined. But then, *What Good can He do, will He do, and how surpassing all Imagination, to them whom He shall bring to Inherit all things!*

The Bee, deserves to be Sung in higher Strains, than ever the most lofty *Georgicks* could arise unto. The *Honey,* which he finds and brings to his well-contrived *Hive,* has Uses in Medicine which cannot be numbred. *A Land flowing with Honey is a Pleasant Land;* and enriched with a Medicine for a Large Catalogue of *Diseases.* But it was also, till very lately, the *Principal Condiment* of our *Diet.* The *Sugar,* which was of old called, *The Honey of the Cane,* and which *Cocceius*[2] thinks is in the *Canticle* of *Solomon* to be mett withal, was little us'd or known in our Nation, as late as Two Hundred years ago.

Millepedes have more *Virtues,* than their Name does assign *Feet* unto them. Was there Ever a more powerful *Opener* of *Obstructions;* and so, a more powerful Releever of a *Thousand Maladies?* Even *Cancers* themselves have been, in the hands of a *Mayern,* conquered by these little Creepers. Poor *Sowbug!* Tho' thou liest in such Obscurity under an old Log of Wood, or in the Bottom of a Dark Cellar; Thou deservest the Honour of a *Title* sometimes inscribed on the gate of a Dead Popes Physician, [Orbis Liberatori.][3] Tis incredible, how much the World might fare the better for thee!

But then, Cantharides; what Wonders have been wrought by their *Epispastic* Applications and Operations! The *Spanish Kings* have never yett Extended their Tyrannies, as far as the *Spanish Flies* have their Benefits; nor have the *Kings* destroy'd so many People, as the *Flies* have rescued. How many Millions of Lives have been saved by them! And how often has *Belzebub*[4] lost his Intention to act as the *Angel of Death,* when these have been skilfully Employ'd in Serving the merciful Purposes of Him who is our SAVIOUR!

It seems, they are plentifully stock'd, with a very hott, subtil, active, and extremely pungent *Salt;* a Considerable Quantity whereof, Entring the Blood on the Application of *Epispaticks,* is there strongly attracted by the Serum, and passes together with it thro' the Several Glandular Strainers; and there acts as a Lymphatic Purgative, or Glandular Cathartic.

And yett tho' these are such Salutary Things, what an Outcry has Dr. *Baynard* made, about the Mischiefs of Unseasonable and Immoderate *Blistering!* However, I hope, he will not object against, the use which I find our *Catharides* of late putt unto. Instead of *Rattsbane,*[5] my Neighbours, with less *Hazard* unto themselves, but with Sufficient *Ruin* to the *Ratts,* lay Balls well stock'd with *Cantharides* for them.

You, *Gentlemen,* that have Encomiastically exercised your Witts and your Pens, on some other Animals, in your, *Dissertationes Ludicrae,* make an Experiment, what you can do in more *Serious Performances,* to Celebrate what a Gracious God has done by such *unlikely Instruments* for the miserable Children of Men.

But being led thus to observe, *That very Diminutive Creatures may become very Profitable Creatures;* And, *Little* Things may be made *useful* ones: Why should not the Observation animate my Wish and Hope, *That so small and mean a Thing as I am, yett may do some Good,* if the Sovereign God please to Accept me and Assist me for it, *in the World!*

My Friend, Tho' thou mayst be a *Brother of Low Degree,* yett sett thyself to think, *what Good my I do?* Lett the *Noble Quæstion* be often, *often!*—considered with thee. If thou mayst have the Wisdome, [and a *poor Man* may have this Despised Wisdome!] to find out *Well-advised Inventions* upon it, who can tell for what a *Doer of Good* thou shalt Stand Registred, in the Book of *Remembrance,* which thy God has *Written before Him!*

Cap. LIX. *Infantilin.*

or,

Infantile-Diseases.

THE *Angel of Bethesda,* will not leave us, till the *Little Ones* [who have their *Angels!*] have had some compassionate Consideration with us.

Poor Infants! Methinks, you did like *Little Prophets,* when you came *Crying* into the World. It is not long before the Occasions for your *Cries* do multiply upon you. Yea, what Vast Numbers of you, go *Crying* out of the World again! *Destruction* and *Death* Siezes you, before you have passed thro' the State of *Infancy. O how unsearchable the Judgments of God, and His Ways past finding out!* The *Lamps* but just litt up, and blown out again!

Parents: When you see your *Infant-Children* Languishing under *Distempers,* Lett the Sad Sight awaken *suitable Reflections* in you.

Think; "Oh! the Grievous Effects of *Sin!* This wretched *Infant* has not arrived unto years of sense Enough, to *Sin after the Similitude of the Transgression committed by Adam.* Nevertheless, the *Transgression* of *Adam,* who had all Mankind *Foederally,* yea, *Naturally,* in him, has involved this Infant in the Guilt of it. And the *Poison of the old Serpent* which infected *Adam* when he fell into his *Transgression,* by hearkening to the *Tempter,* has corrupted all Mankind, and is a Seed unto such Diseases as this *Infant* is now Labouring under. *Lord,* What are we, and what are our Children, but a *Generation of Vipers!* And thus we feel thee in the *Egg* now crushing of us. But there is my *Mediation,* in conveying all this Misery to my unhappy

Offspring. In the Uncomfortable Circumstances of my Child, *My God will humble me,* for the Share which I have in the Sin of our *First Parents.* May my Repentance for our *Original Sin,* be brought unto its *Perfect Work,* by the View of what *My Child* (which is *myself*) is now suffering from it!"

Yea, It will be but a Reasonable Thing, for *Parents,* who see their *Infants* in Distress, to Enquire, *On how many Accounts their Sins may be punished in what befalls their Children;* and how far a Righteous God may be now *visiting the Iniquity of the Fathers upon the Children.* The Moans of your Sick Children, may be Stabs to your Hearts, and pierce and cutt like Daggers there, when you think; *Lo, I have Sinned, and I have done Wickedly; But these Lambs, what have They done!*

At the same time, how Thankfully may you acknowledge the Patience and Goodness of a Gracious God, which has carried you thro' all these Dangers of *Infancy;* and *having obtained Help from Him, you continue to this Day!*

Mothers; How many Weary Days and Nights do you wear away, —e'en worried out of your Lives,—in tending these *Uneasy Children!* But, be *Patient;* Beg of God, that He would Strengthen you with *Patience,* Even to *Long-Suffering.*

Think; "These *Troubles* of the *Married Life,* and the *Sorrows* which attend the Breeding, and Bearing and Rearing of *Children,* are the Portion which a Sovereign, Just and Wise God, has ordered for me. And shall not I patiently take the *Cup,* which my Heavenly Father has ordered for me!"

Think; "The Pains which I am now taking about this *Tiresome Child,* are Employ'd about One of those, that have a part in the *Kingdome of Heaven.* Tis, The Lords: Tis One of those, whom the Blessed SAVIOUR, (who was Himself once an *Infant!*) calls, His Children. If it must Expire in this *Minority,* it shall have a part in the *Holy City* of Him that is a God unto it. But, who can tell? Tis Devoted unto the *Service* of a Glorious CHRIST. It is a *Servant* of God, that I am thus toiling for. Who can tell, but it may Live, and Serve God in its Generation? Who can tell, what it may Live to do in the World! *Lord, I am at Work for Thee, in all that I am now adoing.*"

§ For *the Thrush* in Children, or, a *Sore Mouth.*

Fill an Eggshel with the Juice of *Red Sage;* make it boil in Embers, and Skim it: Then take a Peece of beaten *Allum,* as big as a Pea; and half a Spoonful of *Honey:* Putt this in the Egg, and boil it a little.

So take it off. When tis cold, lett the Childs Mouth be rubbed with it.

Or, crush out the Juice of *Houseleek:* mix it with Honey; add a little powdered *Allum.* Do it about the Childs Mouth with a Feather.

Eldar-Blossom Water, is a notable Remedy for the Thrush.

So is a *Frog* held unto the Mouth of the Child.

§ *Children* commonly abound with *Noxious Acids* in their Bowels; and a great Part of their Maladies, are to be hence accounted for. Dr. *Fuller* observes, Their Cure is to be fetched from *Testaceous* and *Cretaceous* Medicines. He sais, "These are so proper and peculiar to this Age, that I have rarely known them given to *Infants,* in Acute Distempers, skilfully and in sufficient Quantity, but Commendable Success has followed. On the other Side, I confess, I have seldome Seen them do much Good unto grown Persons.

§ Breeding of Teeth.

Our *first Sin* was committed with our <u>*Teeth*</u>. And lo, some of the *First* Griefs and Pains undergone by our Children, are in *Breeding of their Teeth.*

§ Rubbing the Swoln Gums now and then with *Honey of Roses,* often times does marvellously Ease them.

§ Your Dogmatical Philosophers may despise *Innocent Amulets,* as much as they please. But it is very strongly affirmed, That *Calves-Teeth,* formed into Beads for a Necklace, and worn about the Neck, are of real Service to procure an Easy *Breeding of Teeth.*

There is another famous *Necklace,* now in Vogue. I don't know what it is; But I have seen so much, that *I wish you had it.*

§ Worms.

Consult our Fourty-fourth *Capsula.*

Quincy remarks; "*Rhubarb* is good against <u>*Worms*</u> in Children; and is the best Purge that can be given them, to cleanse away those Crudities in the Bowels, which are apt to breed *Worms.* It also gives a Firmness to the Fibres, which from the Slipperiness of their Diet, are generally too lax in those young Creatures; So that its Repetition to them, can hardly be too frequent.

§ Convulsions.

§ Give a *Clyster* in the Fitt, as soon as you can.

§ Bruis'd *Sowbugs* have done Wonders for <u>*Convulsions*</u>.

§ Make an *Issue.* T'wil save the *Witts* as well as the *Lives* of the Children.

§ Many Children have been cured by *This.* Take two or three Drops of the Chymical *Oyl of Rosemary;* putt it into half an Ounce of *Sack,* in an Ounce-Bottel. Stop the Vial; and shake it up into a Whitish Mixture, just before you give it. Give the Child a little Spoonful.

§ Take *Earth-worms;* wash them well in White-Wine; but not so, that they shall dy in the Wine. Then, upon hollow Tiles, or between them, dry the Worms with a moderate Heat, and no farther than they may be conveniently reduced into Powder. To an Ounce of this, add a few Grains of *Ambergris.*[1] The Dose is from a Dram, to a Dram and an half, in any Convenient Vehicle.

§ The Smoke of dried *Lovage-root,* has had notable Effects in Convulsion.

§ The Juice of baked *Turnips,* mingled with a little *Canary* Wine; A Spoonful of this now and then given has done great Cures.

§ Plaisters of *Burgundy-pitch* to the Soles of the Feet (Especially, when joined with Internal Medicines) have had notable Effects.

§ *Willis* mentions it as *A famous Medicine, often Experimented in the Convulsions of Children.*

Take the *Gall* contained within the Gall-bladder of a Sucking *Whelp;* give it the Child, with the Water of *Lime-tree flowers.*

§ He also commends the Plaister *Oxicroceum,*[2] two Parts; *Galbanum* dissolved, one Part; Oil of *Amber,* a Scruple; applied as a Plaister to the Soles of the Feet.

§ He likewise commends, Three Drops of the Spirit of *Hartshorn,* Every Sixth or Eighth Hour, in a Julip of Black-cherry Water.

§ It may not be amiss to purge the Children in the Wane of the Moon, with a Decoction of *Peony-Root,* in which infuse a Dram of *Senna,* and a Spoonful of the *Honey of Roses.*[3]

§ *Baglivi* says, *Convulsions* in Infants, are generally from the Stomach; and gentle Purgatives, particularly, an Infusion of *Rubarb,* give present Releef. Don't give these Children any thing of Spirit of *Sal-Armoniac.* Twil curdle the Milk in their Stomach.

Consult our Twenty Eighth *Capsula.*

§ Scalled-Heads.[4]

Dr. *Quincy* sais, *Pisselaeum Indicum,*[5] or what we call, *Barbados-Tar,* is, *among the Countrey-people in mighty Request for Scald-Heads, which is a thing troublesome enough to Cure, and often puzzles a Good Physician.*

§ A Rupture.

§ The Root and Leaves of *Cranes-bill,*[6] commonly called *Colum-*

binum, finely powdered; Half a Spoonful of this taken Morning and Evening for three or four Weeks together; and washed down with a few Spoonfuls of Red Wine. This is a *Boylaean* Receit, for a *Rupture;* Especially in Childhood.

§ Take Roots of *Solomons Seal*[7] well-cleansed; Scrape an Ounce of them into a Quart of Broth. Take a Poringer of this for a Breakfast.

Or give half a Dram of this powdered in any Convenient Vehicle.

§ The Hooping Cough.

Dr. *Strother* complains of the Neglect with which this *Convulsive Cough* has been treated by Physicians. He says, that he hath quickly succeeded in the Cure, when (after *Bleeding,* and an *Emetic,* and two or three *Catharticks,* in proper Subjects,) he has administred a Spoonful, or a Spoonful and half, or two Spoonfuls, according to their Age, of the following Mixture, thrice a day.

Take, the *Peruvian Bark,* One Ounce; cordial *Milk-water,*[8] Twelve Ounces; *Epidemic* water,[9] Three Ounces: Lett this Infusion Stand a Night. Then Strain it; Add, *Sal volatile oleosum,*[10] One Ounce. Tincture of Castor, Half an Ounce: Liquid *Laudanum,* Half an Ounce; Syrup of *Meconium,* One Ounce. Mix them.

[I doubt, you must have a Pothecary to præpare it for you.]

§ The Rickets.

Tis a new Disease. *Lord, Shew us wherefore thou contendest with us!* What *New Miscarriages* are there among us thus Chastised with *New Castigations,* upon the poor Children of Men.

This Disease was never heard of, till about the year 1630, when it began in the *West* of *England,* and crept away *Southward.* No body knows, who first putt the Name it now wears upon it; but as Dr. *Glisson*[11] observes, Considering how much the *Spinal Marrow* is affected in it, the Name hitts agreeably Enough.

It was not mention'd in the *Bills of Mortality,* till 1634, and there were but 14 for that year. From this time, it increased so that in the year 1660, the Number was 521. Since then, the Number is decreased. And, Some hope, it will Ere Long, Like a Comet, wholly disappear again.

But in our Countrey, it is now a Very Common Malady.

There is in it a *Debilitation,* and perhaps a *Stupefaction,* of the Spirits; with an *Obstruction* on the *Spinal Marrow,* and on the Nerves issuing from it, whence follows an Unæqual Distribution of the *Nutritious Juice,* whereupon one Part grows too big, while another is wasting away.

Tis a Melancholy Spectacle, which the *Rickety Children* afford unto us, when we see their *Heads* growing into an unporportionable Magnitude; with diverse uncomely Protuberances: Their *Breasts* troublesomely straitened, and mishapen; the *Sternum* Sticking out; Their *Bellies* Enormously Swelled; Their *Backs* and *Bones* Crooked; Their *Joints* tumified; Their *Breath* short; an unconquered *Looseness;* An universal *Weakness;* An Indisposition to move; A *Cough;* and the symptoms of a *Consumption* approaching.

Very proper now will be such Thoughts as these, upon the Spectacle.

"All the *Deformities,* and all the *Infirmities,* which afflict the *Body* of this poor Child, make it less miserable, than Those which *Original Sin* has brought upon the *Soul* of it. Yea, I see my own woful Image. For, could we see our *Protoplast,* we might say, O *Adam,* All thy Offspring, as well as that Son from whom all the Offspring thou now hast in the World has issued, is *Begotten, in thy own Likeness, after thy Image.—But* I turn to the Second *Adam; Lord,* Be merciful to the miserable *Soul* of this Child; and by thy Spirit betimes taking Possession of it, Lett all that is in it be Rectified."

And how properly may the Parent now come into this Resolution!

"If I may Live to see this poor Child, grow up into a Capacity for *Institution,* I that am so Sollicitous now to see the *Body* of it, heal'd and help'd, and saved from its Disorders, will have a greater Sollicitude, and use the best Means of *Education,* that the *Soul* of it may be Cured of its Worse Disorders."

But, *O Man,* Tho' thou hast outgrown thy *Infancy,* yett thou art Liable Still unto the *Rickets.* The Christians, in whom *Knowledge* has not *Practice* in any Measure proportion'd unto it; And the Christians, who have a very Disproportionate *Zeal;* mightily concerned about Lesser Things, perhaps Points of *Church-Discipline,* or Modes of *Apparrel,* but having Little Concern and Conscience, about the more *weighty Matters of the Law:*—These are a Sort of *Ricketty Christians.* Beware lest thou be found among them.

§ For the *Rickets,* we commonly bleed the poor little Creatures in the *Ear;* and we find it as *Useful,* as tis an *Easy* Operation.

§ Dr. *Tho. Fuller,* mentions a *Ricket-Ale.*

Take Roots of *Osmond Royal,*[12] (or, for want of it, *Male-Fern,*)

Liquorice, Sassafras, Each one Ounce; Bark of *Ash,* and *Ivy,* Each half an Ounce. Tamarisk-tops,[13] and Harts-Tongue,[14] Each four handfuls; Live Wood-Lice, 150; Raisins 4 Ounces; præpare all for One Gallon. He sais; *It may well go for a Specific in this Distemper.* It should be drunk for a Constancy.

§ Frowardness.[15]

Many Mothers and Nurses are Exercised with *Froward Children.* The poor Little Creatures are frequently and painfully and noisily out of Order, and are unable to tell, *what it is that pains them.*

It were well, if you that are under this Trial of your Patience, would think, *Am not I as Froward as this Child?* But then also think, How *Unacceptable* you render yourselves, when you are *Froward* in your Discontented Murmurs at any Condition wherein the Sovereign God *performs the Thing that is appointed for you;* Or, when you are *Froward,* in your hasty *Passions* and *Speeches,* upon apprehended *Provocations* from those that are about you.

Whereas also, when the Children are *Froward* you don't *sett your Witts against Theirs,* and Childishly grow as *Froward* as *They:* will you not be as much *Superiour* in your Carriage towards *Froward People,* when you have the Unhappiness to be concerned with them? Certainly, you will Scorn to be as *Froward* and peevish and pettish as these *Childish People.* Instead of being *Even with them,* you will be *Above them,* and Scorn it as a Thing *Below* you, to carry on a Quarrel with them.

Well, But lett us now take a Little Care to *Quiet* the *Children.*

Take a Vessel (suppose a *Tea-pott,*) that will hold about a Pint, and fill it with the Herb called *Red-Nettles* (*Red,* because the Bottom of the Stalk is of that Colour:) Then poure into the Vessel, as much Water, as it will receive, when the Herb has filled it. Add, of *Ivory*[16] finely powdered, as much as may Ly upon a Shilling; and of *Saffron,* as much as may be about the Weight of a *Groat.* Make a Decoction, or a Strong Infusion. When you administer it, lett it be Sweetened. A Large Spoonful or more, is a Dose for a Child, a year old. Give it three or four times a day.

Tis a great Medicine for the *Ricketts* in Children; if the use of it be continued for about Twenty Days; and then cease a while; But anon Return to it, if there be Occasion.

Tis also a fine Medicine, to save Children from the *Worms,* which commonly give Rise to most of their Maladies.

But that for which I more particularly produce this Medicine, is This. When the Children are Ill, and out of order, and no body can tell what they Ail, (which often happens,) Then give *This* unto them.

The Medicine must be anew prepared Every Three or Four Days: Else it will grow Sour; in hott Weather Especially.

If the Medicine prove too hott, (which rarely happens,) it is mended by putting in a little Brook-Liver-Wort.[17]

§ For the *Gripes* in Little Children, tis among the *Boylaean* Receits; Take *Oil of Nutmegs,* and of *Wormwood,* of Each a Little Quantity, Mingle them well, and with the Mixture a little warmed, anoint the Childs Navel, and the Pitt of the Stomach.

§ It is a Remark of Mr. *Lock's.*[18] That for CHILDREN a little cold-stilled red *Poppy-Water,* (with Ease and Abstinence from Flesh) often putts an End unto several Distempers at the Beginning, which by too forward Applications, might have been made Lusty Diseases.

§ The *Diet* of Children.

Dr. *Cheyne* says; "The perpetual *Gripes, Cholic, Loosenesses, Hard Bellies, Choakings, Wind* and *Convulsive Fitts,* which torment Half our Children, are Entirely owing to the too great Quantities of too Strong *Food,* and too rank *Milk,* thrust down their Throats, by their overlaying *Mothers* and *Nurses.* For what else do their *Slimy,* their *Gray* or *Chylous,* their *Blackish* and *Choleric* Discharges, the *Noise* and *Motion* in their Bowels, their *Wind,* and *Choakings,* imply, but Crudities from Superfluous Nourishment? This is so certain, that they are universally and infallibly cured by *Testaceous* Powders, which only absorb Crudities; By *Rhubarb* Purges, which at once *Evacuate* and *Strengthen* the Bowels; And by *Milk-Clysters* and *Issues,* which are still upon the Root of Evacuation; and a Thin, Spare, and Nutritive Diet." Be sure, Happy would it be for our Offspring, if we were so *Reasonable,* as to learn from the *Animals* void of *Reason,* how to rear up our young ones!

Dr. *Quincy* sais of *Butter;* "It may be good in Dry and Costive Constitutions; but must be hurtful in Lax, Moist, Corpulent Ones. By the Levity and Tenacity of its Parts, it is also very apt to stop in the Glands and Capillaries; whereby it fouls the Viscera, but particularly the small Glands of the Skin. Hence it is apt to produce Blotches, and all Cutaneous Deformities. And this Opinion is much confirmed by the Experience of all, whose Business has made them much conversant with young CHILDREN, they having much of this in their Diet; Whereby they have been Observed to grow Weakly,

Corpulent, big-bellied, and very Subject to breakings out, and to breed Lice, and such like Uncleanlinesses: But upon Restraining them from it, without any other Visible Means, they have out-grown all those Inconveniences." I know not of what Use this Hint may be, for our poor *Children.* But if they beg that their *Bread and Butter* mayn't be taken from them, they may plead, that for certain, the *Children* had Butter allow'd them, in the Prophet *Isiahs* time; which was more than Four and Twenty Hundred years ago!—

§ A *Purge* for Children.

Take fine *Rhubarb* cutt in Slices, Two Drams. *Liquorice,* and *Anniseed,* of Each two Scruples. Thirty or Forty Stoned *Raisins* of the Sun; putt them into a Quart of Ale.

Dr. Quincy sais: "Tis a pleasant Purge; and Children may be Coaksed to take it, when other more Medicinal Forms cannot be gott down. It cleanses the first Passages, which are generally the Seat of Childrens Disorders; and it destroys *Worms.* The Quantity at first should be Small, and increas'd at Discretion."

Cap. LX. *Paralipomena.*[1]

or

Cures and Helps

for a Cluster [of]

Lesser Inconveniences.

THERE are many *Lesser Inconveniences,* which we Suffer in our Health: So Many, that we may justly Say, *They cannot be Numbred;* But lett us be Thankful, that we need not sadly say, *They cannot be Healed.*

Lett the Afflicted think on the more *Particular Miscarriages,* which his *Conscience* may read rebuked in his Afflictions; And with the *Resolutions of PIETY* humbly relying on the Grace of Heaven, say, *I will not offend any more.*

If he find Releef, by the Method and Medicine proposed, Lett him not think, that no Praises are due to Heaven in so small a Matter; But lett him Study, *With what Acknowledgments ought I now to praise Him who grants this Ease unto me!*

So lett us proceed unto the Offer of Remedies, that shall appear like the *Sporades,* not formed into any Constellation.

§ For <u>Pimples in the Face</u>.

Take Flowre of *Brimstone;* and *White-pepper;* as much as may ly on a Shilling. Mix them well with an Ounce of *Unguentum Pomatum.*[2] Anoint herewith at Night. Wash it off in the Morning, with Water taken out of the Smiths Forge.[3] Continue this for Ten Days.

I have known several Gentlemen very Thankful for the Success of This. *Baglivi* says, A Caustic to the Leg, is a Secret for the Cure of all Redness in the Face.

§ For a <u>Blood-shott Eye</u>.

Shake half a Dram of *Tutty* well-prepared, into an Ounce of Red Rose Water. Drop it often into the Eye.

§ For <u>Eyes inflamed</u> with an hott or sharp Humour.

Take the Tops of *Rosemary,* one Dram. And beat them up with an Ounce or two of rotten Pearmains,[4] or Pippins.[5] Being thus reduced unto a Poultis, warm it, and lay it unto the Eyes, and lett it ly all Night.

§ Or, wash *Red Eyes* with Brandy.

§ For <u>Hoarseness</u> on a *Cold*.

Take three Ounces of *Hyssop-Water;* Sweeten it with *Sugar-candy:* Then Beat well into it, the *Yolk of an Egg*. Drink it at a Draught.

§ For a <u>Canker</u>,[6] in the Mouth.

Boil *Malt* unto a Consistency, and Strain it. Adding a little *Alum,* and *Honey*.

Or, Take *Vinegar* and *Rose-Water,* and Juice of *Plantain:* Mix; and Wash.

Or, Take a few Leaves of *Succory,*[7] and *Plantain,* and *Rue*. Boil these in fair Water with a little *Honey*. So, wash the Mouth.

§ To <u>Cleanse the Teeth</u>.

Nothing like Powder of *Red Coral*. Then wash with Water, wherein *Sal Prunella* is dissolved.

§ To <u>Fasten the Teeth</u>.

Chew Mastick, often.

Or, Take Burnt *Allum,* and *Acorns,* of Each One Dram; *Galls,*[8] a Dram and half: *Red Roses,* half an Handful; Beat these all together; and Boil them in a Quart of good Red Wine, to the Consumption of about a Fourth Part. Then Strain the Decoction. So dissolve in it, good *Acacia*[9] cutt in Small Bitts, half a Dram. Wash the Mouth with this.

Or, To a Pint of *Spring Water,* putt four Ounces of Brandy. Wash the Mouth with it Every Morning.

And roll a little while, a bitt of *Rock-Allum*[10] in the Mouth.

Or, To four Ounces of Claret-Wine, add four Drams of *Terra-Japonica.*[11]

Or Take *Bole-Armenic,*[12] Two Drams; *Myrrh,* One Dram; *Allum,* half a Dram; *Claret-Wine,* a Pint. Boil these gently; use it several times in a day.

§ For *Stuffings of the Lungs,* and a <u>Chin-Cough</u>.[13]

Make Syrup of *Penny-royal,* or of *Ground-Ivy,* moderately tart with *Oil of Vitriol.* Of this take very Liesurely about a Quarter of a Spoonful from time to time.

§ For <u>Costiveness</u>.

Take stewed *Prunes.*

Or, Take Virgin-*Honey;* mix with it as much finely powdered *Cremor Tartari,* as will bring it unto the Consistence of a Soft Electuary. Take a Quantity, to the bigness of an Almond, more or less, as upon Trial you may see Occasion.

Or, Give at Bed-time, Eight or Ten Grains of *Saffron,* in any proper Syrup or Conserve. This is good also for dry or convulsive Asthmas.

Take *Sage* pulverized. Mix it with Grease. Anoint the Navel with it. Nothing so Safe.

§ For a <u>Strain</u>.

Take the Strongest *Vinegar* you can gett, and boil in it a Convenient Quantity of *Wheat Bran,* until you have brought it unto the Consistency of a Poultis. Apply this as Early as may be to the Part affected; and when it begins to grow dry, Renew it.

My Lord *Bacons* Experienced Medicine was. Take an Handful of Fresh *Wormwood;* Boil it in Strong *Ale,* to the softness of a Poultis. When you apply it, which is to be done, while it is very hott, putt in a Spoonful or two of Brandy.

§ For a <u>Stinking Breath</u>.

Wash the Mouth often with a Decoction of *Myrrh* in Water.

§ For a <u>Contracture of Limbs</u> by keeping them too Long in an undue Posture.

Anoint well the Part affected once or twice a day, with *Dogs-grease;* Chafing it in with a Warm Hand; and keeping the Part warm afterwards.

§ For a <u>Tenesmus</u>.[14]

Mindererus bids you; take a Burnt Brick out of the Hearth. Heat it thoroughly. Wett it with Sharp Vinegar. Lett a Linen-Clothe be wrapt about it. Lett the patient sitt on it, as hott as he can bear it.

§ For <u>Untiring</u> a Souldier after a Long March, *Willius* writing *De Morbis Castrensibus,* præscribes, A Decoction of *Mugwort,* and washing the Feet with it: Or, Dissolving some Gun-Powder in luke-warm Water.

§ For <u>Chilblains</u>.[15]

Take a *Turnip;* Roast it well under the Embers; Beat it unto a Poultice. Apply it hott. Keep it on three or four Days; in the time shifting it once or twice, if Occasion require.

§ For <u>Kibes</u>.[16]

Take the Ashes of the Soles of *old shoes;* mix with *Oil of Roses,* and apply to the Heels.

§ For <u>Stinking Feet</u>.

Be not slovenly, wear Socks, often shifting 'em. Keep your whole Body in Health.

§ For the <u>Cramp</u>.

Use *Cotton-Wick,* as a Garter.

or, Take Leaves of *Rosemary:* chop them small; sew them up in fine Linen, or Sarsnett,[17] so as to make a Garter, to be worn about the Bare Leg.

§ For a <u>Pleuresy</u>.

Riverius bids you: Take an Apple; open the Top; Take out the Core; Fill it with white *Frankincense:* Stop it again with the Peece you cutt out; Roast it in Ashes; Beat it to a Mash; Lett the Patient Eat it.

Baglivi says "The Exhibiting of hott Liquors, is to me a Secret, for dissolving Stubborn Viscosities, in Epidemical, and Malignant Pleurisies, as well as all other Diseases of the Breast, proceeding from a like Cause—Draughts of a pectoral Decoction, taken down very hott."

§ For <u>Spitting of Blood</u>.

Take *Yarrow* bruis'd, and dried in the Sun, and finely powdered: from half a Dram, to a Dram, twice a day, in a proper Vehicle.

§ For a <u>Whitloe</u>.[18]

Take *Shell-snails,* and beat the pulpy Part of them very well, with a Convenient Quantity of chopt *Parsley.* Apply it, and shift it once or twice a day.

or, Take a little *Green Sorrel:* covering it with Paper, putt it a Minute into the hott Embers; and it being Roasted there, apply it unto the *Whitloe;* It will Ripen it, Open it, Heal it; All in a few Hours time.

§ For St. <u>Antonies Fire</u>.[19]

The *Blood* of almost any Living Creature, is found a Specific, against an *Erisypelas;* being often anointed upon it; or a Clothe dipt in the same, laid upon it.

§ For Extreme <u>Fatness</u>.

Many Remedies have been advised, whereof the Learned *Borellus* gives this Caution: *ex ijs pauca tuta et certa esse existimo.*[20] Too much *Abstinence* has been mischievous. *Vinegar* taken in too great Quantities, may hurt the *Stomach* and the *Bowels.* Yett he tells of a Spanish General, who found a wondrous, and harmless Imminution of his *Obæsity* by it; abating Eighty Seven Pounds of his Weight. He elsewhere tells of a very corpulent Nobleman reduced only by chewing *Tobacco.*

It may be a Diet of *Milk,* with *Dry Bread,* under due (progressive) Limitations, may do the Business.

After all; There [is] nothing like an *Obstinate Abstinence* from all Sorts of Liquors; from *Drink* of all Kinds.

§ For any <u>Green Wounds</u>.[21]

A most Excellent Balsame.

Take Oyl of St. *Johns* Wort, and *Venice-turpentine;* of Each a like Quantity. Sett them over the Fire, in a gentle Heat, Half an Hour or less, that they may incorporate. Putt it up; and *keep it* (sais the *Boylaean* Receit) *as one of the best of Balsams.*

§ For a <u>Fistula</u>.

The Illustrious *Boyl* mentions, a Drink taken twice or Thrice a day. Take *Wormwood,* and *Mint,* and Three Hundred *Millepedes* well beaten in a Mortar (after their Heads pulled off:) tunned[22] up with the Herbs; which are to be suspended in four Gallons of small Ale, during its Fermentation.

Syringe Burnt Butter, Exceedingly Hott, into the Sores.

§ For <u>Lowsiness</u>.

Aboard Ships (and in Prisons and Garrisons, and the like Sordid Places) they are much troubled with <u>Lice</u>.

Lett a Man Eat a Little Bitt of *Brimstone,* as big as a Pea, Every Day, or Every other Day; Tis affirmed, No *Louse* will dare, or can bear to be about him. Yea, twil bring him to be of such a Constitution, that long after he has left off the Practice, a *Louse* being putt upon him, will Swell and Dy.

Mindererus directs the poor Souldier. Take *Wormwood,* and the Inner Cuttings of *Horse-hoofs* cutt out in the Shoeing of Horses. Boil these together in Half Lye, half Water. Putt the Shirt into it. Afterwards dry it in the Air. No Louse will come into it; or if any one were in it he would not stay there.

§ For <u>Warts</u>.

Rub them three or four times a day, with the Juice and Mash of Green Leaves of *Marygold,* beaten.

or, Touch them with the Juice of *Celandine.*

or, With the Juice that comes from *Shell-snails* on pricking of them.

or Take *Beef,* or *Bacon,* and rub the *Warts* with it; Then bury the Flesh in the Ground; or, hang it up to dry in the Air.

or, Wash the Hands with Water wherein a little *Sal Armoniac* has been dissolved. A great Physician, *Millies Expertus est.*[23]

§ For <u>Corns</u>, you need only Soak your Feet in Warm Water; Anon you'l be able not only to pare them down, but Entirely to Extirpate them.

or, Lay on a Plaister of *Gum Ammoniacum.*

or, Wett them often with a *Cows Gall.*

or, Bind a *Snail* gently on the *Corn,* when you go to Sleep. Hee'l feed upon it; and you'l no more be troubled with it.

Mersennus[24] writing a Mathematical Book, in a Chapter of *Arithmetical Combinations,* cannot forbear bringing in a Remedy for *Corns;* which is, To apply and Renew for diverse days together, the middle Stalk, that grows between the Blade and the Root of *Garlick,* bruised.

§ For *Tumours* that are like to prove *Wens* of a Troublesome Tendency.

Take an old *woodden pott lid,* which most Kitchens can supply you withal. By holding it unto the Fire, melt out the grease; and with this Grease anoint the Part affected.

Fasting Spittle; or, a *Dead Hand* will do Wonders in such Cases.

§ For any *Roughness* of an Inflamed <u>Skin</u>; Especially on the *Lips.*

Anoint the Part affected, with fresh *Cream.*

§ To take out the *Marks* of <u>Gunpowder</u>, Shott into the *Skin.*

Take fresh *Cow-dung,* and having warmed it a Little, apply it as a thin Poultis, to the Part affected. Renew it, as the Case may require.

§ For the Running of the Reins.[25]

Take two Ounces of ripe *Laurel-Berries,*[26] and infuse them for a Day, in a Quart of good *Whitewine;* of this, Lett the poor Creature drink two or three Spoonfuls twice a day, for a pretty while. Only intermitt once in three or four days, to take a gentle Purge.

or, Take a sufficient Quantity of *Mastich,* finely beaten; Take about half an Ounce of this at a time, in the Yolk of a New Laid Egg. Wash this down, if need be, in any Convenient Liquor.

or, Take choice *Amber* and *Mastich,* both finely powdered. Give half a Dram of this Mixture, in any proper Vehicle; or in a Dish of *Chocolat.* Continue this for a few Weeks. Purge the Day before its begun to be taken; and once Every Week afterwards; and once at leaving off.

§ For Burns and *Scalds:* Nothing like a Poultis of our *Indian Meal,* applied immediately.

or, Beat *Onions* into a Soft Mash; keep it on till it begin to grow Dryish. Then if need be, Renew it.

or, Drop *Hoggs fat* boiling, on Leaves of *Laurel.* Anoint the Burnt Place with this Ointment. *Borellus* tells you, Twil be cured in Three Days; *quasi quodam Incantamento.*[27]

For Burns and Scalds, We have a Balsame compounded of Sallet-Oyl, and Bees-Wax, and *Lapis Calaminaris,*[28] with which our Good Women do abundance of Good.

Nothing so soon and so well takes out *Fire,* as dried *Clay* and *Vinegar.*

§ For Ulcers.

Take a Quantity of White, and of *Roman Vitriol.*[29] Dissolve it in as much Water as may be sufficient. Then add a third more of Water. Lett it Simmer over a Fire, till a Third be boiled away.

This was the *Arcanum* of a Gentlewoman, famous for the Cure of *Ulcers,* (even of *Scorphulous* ones) that has been given over by Physicians.

§ For fresh Wounds and *Cutts.*

The Juice of *Celandine* will be a Balsame.

or, plunge the Part with *Brandy,* or with a Sponge apply *Brandy* to it.

§ For Stenching of <u>Blood</u>; Especially in <u>Wounds</u>.

Take those round *Mushrooms* which they call, *puff-balls,* when they are fully ripe; and breaking them warily, save carefully the flying Powder, with the rest that remains, and strew this Powder all over the Part affected; binding it on.

or, Strew over a little *powdered Allum.*

or, Strew upon the Part, the Powder of *Rosin,*[30] beaten very small.

or, Use *Colcothar of Vitriol.*[31] For Stanching of Blood scarce any Thing exceeds it.

§ To draw out <u>Splinters</u>.

Stamp *Southernwood* with Grease; and Lay it on.

§ For Outward <u>Bruises</u>.

Apply to the Part affected, skim'd or purified *Honey;* Spread upon cap-paper. Keep it on with a Convenient Bandage; and shift it once or twice a day.

or, Fresh *Butter* and *Parsley;* A Cataplasm.

or, Black Soft *Soap,* with Soft Crumbs of *White-bread*. A Paste.

§ For the Resolving of <u>Extravasated Blood</u>.

Grate the Root of *Burdock.* Spread the Powder on a Linen-clothe; Bind it on the Part affected: Renew it twice a day.

§ <u>Sinapisms</u> are of Wonderful Consequence,

To *call back* the Spirits and Humours to a Weak Part, and restore the Tone thereof:

To attract matter which lies deep, unto the Surface; and so they are good in Pains remotely scituate;

To revel from the Part affected, and thereby draw away Pains of the *Head* and of the *Teeth,* and Rheums from *Sore Eyes;* and so to disperse the Tumultuous Clusters of the Spirits, when one particular Member is Hysterically, or otherwise Spasmodically affected.

Here's a Good One.

Take the Crum of *White-bread,* Two Ounces: Fine Meal of *Mustard-seed* Searced, One Ounce; Oil of *Cloves,* thirty two Drops; *Vinegar,* three Ounces; *Honey,* as much as needful. Bring all to the Consistence of a Cataplasm.

A noble *Drawing-plaister!*

Memorandum.

§ An Handful of *Crows-foot Flowres*[32] with half a Spoonful of Mustard, beaten into a Poultis, is (a *Slower,* but) a *Safer* Blister, than that of *Cantharides.*

CAP. LXI. *Medicamenta sine quibus.*[1]
or, certain Remedies, that People of any Condition,
may always have ready at hand, for themselves and their Neighbors.
A Family-Plaister.

THERE is a certain PLAISTER of Such Extensive Benefit, that it is a Pitty any *Family* should be without it. It very little differs from what has gone under some other Names; But, for the Cause I have mention'd, I am willing to have it called, <u>The Family Plaister.</u>

Take Two Pound of the best *Oil Olive;* of good Red Lead, One Pound; White Lead, One Pound; well beaten to Powder: Twelve Ounces of *Castile-Sope:* [good old Mrs. *Eliot,*[2] from whom Hundreds of People had it, and had good by it, under the Name of her *Spleen-plaister,* added a little Oyl of *Bayberries:*] Incorporate all these together, in an Earthen Pott well-glazed. After they are well Incorporated, and the Sope comes upwards then putt it upon a Small Fire of Coals, and keep stirring it there with some convenient Instrument, for about an Hour and half; Then increase the Fire, till what was Red grow Gray, and then also leave not off till it grow a little dark. Drop it then upon a Woodden Trencher, and if it cleave not unto your Fingers, tis done Enough. So make it up into Rolls. It will keep Twenty years: the older the Better.

A World of People are Labouring under Disorders, which they commonly ascribe to, *The Spleen;* Few are Entirely free from them. To Remove or Suppress these Disorders, would restore the *Comforts of Life,* to thousands of People, that are overwhelmed with Vapours, and with the *Splenetic Maladies,* which may say, *Our Name is LEGION,* as well for the *Number* of them, as for much of the *Devil* often in them. This *Plaister* is peculiarly Calculated for these *Vexatious Maladies;* and a vast multitude of People far and near have with notable Success found it Serviceable to them on these accounts. I have already mentioned one in this Countrey, who charitably dispensed it unto hundreds of People, that gave Thanks unto Heaven for the advantage they received from it. Apply the *Plaister* to the Region of the *Spleen;* and Renew it, as there may be Occasion.

This *Plaister* Laid unto the *Stomach,* is very good for a Weak Stomach; Will notably Assist and Excite the Appetite. And Every body knows, that all the *Wheels of Nature,* are kept in the better Trim, when this *Great One* is well provided for.

This *Plaister* Laid unto the Belly gives Ease in the *Cholic*. I knew a Practitioner, who used it as a Secret with such Success in *Cholical Affects,* that People sent from very Distant Parts unto him for it.

This *Plaister* Laid unto the Region of the *Kidneys,* it Stops the Bloody Flux, and the Running of the Reins, and Præternatural Heats in the *Kidneys.*

It is an admirable Plaister for *Sores,* and *Swellings,* and *Aches,* and *Bruises,* and *Chilblains,* and *Kibes,* and *Corns.*

It breaks *Boils,* and *Felons,* and *Impostumes;* and it heals them when it has broken them.

If the *Skin* be rubb'd off the *Legs,* Our *Plaister* commonly cures. It will also draw out *Running Humours* in the *Legs,* without breaking the skin.

And they that have *Issues,* can't Easily dress them with a better thing: Take a Little Square Peece of *Brown Paper;* on the middle of which you may rub a Little of this Plaister, holding the End of the Roll to a Candle for that Purpose. You may prepare an hundred of them in a few Minutes; and as often as you dress your *Issue* Renew them.

There are many other Uses of this *Plaister*. But here is Enough to Recommend it.—

Since I wrote this, I find this *Plaister* among the *Chymical Receits* of Sir *Kenelm Digby;* who cries it up, for all the Virtues aforesaid; and adds: Being applied unto the *Head,* it Strengthens the *Eysight.*

II I am well aware, What sharp *Satyrs* have been written against WOMEN pretending to practice *Physick:* "The *Hae Galeni*[3] [say, Master *Whitlock!*[4]]—*Nam Genus Variant.*[5]—The Quacking *Hermophrodites;* the *Physician* and *Physic,* both *Simples,* compounding the Destruction of the Patient: Applying their *Medicines* (as the *Athenians* their Altar, *unto an unknown God*) *unto an unknown Disease.*—In the *Bills of Mortality* [quoth my *Satyrist,*] we may justle in She-Physicians among the S's for a Disease, as surely killing as *Stone* or *Surfeit.*—A practising *Rib* Shall kill more than the *Jaw-bone* of an Ass, and a Quacking *Dalilah* than a Valiant *Sampson.*"

It was reckoned a Sad Story: and, *O Miserae Leges!*[6] was cried out upon it.

> *Fingit se Medicum quivis Idiota, profanus,*
> *et Distillator, histrio, Tonsor, ANUS.*[7]

But yett after all, In the most Ancient Writers, we find *Women* celebrated as Eminent in the *Art of Healing. Homer* in his Eleventh *Iliad,* mentions *Agamede,*[8] in Terms almost like what we read of *Solomon:*

> *She that all Simples Healing Vertues knew,*
> *And Every Herb that drinks the Morning Dew.*

And in his *Odysses,* he mentions *Polydamne*[9] as Excelling in this Way of usefulness.

I call to mind also Mr. *George Herberts*[10] Advice, That the *Wife* of the *Countrey-Minister,* should have Some Skill and Will to *help the Sick.* More particularly, he adds what I shall not Judge it amiss to transcribe. "Accordingly For *Salves,* his *Wife* seeks not the City, but prefers her Garden and Fields, before all outlandish Gums. And Surely, *Hyssop, Valerian,*[11] *Mercury, Adders-tongue,*[12] *Yarrow, Melilot,*[13] and St *Johns Wort,* made into a *Salve;* And, *Eldar, Camomil, Mallows, Comfry* and *Smallage,*[14] made into a *Poultis;* have done great and rare Cures." 'Tis true, there was a Law among the *Athenians,* which forbad *Women* to meddle with *Medicine.* The Young Lady *Agnodice,*[15] to gratify her Inclination that way, disguised herself in a *Masculine Habit.* The Court of *Areopagus* upon the Discovery would have punished her upon the Law of *Athens.* But the Dames of the City made an uproar, and procured an Abrogation of the Law.

We will then venture to proceed, and say, it would be a Laudable Thing for our <u>Gentlewomen</u> to have their Closetts furnished with several Harmless, and Useful, (and Especially *External*) Remedies, for the Help of their poor Neighbours on Several Occasions Continually Calling for them.

Such more particularly would be,

Ointment of *Tobacco;* for Sores.

Ointment of *Marsh-mallows,* for Pains.

And Several of the Remedies, mention'd in several of the former *Capsula's.* Take your Choice, *Ladies!*

But, be sure, don't forgett the *Amarum Salubre*[16] in the *Capsula* of, *Help for the Stomach depraved.*

An Appendix.
What is your Occupation?
or, *The Trades-mans* Præservative.

At the Bottom of this *Capsula,* the Reader must find Lodged, a Short *Advertisement* about the *Maladies,* which the Several <u>Trades</u>, that People subsist upon, do most meet withal and most lead unto.

I will in the first Place, readily acknowledge, That one of the *Worst Maladies,* which a Man in any Trade, or Way of Living, ever can fall into, is, *For a Man to be Sick of his Trade.* If a Man have a *Disaffection* to the *Business,* that he has been brought up to, and must live upon, tis what will Expose him to many and grievous *Temptations,* and hold him in a sort of *Perpetual Imprisonment.* MAN, Beg of God, an *Heart* Reconciled unto thy *Business.* And if He has bestow'd such an *Heart* upon thee, as to take Delight in thy *Daily Labour,* be very Thankful for such a Mercy! There is much of the *Divine Favour* in it.

But then, There are more *Special Maladies,* which the *Various Employments* of Men, do more peculiarly Expose them to. And, they that are wise, will consider how to guard against them.

Some Learned and Holesome Things have been written *De Morbis Artificum.* What *Ramazzini*[17] has done upon this Head, is well worthy to be more known among *Artificers.*

Yett more particularly. Seeing how liable <u>Mariners</u> are to the *Scurvy,* One cannot but Encourage them to their *Pease-Diet,* and the use of *Limons,*[18] and the Drinking of the Best Fair *Water* they can come at, and feeding on as much *Fresh Provisions* as tis possible.

Seeing how liable the <u>Blacksmiths</u> are, to Impairments of their *Eyes,* One cannot but recommend much Use of *Ey-bright* for them. And Since they are so prone to be very *Costive;* One would invite them to Suppers of *Barley-gruel,* with Raisins and Corints.[19]

When we see how the Caustic Powder of the *Lime* they deal in, brings *Consumptions* upon <u>Masons,</u> One would Exhort them to Drink much *Water,* and Eat abundance of *Almonds.*

When we see, how <u>Millers</u> and <u>Bakers</u>, contract *Asthma's* by the Flowre Entring into their Breasts, One would wish them, Some Ingenious Contrivances, that the Air may be inspired without it.

The poor <u>Potters</u>, and <u>Plumbers</u>, and <u>Painters</u>, who are poisoned with mineral Fumes; and the People, whose Work is much about <u>Quicksilver</u>; What shall be done for these, that they may not find their *Death* in their Way of *Living?* Proper and Early *Antidotes* must be thought upon.

<u>Scriveners</u>, <u>Tailors</u>, and Others that *Sitt Still,* with little Motion of their Bodies, in the *Work of their Hands,* must think on frequent *Exercise,* to Stir their Limbs.

Be sure, <u>Students</u>, and Men that lead *Sedentary Lives,* will do well to be on *Horse-back,* as much as they can.

For the rest,—Consult a Wise *Physician.*

Ⅱ Since we are proposing Remedies to be always ready *at hand,* a Collection of Easy *Emeticks,* and of Easy *Catharticks* to be had always ready *at hand,* may be neither unserviceable nor unacceptable.

Data Tempore Prosunt.[20]

I. For Easy *Vomits.*

§ Take Lukewarm *Water,* One Pint; *Oil* (of *Olives,* or of *Almonds,*) four Ounces. Mix for a Draught.

§ *Green Tea,* half an Ounce: Boil it in Water, (or, Ale) from one Pint to half a Pint; For a Draught.

§ *Oxymel of Squills,* three Ounces; Drink it in a Draught of Posset.

§ *Emetic Tartar,* from one Grain, to five or six. Of this, I can Scarce forbear Saying, *There is none Like it.*

§ *Salt of Vitriol,*[21] from one to two or three Scruples; given in a Draught of Posset.

§ Syrup of *Peach-Blossoms.* There is hardly a better or safer. It may be given to Infants; yea, as soon as they are born.

§ Powdered Root of *Ipecacohana;* From half a Scruple (for a Child:) to half a Dram, or two Scruples, (for a Man.) Sir *John Colbatch* says, *Tis the safest, and perhaps the best Vomit, that ever was made known to the World, barely as a Vomit, to cleanse the Stomach.* This is now in its Reign; The most *Fashionable Vomit.*

§ Penetrate the Throat with a *Feather: Borellus* writes, That his Father (and some other Gentlemen) lived unto a great Age, by Vomiting once a Month, no other way.

§ You'l pardon me, that I don't recommend another famous Vomit; but rather transcribe the Words of an Eminent Physician. "It is well known [*he says,*] that a pretended Chymist, who calls himself *Lockyer,*[22] hath gained by a *Pill* many thousand pounds, which is one of the Vilest and most Contemptible, among all the Mineral Præparations I ever yett knew tried in Medicine."

I am not sorry, that *Antimonial Emeticks* Begin to be disused.

Instead thereof, I will recite the Words of honest *John Smith,* in his Essay upon *Common Water.*

By means of *Water,* all *Sickness at the Stomach* may be cured. It is done thus. Take four Quarts of Water; Make it as hott over the Fire as you can drink it: Of which Water lett a Quart be taken down at several Draughts. Then wrap a Rag round a small Piece of a Stick, till it is about the Bigness of a Mans Thumb; Ty it fast with some

Thread; and with this, by Endeavouring gently to putt it a little Way down your throat, provoke yourself to Vomit up again most of the Water. Then Drink another Quart, and Vomit up that; And Repeat the same, the Third and Fourth time. You may also provoke Vomiting, by tickling your Throat with your Finger, or the Feather-End of a Goose-quill.—By this way of Vomiting, which will be all performed in an Hours time, that viscous and roapy Flegm, which causes the Sickness, will be cast up, So that the party in that time will be free from all that Inward Disturbance, if you use the Remedy at first. But, if the Sickness hath continued for a Time, it will require the Same Course, Once or twice more: which may be done in three or four Hours, one after another.—This Remedy, by Forty Years Experience, I look upon to be Infallible, in all Sickness at the Stomach, from what Cause soever, and for all Pains in the Belly, that seem to be above the Navel; which Pains are generally Counted the *Cholic,* but they are not so. By this Means I have Eased very great Pains, Caused by Eating *Mussels* that were poisonous. And it is also a certain Cure for all *Surfeits,* or Disorders that follow after much Eating; So that the Lives of multitudes might be saved by this Means, who, for want of Expelling what offends, do often dy in Misery: For by this cleansing of the Stomach at the first, the Root of Diseases proceeding from Surfeiting, or unwholesome Food, or any Viscous Humours from a Bad Digestion, are prevented: The Stomach being the Place in which all Distempers do at first begin.—Tis not a nauseous Remedy; It does not make the Patient sick; as the best of all Vomits do. And then, tis a Vomit which is at our own Command; Since we can leave it off when we please.—As for People who are troubled with *shortness of Breath,* tis certain from Experience, that Vomiting with Warm Water three or four times will afford Certain Relief.—Dr. *Cook,*[23] in his *Observations on English Bodies,* does præscribe for the *Cure of Fevers,* first a *Vomit,* and afterwards as much *Cold Water* as the Patient can drink.—*Rest, Fasting,* and *Drinking much Water,* after a Vomit or two, is a Course that hath never failed to cure *Fevers;* by clearing the Stomach of that Sordid Filthiness, which causes the Distemper.

II. For Easy Purges.

§ Take a little *Manna.* From two Drams to an Ounce, for Children. An Ounce or two, or more, for Grown Persons. It must be remembred, That Old *Manna* sometimes has proved as bad as Poison.

§ A little *Senna.*

§ Syrup of *Roses.*[24]

§ An Infusion of *Senna, Liquorice, Anniseed,* of Each Half an Ounce; with *Salt of Tartar,*[25] a Dram; in a Pint of Water scalding hott, for half an hour. Take four Spoonfuls of this Every Hour, until it begin to work.

§ Fresh *Damask-Rose Buds,* one Ounce. Putt them into a Quart of *Whey* over night. Strain it, and drink it, the next Morning.

§ Slice *Liquorice;* Beat *Anniseeds;* Shred *Hysop;* and Boil these in *White-Wine.* Strain it. Take from half an Ounce to an Ounce, or more. Tis a Purge for Tender Children.

§ Syrup of *Violets.*[26] *Infants* may take this gentle Purger. And indeed it is most proper for *Them.*

§ Two Ounces of *Rhubarb;* Four Ounces of *Gentian;* A Quart of Good *Anniseed Water.* Infuse the Roots in this Water. Two Spoonfuls is a Dose.

§ *Pillulae Ruffi.* Especially, when Chalybeated with adding about a Third Part, *Sal Martis.*[27]

§ An Ounce of choice *Rhubarb,* finely powdered; Eight Ounces of good *Currants;* pick'd and wash'd; and rubb'd dry. Beat these together in a Glass, or Stone Mortar, for near two Hours. Take about the bigness of a Chestnutt in a Morning. Tis a pretty Purging Electuary; Especially for *Children.*

§ Or, Keep in the House a Bottel of *Anniseed Water,* with a Convenient Quantity [a *Dram* or two] of *Rhubarb* steeped in it. It is an Excellent and Ungriping Purge; useful on a thousand Occasions. Especially to stop *Fevers,* and cure *Fluxes.* It has been thought by some, *It can't be cried up too much.*

§ It is a General Caution for Purges: That they be very sparingly used in the Decline of the year; Especially after an *Hott Summer.*

Super-purgation is presently Cured with a Scruple of *Venice-Treacle.*

Cap. LXII. *Fuga Daemonum,*
or, Cures by CHARMS
considered,
And, a SEVENTH-SON Examined.

THE *Wicked Spirits,* which are the *Power or Army of the Air,* under the Command of a *Prince* that Headed them in their *Apostasy* from God, are doubtless very *Many;* No Man alive can tell how *Many.* They come down upon us, *As Grasshoppers for Multitude,* and the *Frogs* or *Flies* in the Plagues of *Egypt* Swarmed not in such Inexpressible Numbers. They and their *Hosts,* are *much People even as the Sand that is on the Sea-shore for Multitude.* A *Dæmon* who comes to possess and molest one poor Man, may have a *Legion* attending on him. These *Evil Spirits,* are poisoned with, and confirmed in, a Disposition to affect the *Honours,* which are due to none but the Infinite God: And among those *Honours,* there may be none that their Affectation may be sett more upon, than to have paid unto them the Regards which belong to, *The Lord our Healer.* Yea, they may apprehend, That if the poor Children of Men apply unto *Them* for their *Health,* it may not only gratify them in their *Usurpation,* but we shall thereby provoke the God of Heaven to deliver us further up unto the *Power* of those to whom we have so Impiously Resigned ourselves, and permitt them to Inflict some greater *Mischief* on us, after they have done what seem'd a *Kindness.* Now, as the *Kingdome of Heaven,* So the *Kingdome of Darkness,* has the *Sacraments,* in the Observation whereof, we declare our *Subjection* thereunto; and Subscribe ourselves, *The Children of the Kingdome.* And the *Sacraments of Hell* are particularly observed, in the *Sorceries,* wherewith many ungodly and unhappy People seek the Cure of their *Diseases.* Upon the Practice of certain *Sorceries,* People often find a strange Releef of their *Maladies:* and upon Use of odd and mad *Charms,* the Spirits of the *Invisible World,* some or other of which are always at hand, and are, no doubt, very *Skilful Physicians,* help them to some Ease of their Distempers. It is doubtless a Mistake in a Great Philosopher, *Diaboli potestas eo se non Extendit, ut Claudum Pediculum restituet.*[1] By the *Charms,* of *Words* and *Marks,* and the like, which tis plain can be of no *Natural Efficacy* for the Cure of Diseases, People in short plainly *go to the Devil* for a Cure; And how tremendous must be the Consequences!

But this Impiety, how commonly is it practised: Even among those who have been *Baptised* for God, and in their *Baptism* have renounced all Dependence on the *Devil!*

The Learned *Borellus* who has collected many Exemples of such Things, passes this Judgment upon them; *Latet ut opinor, aliquid Diabolici in his Curis, seu pacticimpliciti cum Daemone, ut fere ab Omnibus notatum fuit.*[2] In short, Theres the *Devil* in them; yea, an *Implicit Covenant* with the *Devil.*

In what *Fernelius* has written, *De abditis rerum Causis*,[3] the Curious may read more of these Things. But I would not have Quoted these Authors, if I thought our *Common Fools* could come at them. The *Learned* will not be *Such Fools,* as to try the cursed Experiments.

Indeed I am Lothe to *Describe* any of these *Charms,* Lest I should unawares *Instruct* some Vicious Minds, and Furnish them, for a criminal Employment of them; As the Excellent *Hemingius*[4] relates, That he pleasantly reciting to his Pupils, a Distich of *Unintelligible Terms,* which being written and eaten, by one at a Time, on a Peece of Bread, would cure an Ague, by the Time that all the *Terms* had been so swallowed; a silly, but an honest Youth, taking him in Earnest, made the Experiment, with such Success, that he quickly cured a notable Number of Patients.

I know very well, that *Austin*[5] reports, that *Charms* are no Longer efficacious, after they come to be divulged. But yett I think, the Divulgation of such Things, as for Instance I find foisted I guess, by the bold Whimsical, Maggoty Bookseller, into a Book of, *Remarkable Providences,*[6] to have been a very Indiscreet and Pernicious Action.

The Wise Reader will but Smile at the Old Cure for a *Quartan Ague,* which yett was very seriously præscribed by *Serenus Sammonicus,*[7] a Physician, and Præceptor to the younger *Gordian,*[8] the Roman Emperour.

Maeoniae Iliados quartum Suppone Timenti.[9]

However, I may venture to complain of such Things, as the *Nefandous Abuses,* which many Jews putt upon the *Psalms* in our *Psalter,* when they employ these and those Passages in them, as *Charms* for the *Cure of Diseases,* in such ways, as have been related by *Amama,*[10] in his *Antibarbarus Biblicus.* Even the Plant called, *Fuga Daemonium,*[11] has been so employd by People, that the Power and Service of *Dæmons* has been therewith brought into Operation.

How frequently is *Bleeding* Stancht, by writing of Something, with Some Ceremonies, on the Forehead!

How frequently is a *Toothache* Eas'd, and an *Ulcer* Stop'd, and an *Ague* Check'd, by Papers, with some *Terms* and *Scrawls* in them, sealed up and worn about the Neck.

Famous is the Operation of *Abracadabra:*[12] a Word wherein some Learned Men suppose a reference to the *Chaldee* Names for the Three Persons in the Eternal Godhead: Tho' our *Selden*[13] supposes it may refer to *Abraxas*,[14] a Certain Deity about which *he*, and *Beyerus*[15] and *Saubertus*[16] and others have Entertained us with some Strokes of Erudition.

Others besides *Langneus*,[17] have done Strange Cures, with a *Magical Staff*, made with foolish Regards to the Aspects of the *Stars*.

The *Sigils*[18] of *Paracelsus* being worn, have been follow'd with Strange Cures, on some that have been too willing by wearing them to list themselves among the Votaries of the *Devil:* and become *Sealed* for Perdition.

The *Curatio Morborum per Mensurationem*,[19] reported by the most Learned Pen of the North, is one of these *Transgressions* wherein the *Wicked say, There is no Fear of God before their Eyes*.

But that which has been *Wicked* in this Kind, *cannot be numbred*.

It is not for my Purpose, to make any Delibations here from the *Scrutinium Amuletorum*, published by *Jacob Wolff*,[20] which has in it a Vast Amassment of Things, that occurr in the Writings of the Learned, about the many Sorts of Superstitious *Amulets*, wherewith millions of unadvised People, have surrendered themselves unto *Satan*, and confessed themselves the *Children of the Wicked One*.

I will only Exhibit a Couple of Relations, wherein I think, I may venture to mention the *Charms:* I need not fear, that any will venture to Repeat them.

The One shall be, What *Gotschalcus*[21] has given us, as what he himself knew to be True. A Woman grievously troubled with *Sore Eyes*, Engaged a Liberal Reward unto any one that would help her. A Scholar, who was altogether unskilful in Medicine, yett undertook to do it. He gave her a *folded bitt of paper*, which he wrap'd up in a Bag, and order'd her to wear it about her Neck. She did so, and found upon it, a marvellous Releef of the Infirmity. After a Year or two, her Curiosity led her to pry into this Wonder-Working *Paper*. Opening of it, she found some Characters of no Regular or Intended Shape, and this filthy Sentence under-written, *Diabolus Eruat tibi Oculos, et foramina Stercoribus impleat.*[22] She threw it away with Indignation. But, which is very surprizing; her Infirmity immediately returned upon her. My Author adds; *Unde efficacia, nisi a Daemone, qui ista fraude delectabatur?*[23]

The other, shall be of a Late Sorrowful Exemple. A Gentlewoman in the City of *London*, that shall be nameless; being troubled and much tired, with an *Ague*, at Length, came to the Remedy of wearing a *folded Bitt of Paper* about her Neck. She found her Sickness releeved and removed upon it. But after some Time, She must needs Enquire into the Contents of the Fever-frighting *Paper*. Opening of it, she found that fearful Sentence written in it; *Ague, Farewell, Till thee and I meet in Hell.* It struck her with horrible Consternation. She fell into *Horror of Conscience.* Her Soul was fill'd with the Terrors of God. She never saw good Hour more in the World. She died in a Despair, that was very Lamentable.

My Friend, Be warned against such *Impiety!* Rather undergo any Miseries, as long as an Holy God may please to lay them, and keep them on thee, than repair unto *Devils* to take them off. They may have Leave to Gratify and Encourage thy *Impiety,* with a present *Show of Success;* but it will be only that they may afterwards Exercise a more dreadful *Tyranny* over thee, and have thee fall as a more certain and woful *Prey* unto them.

It is Old and Sage Advice, that we find in the *Thirty Eighth* Chapter of *Ecclesiasticus: The Lord has created Medicines out of the Earth, and he that is wise will not abhor them.* Certainly, far from *Wise,* are they that will go to *Hell* for *Medicines:* If we are *Wise* we [worn off]

Mantissa.

We have a Fancy among our Common People, That a SEVENTH SON, among Brethren that have not had a Sister born between them, is endued with I know not what, *Power of Healing* Various Distempers, with a Touch of his Hand upon the Part affected. But may we not be afraid lest some *Unlawful Fellowship with the Invisible World* may ly at the Bottom of it? If we suppose the *Matter of Fact,* I would Enquire:

First; Can any Reasonable Man imagine, that a *Seventh Son* should be distinguished *Naturally,* with such a Sanative and Balsamic Vertue in his Constitution, that he should be like the *Miraculous Pool,* when an Angel made his Descent into it? Why should the Intervening of a *Sister* deprive him of this *Distinguishing Prærogative?* Why should the seventh have it any more than the *First-born,* to whom there belongs *the Excellency of Dignity and the Excellency of Power?* Yea, is not the *First-born* as really the *Seventh* as the *Last?* Or, Is it requisite, that all the *Seven* have the Same Father and Mother? Or, may the Father have the *Seven Sons* by different Wives? Or, The Mother of these *Maccabees,* by different Husbands? Or, *How?*

Or, Secondly; Is it possible to resolve the Matter into any other than a *Sacramental Original?*

Either we must Suppose, that the Glorious God, before whom we are *as the Clay before the Potter,* has Endued the *Seventh Son* with a *Gift of Healing,* Like that which in the primitive times of Christianity, recommended some *Favourites of Heaven* among the First Preachers of the Gospel unto the World; or at least, Like that which the famous *Greatreats, the Stroker* in *Ireland,* was for a While an unaccountable Instance of. But where have we been *Taught of God* any thing of this Importance? Or, what if the *Seventh Son* should be a *Vile Person; a Child of Belial; a Devil Incarnate?* and one belonging to the Tribes that are the *Abhorred of the Lord?*

Or, we must Suppose, (what is most likely) That in the *Kingdome of Darkness,* there is a Surprizing Imitation of many Things that occur in the *Kingdome of God.* And as the Number Seven, has been Strangely Considered in the Affairs of the Heavenly World, (as well as the Number, *Twelve,*) So, in the *Kingdome of Darkness,* it is affected, for the Number *Seven* to be brought into a peculiar Consideration, (as well as the Number, *Twenty five!*) And more particularly, an Application to a *Seventh Son* for a Cure, shall be a *Sacrament,* wherein the *Dæmons* that attend him, shall reckon themselves acknowledged, as the Dispensers of the *Cure,* that is here Looked for!

That the *Dæmons* are very officious to Convey *Cures,* unto the Patients, that with *Cæremonies* approved by *Them,* do seek unto them, is notorious from the Experience of all Ages, and of all Places, as well as from the *Dreams* of old obtained in the Temple of *Esculapius.*

If the *Healing Vertue* be not in the *Natural Constitution* of the *Seventh Son,* must it not needs be in the Operation of some assisting *Dæmons?* And the Homage, or the Regard, that is paid unto the Number *Seven* in this Way, is the *Sacrament* that brings the Patient under the Efficacy of it.

But what an *Enchanted Field* are we now brought into: And what a Door is opened unto Ten Thousand *Sorceries!* If *Numbers* are to be Esteemed for the Healing of Diseases, why should not *Figures* be so too? And from *Figures* let us pass to *Letters,* yea, to all the *Ephesian*[24] ones. And why should not the *Seventh Son* pronounce *Words,* and use his *Lip* as well as his *Hand,* for a Cure? And why not also manage the *Motions* of his *Hand,* in the Way of *Magical Cæremonies?* And would not a Cure be wrought as effectually, if he should only pronounce Words, and make no Use of his *Hand* at all? Would not a *Spell* from him do as well as a *Touch?* I doubt it not!

Indeed, I have read concerning the *Seven Sons* of one *Sceva*[25] a Jew, among certain Exorcists and Vagabonds, who did some *Notable Things*. But among these, *all the Seven,* for ought we see, were as potent Knaves as the *Seventh*. And I make no Doubt, That if People would once take up the Fashion of applying to a *Sixth Son,* they would find *him* do as *Notable Things* as now they think the *Seventh* can do for his Ill-advised Patient.

I pray, Lett us not foolishly leave the *Ordinary Ways of Cure,* and run into impertinent, yea, very *Unwarrantable* Superstitions.

In my Opinion; One setting up for, *An Healer,* no otherwise Qualified and Empowered for it, than as being, *A Seventh Son,* deserves little better Usage than a *Quack* was wont formerly at *Montpelier*[26] to meet withal. *Is apprehensus Asino imponitur, Et urbe Pellitur, Ovis putridis et alijs Sordibus, sit Venia dicto, quae in ipsum Conjiciunt, donec per urbem magno dedecore deductus sit, alium locum Petiturus.*[27]

An Appendix.

Popery ridiculed.

PROTESTANTS, Be ye Thankful that a Gracious God has rescued you from the *Strong Delusions* of *Popery,* and that You are no Longer under the *Fascinations,* which the *Man of Sin* had Laid upon a Woful World. How Ridiculously foolish is the *Revived Paganism* in the *Popish* Idolatries and Superstitions, applying to such and such particular Saints, for the *Cure* of these and those Diseases! One can hardly recount the Follies of the Miserable Papists in this One Article, without Some Thought on St *Medard,*[28] the Saint which they say, helps to *Smiling* or *Laughing*. Most certainly, if St *Maturin,*[29] whom they make the Psysician for *Fools;* or St *Acaire,*[30] who cures the Furious, or St *Avertin*[31] who cures the Lunatic, would Exert their pretended Energies, these Follies would soon be Cured in their Votaries. Doubtless the Saints of *such Names* were Stumbled on for *Such Cures,* because of Some Signification in the Names leading thereunto: As *Maturin,* the Saint for *Sotts;* [But if, to all such, *How Large his Diocese!*] from the Italian *Matto,* which comes from the Greek Ματαιθ. But how blundred were they, when they made St *Eutropius*[32] the Physician for a *Dropsy,* if they confounded *Eutropius* with *Hydropicus?* There is more of *Homonymie,* in making St *Mammard*[33] the Physician for Distempers of the *Paps:* and St

Main[34] for those of the *Hands;* and St *Phiacre*[35] for the (*Phy,* or) Emrods; and St *Genou*[36] for the *Gout,* which is often in the Knee. There was a grievous Trespass on Chronology, in making *Job,* the Physician for the *Foul Disease.* It seems, the *Heavenly* Physicians in this differ from our *Terrestrial* ones: *They* don't profess the Cure of all Diseases as *ours* do; But St *John*[37] and St *Valentine*[38] cure only the *falling Sickness,* (which is called St *Johns Evil:*[39]) St *Sebastian*[40] cures only the *Plague:* [and worthy to be a *Saint,* could he do That!] St *Roch*[41] cures only the *Scab;* (no doubt making People *Sound as a Roche:*) St *Petronelle*[42] (St *Peters* Daughter) cures Fevers. St *Romain*[43] dispossesses Devils. But St *Cosmas* and St *Damia*[44] are only Cheirurgeons. If St *Claire*[45] a Woman-Saint cure Sore Eyes, here again there was doubtless an Eye to the Etymology of the Name; For they tell us, there is no better way to cure the *Eyes,* than to make them see *Clearly.* But sometimes there are Several Saints, that stand Competitors for the Office of curing One Disease. And St *Quintin*[46] can't peaceably alone Enjoy the Office of curing a *Cough.* And some have pleaded, that St *Christopher*[47] may come in with St *Apollonia* for the Cure of the *Toothache,* considering the Size of his *Tooth,* which they show among their adored Reliques.

But I will stop; not for the Reason given by the witty *Henry Stephens,*[48] Lest I should *purchase the Displeasure of the Colledge of Physicians; in the Peoples leaving them, and going to the Saints, and I be accused of marring their Market.* Nor need we be afraid, That the *Saints* who may be overlooked, will take the Vengeance of a St *Anthony*[49] upon us.

We are by our happy Instruction in the *Protestant Religion* Emancipated from these Fooleries; And instead thereof, we have so *Learned CHRIST* as to understand, That we have an Admirable SAVIOUR, in whom Alone we shall truly find All the Scattered *Powers* and *Favours,* for which the Deluded Gentiles have look'd unto their Several Idols. And HE is a God who will *hear them that call upon Him.*

Yea, and by hearkening to the *Maxims* of this *Religion,* and following and obeying the *Holy Author* of it, a Man will himself become a *Saint,* by which there will be greater Cures wrought on him, and Things done for him, than could be Expected from all the *Saints* that are the *Inhabitants of the Heavens.*

But that we may yett further depreciate the *Healing Vertues* of the *Saints;* I have been told, that when a Languid Pretender to the

Crown of *Spain* to whom the Queen of *England* lent her Assistances, expressed his Hopes in the *Blessed Virgin* for his obtaining of what he desired, an English General freely and wisely told him, That if his *Royal Mistress* did him not more Service than St *Mary,* he would have no great Harvest of it.—This I will Say; a Skilful and Faithful Physician will do more for a poor Patient than all the *Saints* in the *Romish Kalender.*

I will take leave to add this one thing more. The Assigning of particular *Plants* to particular *Planets,* or to say, as your *Culpepper*[50] continually does, that such an Herb is governed by *Saturn,* and such an one is under the Dominion of *Jupiter,* and the Rest; It is a Folly akin to the Idolatry and the Superstition of the *Roman-Catholicks,* in looking to *Saints,* for their Influences on our Several *Diseases.* Tis amazing to see Mankind so *Planet-Struck;* and Men that can *handle the Pen of the Writer* become so very Impertinent and Ridiculous.

CAP. LXIII. *Misocapnus;*[1]
Taking the Use of TOBACCO
under Consideration.
with a *Pinch* upon the *Snuff-box.*

TOBACCO; Tis a Plant, the Use whereof, in *Two very Impertinent Ways of using it,* has extended itself over the Face of the whole Globe, at a rate that may be justly wondred at! The King[2] from whose *American* Dominions it was first introduced, has not Extended his Dominions, tho' he boast of the *Sun* Rising and Setting in them, So far as the Plant they have afforded us. The Idol in the Plain of *Dura*[3] never had so many Votaries to partake in its *Burnt-Offerings!* No *Tamerlane*[4] ever had so Vast an Empire! An Emperour with a *Stalk* of *Tobacco* for a *Sceptre,* Commanding all that the *Leaf* intoxicates, would have a Claim to Titles, which no vainglorious Monarch of the *East* ever yett had Vanity Enough to pretend unto. O! Had the *Religion* of our SAVIOUR near so many Disciples, as a silly and nasty *Custome,* in which so many Professors of *His Religion,* have *Learnt the Way of the Heathen!*—Our King *James* I. when he allow'd a *Counterblast upon Tobacco,* to go abroad under his Name had the *Spirit of Prophecy* as little in *that,* as in some other Things: and foresaw not, that one *Lane,*[5] who (being brought over from

Virginia, by Sir *Francis Drake*) brought with him the First of the *Tobacco* that ever had been seen in *Europe,* came furnished with what would shortly bring in Four Hundred Thousand Pounds yearly Revenue into the public Treasury. *Avidius Cassius*[6] had the Honour of Inventing the Punishment of *Smoaking men to Death.* And thou, *Lane* shalt have the Honour of bringing over the Invention of thus *Dying* in the English World. But, alas, we *Love Death.* And the Way of Dying by such a *Smoke,—*the *Weed* that gives it, may say, *my People do love to have it so.* We will proceed in the way of Distinct *Remarks* upon it.

I. The Plant, which has its Name of *Tobacco,* from a Province (an Island)[7] of *New Spain,* which is of such a Name; Tis a Plant of so many Vertues, that if *Nicot*[8] the French Embassador at *Portugal,* or, the Queen of *France,*[9] could have gott the Name of *Nicotiana,* or, *Medicea,* or other Competitors have gott their Names more lastingly fixed upon it, it might have been a Subject which among the Pursuers of that *Smoke* we call, *Honour,* might have been thought worth contending for. It has passed for a Sort of, *Panacaea;* Whole Treatises have been Written, with much Ostentation of Erudition upon it; and Several under the Title, which *Neander*[10] has given to his, *Tabaco-Logia.* The Epigram of *Castor Durant,*[11] upon the Vertues of *Tobacco,* tho' it sum them up in a few Lines, yett they are too many to be *Recited,* if not also to be *Beleeved.* However we will hear a Distich of *Johannes Posthius.*[12]

> *Nulla Salutifero se comparet Herba Tobacco;*
> *Viribus hoc Omnes Exsuperat reliquas.*[13]

Among other forms of Exhibiting this Plant unto the Service of Mankind, there is, the Tobacco-Ointment, of which the *Dispensatories* teach Every body the Præparation. Old *Culpepper* is in a Rapture upon the Mention of it; He would have nothing but the *Philosophers Stone* to be more valuable; He would have *Jubertus*[14] famous as long as the Sun and Moon Endures for inventing it. Be sure, The vertues of that Ointment, are very many.

II. But then there is an *Abuse* of this Plant, which requires, that some Notice be taken of it. The Incomparable *Alsted*[15] shall Express the Matter; *Maximus Tabaci Abusus est, quotidiano Ejus usu, Semet ipsos et bonas Horas perdere, et ex Cerebro, Mentis nobilissima Sede, Caminum et Cloacum Efficere.* In plain English; Tis a most *Vile Abuse* of *Tobacco,* for People by the *Daily Smoking* thereof, to Hurt themselves, and throw away their *Precious Hours,* and make a *Chimney,* or a *Dunghil,* of the *Brain,* where the *Soul* should have a most Noble Habitation. I am not so Vain, as to think of driving this *Foolish Custome* out of the World; No, tis too *Bewitching* a Thing, and the Lady *Circe* has too much Power over her Votaries, to leave any Room or Hope for *Hearkening to Reason* in the Matter. The *Flies* that are entangled in the *Spanish Cobweb,* are not easily disentangled. I don't know what may be done when *it has had its Day.* Nor would I absolutely Decry the Practice of *Smoking Tobacco. Smoke on,* Good People, You that can Really Say, *That you Really find Good by it.* But how few *can* say So! And what *Fools* must they proclame themselves, who *Smoke,* and *cannot* say so! However, This I will *take* Leave (Whether the *Smokers* will *give* it or no!) to say, That as it is commonly used, it is a *Custom,* which if People were *well-advised,* they would have the *Wisdome,* to decline it. I will not be so *Poetical,* as to say with our old *Laureat,*[16] *That the Destroyer* has in these last Ages plaid upon the World, with Two *Smoking Engines,* namely, *Guns* and *Pipes,* out of the *Mouths* whereof *issue Fire and Smoke,* and, *By these the third Part of Men are killed;* adding,

> *We may be bold to think, the last the worst;*
> *However Both in their Effects accurst.*

But I would argue most *Seriously* upon the Matter. The *Tobacconists* do *Speak* sometimes, [But will they truly *Take!*] of a *Serious Pipe.* I wish they would allow a *Serious Pen,* to Reason with them.

III. I must and will insist upon it; That a *Slavery* to the *Custome* of *Smoking Tobacco,* is a Thing, by no means Consistent with the Dignity of a *Rational Creature;* and much less, of a *Vertuous Christian.* The *Nature* of *Man* is debased and is disgraced by such a *Slavery;* and much more the *New Nature* of one that is *Born again,* has a Contumely Cast upon it. There is a *Slavery* to it, when People *cannot live without it;* when they are insatiably *Craving* after it; when the Best *Exercises* that give a long Interruption to it, seem therefore Tedious to them; And, in short, when *Better Business,* must give way to it; and Things of more Importance must be Superseded, for it. My Friend, If this be thy State, thou throwest away a *Liberty,* with which thy Maker and Saviour has dignified thee; and thou art *Entangled with a Yoke of Bondage* to an *Appetite,* which is not of *His,* but of *Thy own* Creating, and, when thou art *come to thyself,* thou wilt *groan to be delivered from this Bondage of Corruption.* Thus to be Enthralled, in so mean a Slavery; Do but *Show thyself a Man,* and thou wilt Scorn it! *Poor Slaves;* The more *Sober* Part of Mankind, Enjoying the *Liberty,* which is our *Birthright,* and which you have *Despised,* they cannot but look upon you with a *Pitty,* not altogether unlike what they would employ, if *Galley-Slaves* were made *Spectacles* unto them: it appears to them not altogether unlike the *Habit* of the *Galley-Slaves* upon you. *Ignominious Captivity!*

IV. It were to be wish'd, That many who Should *know Better,* and particularly, the *Ministers* of the Gospel; were less *Excessive* this Way, than too many of them are. Syrs, You know very well, that Incontestible Rule of PIETY; *Whatever you do, do all to the Glory of God.* You should forbear doing of any Thing, whereof you cannot say, *Tis a Service to God;* and, *I am yeelding some Obedience to God in the doing of it.* But can you say so, upon all the *Excesses* which you run into! Some have used the *Formality,* of letting the Standersby observe, That *they crave a Blessing on Every Pipe.* This I press not for; It may look too *Formal.* But this I will say; *Smokers,* Can you comfortably *Pray* over what you do, and with Confidence ask a *Blessing* on it, as an Action wherein *God is Glorified?* I beseech you, Lett the *Candle of the Lord,* make a True Discovery to you; and lett not your *Smoke* so blind your Eyes, as to hinder your discerning, *Whether it be not become a Lust that you are Serving of?* A *Lust* that aims meerly at the *Pleasure,* that is tasted from the *Salt of the Smoke,* tickling the Glands that are affected with it! You *must have* this most sorry *Pleasure,* it seems; you *can't bear* to go Long without it! Is *this* your Principle? *Declare Honestly!* Is *this it?* Alas, To be given up unto such a *Vile Affection!*—[And, You Gentlemen, who say, *It helps your Studies;* Are you sure, you can say so? Or, do the distinguishing and superior Effects of your *Studies,* convince your Hearers of it?]

But the most by far of them who have their Minds *Beclouded* with the *Smoke* of *Tobacco,* are People incapable of receiving Impression or Instruction from *Such* Considerations. They are only the *Heart-String made of the Finer Clay* that will be sensibly touched by *such* Considerations.

V. These Inhabitants of the *Terra del Fuogo*[17] and the People that out-do the *Salamander*[18] for thus *Living in the Fire,* may do well, to Examine, How much *Time* out of a Short Life goes to the Impertinent and Unprofitable Employment of *Smoking* with them! And examine whether by Drying and Parching their Glands, with *Smoking* they don't Superinduce a Necessity of *Drinking* much more than else they would have done! And Examine, Whether it leads them not into the *Temptations,* and *Pollutions,* which *Vain Company* uses to be attended withal! And if it be enquired, whether (at the *Tavern* Especially) it may not often produce those things, for which it has worn the Name of, *Herba Rixosa,* or, *Clamour-wort,* among the *Germans,* who are well-acquainted with it! Say also, Whether it be not Commonly made the Instrument of *Diverting* and *Confining* of *Conferences* from Subjects, that are infinitely more worthy to be discoursed on! If so: *Do this now, My Son: Deliver thyself as a Bird from the hand of the Fowler.*

VI. The Custome of *Smoking,* is brought on, and kept up, with such *Disreputable Circumstances,* that all who come to it, and keep at it, should be able to give a Good Account, *Why they take it up!* *O ad Servitutem nati,*[19]—it putts you unto abundance of *Trouble* ordinarily, and it Costs you many a *Qualm,* and many a *Sweat,* that you may *Learn to Smoke.* And when you have Learnt the *Mystery,* and gott the *Mastery* of your *Pipe,* you have added unto the Number of *Necessities,* which you must Submitt unto; as if you had not *Enough before*; and there is a *New Thing* after which you will *Daily,* if not *Hourly,* feel at least an *Uneasy Hankering!* When you come to Exercise your Noble Skill in Company, to say nothing of the Rudeness, with which you make the Rest of the Company to *Stay* for you, when they have Nothing else to stay for, but for you to Lay by your Pipe, (for which Cause, tis called, *The Stay of the Countrey!*) and we that are *Free-men* must be made the *Servants of Servants,* because it is not your Pleasure to Release us, or; I will rather note, how *Uncivilly,* and how *Indecently,* do you treat the Company, with *Puffing* and *Spitting* and *Spawling,* before them! Should any One without a *Pipe* in his Mouth, *Spitt* and *Spawl* before other People in a Room, as you do, would they not be Look'd on, as *Unpardonable Slovens?* The *First,* and indeed the *Sum,* of all *Good Manners* is, *To do nothing Offensive.* There are many, whom the *Smoke* of *Tobacco* is always *Offensive* to; and, if they are in a *Close Room* with many *Smokers,* they grow *Sick* upon it. But, it may be truly Said, That you *Take Physic* in the Presence of them, whom you Sitt withal, and you *Discharge your Excrements* before them. You would be Loth to call for the *Vessels of Dishonour,* or do the Business of the *House of the Secret Seat* in their Presence. This Action indeed comes not up to *Those;* But yett, methinks, it is not *without offence;* tis too *Nauseous* to be done before those whom we would pay Respect unto. I say then, *Some Account* should be given of the Action, that may be a *fair* and *clean* Defence for it. You must permitt us to call what you are *Smoking,* by the Name of *Goose-grass;* until you can do what we now demand of you.

VII. It was a very just Caution, given by a Writer always worth hearkening to: *Ad Necessitatem, non ad Libidinem, hunc Fumum Sorbeto.*[20] It is by no Means to be allow'd, That you Sufficiently Defend what you do, by Saying, *I Learn to Smoke, that I may be Sociable, and fitt Company for them who do it.* A most Empty *Complement,* a *Complement* that has *Nothing* in it. Nor can such *Company* be worthy of such *Complaisance!* Nor can you Sufficiently Defend it, by Saying, *I do it as an Amusement, that, like a Turk at his Opium, I may dream the Time away.* An *Amusement* that carries in it a *Besotment* very Ill Beseeming one that has but a little while to live in the World, and for whom, *Here is no Abiding.* A poor *Nepenthe!*[21] 'Tis impossible to defend it any way, but by being able to plead, *My Health requires it.* But you had need be well Satisfied for *This;* 'Tis a Plea, of which it may be remonstrated, *How few can truly make it!* I am very positive in it; Every other *Plea,* will in the Balance of Reason, be found *Lighter than the Light Dust of the Balance;* and even Lighter than the Seed of *Tobacco,* whereof it is found, *That there is not the Weight of One Grain in a Thousand of them.*

VIII. If you want an *Hydrogogue,* or, Something to draw off a *Rheum* or *Flegm,* which you fancy that you abound withal, would you not be accommodated with one much more præferrible, in chewing a Bitt of *Mastick?* This would also, whiten your *Teeth,* and Sweeten your *Breath:* whereas by *Smoking,* your *Teeth* become Filthy and Sooty and Rotten; and it is well if you don't gett such a Stinking *Breath,* as that it may be wondred how your *nearest friends* can Endure you. Those whom you *talk* withal, can't bear your *Approaches* to them; tis an *Irksome Scent* they suffer from you; they are well-nigh Struck *Backward* with it: You are little better, than *Abdal Melek,*[22] the *Saracen General* you may have read of, before whom the flying Insects would fall down dead if they came within the reach of his breathing on them.

IX. It has been Enquired, Which were the *Greatest Number* of People, They that gott *Good,* or they that gott *Hurt,* by the *Smoking* of *Tobacco?* Some have answered it, That the *Greatest Number* is of those who may say, *They gett neither Good nor Hurt by it.* If it be so, then the *Greatest Number* do not well to practise it; It is a *Needless Mispence of Time,* that they are to be charged withal. But it may be feared, whether this Answer may not be too Favourable.

It is probable That for them who have to do with Persons and in Places, where Infection may be feared, the *Smoking of Tobacco* may be a very Excellent Præservative. And it is possible, that in some *Damp,* and *Cold,* and *Coarse* Employments, the *Pipe* will be a good Companion.

But for the most Part,—

There is a *Caustic Salt* communicated unto the Mass of Blood, by the too frequent *Smoking* of *Tobacco:* From which there cannot but follow many Infellicities. And I pray what will the *Flesh* be the better for being so *Baconized?* It is thought by Some Judicious Observers, That it has been one Main Cause of the *Scorbutic* Humours, which infest our Bodies more than they did our Ancestors. The Learned *Pauvius*[23] and *Falkenburgius*[24] and *Raphelengius,*[25] affirm, That the *Brain* Sometimes Contains a *Black Soot* from it; which Cannot but be of Evil Consequence. Our *Strother* warns you, that nothing will contribute so much to Abate the Appetite and Concoction, as to rob the *Stomach* in this Way, of the *Salival Juice,* which is to assist the Digestion there. If smoking may be useful in some Defluxions? yett under these *Tobacco* should not be (illegible) tampered with. Yea, *Magnenus,*[26] tho' so great a Friend as he was unto it, yett acknowledges, "That it is not Easy to relate what are the *Damages* which the Inordinate and Immoderate Use of this *Fume,* does bring to Men. For besides the insatiable and greedy *Lust* of taking it, by its *daily use,* the *Memory* is impaired, the *Stomach* Violated, the *Brain* Exiccated, and the *Life* Shortened; and if they have *Children,* they are frequently not long-lived but Consumptive Children." And this very *Magnenus,* in the midst of the Expressions which he makes in his *Exercitations,* of his Friendship for this *Fume,* yett gives it as a Maxim, *That the frequent and familiar Use of it can be good for no Man.* There is indeed so much *Poison* in it, that our *Botanists* have called it, The *Henbane of Peru.* And among our Physicians, who know what is for their *Own Health,* how few great Men list themselves in the Tribe of *Smoakers.* Our very Learned *Gale,*[27] from his own Experience, taxes the *Smoke* of *Tobacco* with very *Noxious Qualities.* He sais, That he found it *made* more Humours than it brought away; and tho' it *opened* his Body for the Present, it made him the more *Costive* afterwards; and Nature was but the more sluggish and feeble anon, for the *Force* in this way often putt upon it. He sais, At last, *I came under a fixed Resolution to deliver myself from this Vassalage: And this I account not the least Deliverance of my Life.* He that *now* writes may join with him, in such an *Acknowledgment.* He concludes; with desiring the Reader to pardon his Discourse, which might *Seem Severe;* and which, he sais, *Nothing but Sincere Love to the Good and Honour of my Nation could have Extorted from me.* And he that *now* writes may again join with him in such an *Apology.* A Doctor no less worthy to be hearken'd to, than our *Cheyne,* sais, *To Thin, Meagre, and Hectic* Constitutions, it is highly Pernicious. Its Heating the Blood; Its Drying the Solids; Its Defrauding the Food of the *Saliva* so necessary towards *Concoction,* procures from that just Judge a Sentence of Banishment upon it.

To See so many Thousands of People accelerating upon themselves a *Death* like what the Emperour *Severus*[28] (perhaps not over *Severely*) doom'd a *Bribe-taking Judge* unto!—This has moved the Compassion, which now calls upon them that have made their Souls *Prisoners* in the *Tobacco-Box,* as the Apostle called upon the *Gaoler, Do thyself no Harm!* This tis that has made me ready to say with D. *Lebenwald,*[29] *Eliminarem sane et proscriberem hanc Herbam sin in mea potestate esset,*[30] (that it, for the use of it.) But that there are so many Pleaders for it, *Cuique Ergo placeat Fumus Odorque suus.*[31]

X. I don't Suppose, that many Captives of the *Pipe,* will Easily Emancipate themselves. But if any should with a proper Indignation at the *Stupefaction* which has been upon them, think of escaping from their Captivity, [will there be any such, *Prisoners of Hope?*] it is a *Wholesome Caution* for them, *Non temere nec Subito mutanda est Consuetudo;* Lett 'em not Reform *All at once,* but leave off *by Degrees.* A *Sudden* Change may be *Dangerous.* But for them who continue in the Practice, the most *Wholesome Counsil* that can be given them, will be to Use the *Direction* and the *Discretion* of the Word, which I have seen Written on the Lid of a *Tobacco-Box,* Moderation. Beware of *Over-doing.* Be not a *Servant* of it; *For, of what a Man is overcome, of the Same is he brought in Bondage.*

Yea, I will proceed so far, as to propose; why may not Good People *Exercise themselves* to Something of *Godliness,* in Exercise of *Smoking Tobacco?* In the Way of *Occasional Reflection,* why may not the *Vanishing Smoke* lead them to Thoughts on the *Vain Appearances* of the *Sublunar* Things, wherein Man *Walks in an Empty Show?* Why may not the *Discharge* which they make, Lead them to Thoughts, on what we have *within us,* that we shall do well to *part withal?* Cannot the *Period* of their *Tobacco* putt them in Mind of what the general *Conflagration,* shall bring on a World, that shall one day be *Burned as a Witch?* Why may not the *Ashes* which they soon reduce their *Weed* unto, Lead them to Thoughts on what will quickly be done by *Mortality* upon us all? Yea, to Confirm and Repeat this no less *Useful* than awful *Meditation,* Methinks, there is a further Inducement, in the *Confession* which the *Smoakers* ordinarily make, That they have a *Need* of what they do, and need more *Means* to preserve their *Lives,* than their Neighbours who see no Occasion to *do as they do.* Tis a Peece of an old Song:

> *An House that must have many Props, and Stayes,*
> *Is near its Fall, and faster it decays.*

Tobacco was by *Swenckfield,*[32] and others, called, *Herba Sancta.* This Way of using it, will the best of any render it worthy to be called so. We may Speak of *Sweet-Scented Tobacco,* when Such Thoughts give a Flavor to it. But, what shall be said unto them, who have hitherto Escaped the *Epidemical Contagion,* and are not yett come into this *Way of all the Earth?* I know no better Terms to advise them in, than these: *It is good for them, if they abide, Even as they are.* Add, *If thou mayst be kept Free, use it rather.*

Parents, Tutors, Teachers of all sorts; Advise your Children against it. Young Man, Be not rashly drawn into it. *My Son, Be wise for thyself.* And, *If they Entice thee, Consent thou not.* It is Good Advice. Take it, and thou wilt one day thank him that gave it.

The *English* Reader may do well to read what *Hall* on *Timothy* sais on *Tobacco.*[33]

And lett Scolars turn into *English,* this *Latin* of the great *Voetius.*[34]

Quamvis in se omnis Tabaci usus illicitus non sit, minime tamen Convenit Viris honestis et gravibus, (nominatim Ministris et Ministeris Candidatis) in Conspectu et Consortio aliorum; quod hominum otiosorum et Voluptuariorum non tam cibus quam Fumus, et Vanitas vulgo Indixetur.

Usus ejus, praeter Medicinalem, Si quis praetexatur; ad Tempus scilicet fallendum, aut ad Sentinam humorum Corporis Exhauriendam, ut cetevissa ac Vino impleatur; aut tantum Consuetudinis Ergo, aut Conformitatis cum famosis Tobacco helluonibus, omnis est a Malo.[35]

Coronis.

I have Something further to say:—

The Practice of taking *Tobacco,* in the Way of *Smoke,* may have Something said for it. But the Practice of taking it in the Way of *Snuff,* is altogether *Inexcusable.*

It is a Thing, which must I say, more *Sorrowful,* or *Provoking?* —to See so *Foolish* and *hurtful* a *Lust,* So ridiculously *drowning* so many People in *Perdition!* So many buried Alive in *Pungent Grains of Titillating Dust.*

The *Mean Delight* of Tickling the *Olfactory Nerves* a little, is all that can be pretended for this *Practice.* But how *shameful* a Thing is it, for *People of Reason* to confess, that they can't live Easily half an Hour together, without a *Delight,* so Sensual, so Trivial, so very Contemptible! Poor Creatures, you *Glory in your Shame!* And your Dirty *Upper Lip,* does but proclame the *Meanness* of your Souls! Tell us not you do it, that you may discharge your *Brain:* Tis a Whimsey, *That!*—your *Brain* is not overstockt.

Or, Is *this* Enough? *Tis the Mode.* This is what we complain of. —And why must it be the *Mode?* If it be an Irrational *Mode,* and an Indefensible *Mode,* you ought not then to *Follow the Multitude.*

But what is yett more Unaccountable, is, That you are all this while doing the Part of *Self-Destroyers.*

Whatever you think of it; The Passage thro' the *Os Cribriforme,* tho' it may not admitt the *Grosser Powder* of your Snuff to pass into the *Brain,* yett there are some very Thin and Fine Parts of it, that find their Way thither; And what Mischiefs must needs follow upon a *Brain* so poisoned?— Nay, One would think, your *Brain* were already touch'd, or you could not act so sillily, as you do, and be so Violently and Obstinately Attached as you are, to the *Evil Habit* that you have brought upon you. The *Snuff* more openly and readily finds a way down into your *Lungs,* and *Stomach:* And how many *Early Deaths* have you seen brought upon the miserable Children of Men, by this *Unreasonable Vanity?* A very just Motto for the *Snuff-box* might be, A Leader to the Coffin.

Our Ingenious *Quincy,* among others has Condemned this Practice particularly for *Spoiling of the Appetite.* His Words are, "Most of the Common *Snuffs* are *Tobacco;* Whereof Some will pass down the Throat, into the Stomach; Especially in those who take much. Whence it destroys the Natural Appetite, as many confess to find by Experience, altho' they cannot be prevail'd with, to leave it off." And I know not why the Words of the Judicious *Cheyne,* may not be thrown into the Scale. "The ridiculous Custome of perpetually Suck-ing in Sophisticated Powders and other foreign Drugs sold for *Snuff,* cannot but be prejudicial, both to the *Eyes,* and even to the *Stomach;* at least, if we believe the Reports of those, who say, They have brought it up from thence." Yea, a Learned Physician of the French Nation, has demonstrated, That the *Vellication* given to the *Olfactory Nerves* in the *Titillation* which the *Snuff* gives unto them, is really commu-nicated unto the Whole System of the *Nerves* all over the Body; And the very frequent Repetition of this Commotion and Convulsion to them, anon weakens their *Tone;* and so there are brought on, those Cruel Diseases, wherein the *Genus Nervosum* is affected. *Scurvies, Rheumatisms, Belly akes,* and many more such fearful Distempers break in upon People; and they are not aware, that they came out of that *Pandora's Box,* which they so fondly dote upon.

Away with it! If you would act like People of Reason; *Away with it!* Yea, If you Love your Lives, *Away with it!*

Cap. LXIV. *Restitutus.*

or,

A Perfect Recovery,

in the wise and good Conduct of one Recovered from a Malady.

THE *Jews* have a Reasonable Saying: That there are Four Sorts of Men who are bound above others, to Confess the Goodness of God in what is done for them; *Travellers* that are come to a Settled Habita-tion; *Prisoners* that have obtained their Liberty; *Mariners* that have performed their Voyage; and, *Sick People recovered out of their Sicknesses.* No doubt the *hundred and seventh Psalm* taught them so much Christianity.

It is to be hoped, That many *Patients* have gott some Good by our *Angel of Bethesda;* whether it be so or no, yett there are many who some Way or other, are gott out of *Maladies* that were grievous to them. A Solemn Address is now to be made unto these, That so the *Work* may be brought unto *Perfection,* and that the *End* of it may be attain'd, without which it will not be a *Perfect Recovery.* Certainly, There is no Need of quoting Aquinas for it: *Finis Exterioris Cura-tionis per CHRISTUM facta, est Curatio Animae.*[1]

Wherefore, *O Recovered Man;* You will consider the Glorious

God your SAVIOUR, as the Author of all the *Good* that has been done for you, and give Him the *Glory* of it; with such Acknowledgments as these: Psal. XXX. 1, 2, 12. *O Thou Eternal God, Thou art // my God; I unto thee // have made my Cry* in my Distress; // *and thou hast healed me.// Thou, O Eternal God, hast brought // my Soul up from the Pitt;// Thou hast made me to Live, that I // descend not to the Grave.// Glory shall therefore Sing to Thee,// and shall not hold its Peace;// O Thou Eternal God, my God,// Thee I'l forever Praise.*

It was an Ill Thing in a Good Man Recovered from Sickness, of whom we read, *He rendred not again according to the Benefit that was done unto him.* His Recovery was accompanied with a *Retrograde Motion of the Earth,* So that the Shadow of the *Sun* went back diverse of those *Points,* by which they distinguished the Difference between the *Summer Hours,* and the *Winter Hours,* on the *Dial;* A Thing that was as far off as *Babylon* wondred at. When the *Babylonian* Embassadors, who were worshippers of the *Sun,* Came to be Satisfied about it, (it is reported) he did not now so freely, so fully, so ingenuously as he should have done, assert his Glorious JEHOVAH, to be the Maker of the *Sun,* and the *Author* of his *Recovery.* He did better, a little before This; when in his *Writing after he had been Sick, and was recovered out of his Sickness,* he had these Passages: *ETERNAL, Thou Recoverest me,// and makest me to Live;// The Living, the Living, shall Praise // Thee, as I do this Day.//*[2]

But herewithal; Consider, how *Mercifully* the Glorious God has dealt with you, in thus *Recovering* of you; and lett *Mercy* have the *Glory* of it, *Undeserved Mercy!* For you may Say, *Lord, Thou hast punished me less than my Iniquities deserve.* Yea, *Distinguishing Mercy!* And you may Say, *Why am I so distinguished, when so many others are left unrestored!* And, O *Redeemed of the Lord,* if the Great and Last *Enemy* have been laying his Hand upon you; Be sensible of This, He would have carried you off, if the Blessed JESUS had not by pleading his Purchase for it, *Redeemed you from the Hand of the Enemy.* GOD has been *Gracious* to you, and you have been *Delivered from going down to the Pitt,* because this *Advocate* has *Produced His Righteousness* on your behalf, and so, *A Ransome has been for you.*

The Pagans had a Goddess, which was called, Ὑγιεια, SALUS, or, HEALTH. *Temples* were Erected for Her, wherein *Prayers* were made for *It.* Her *Coins* were often Struck, on the Recovery of Some Great Person; But, O CHRISTIAN, tis thy JESUS, Who must have thy *Praises*. If there be, and why should there not be?—Some *Coin* in the Case, Lett it be in gratefully disbursing a due Quantity of *Coin*, upon *Pious Uses*.

Above all; You must be sollicitous, that the *Declared Ends* for which the Glorious God Sent your *Malady* upon you, and now sends you a *Recovery* from it may be complied withal: that *by this, Iniquity may be purged, and all the Fruit may be to take away Sin:* and That it may be according to the Saying of the Ancients, *Ægritudo carnem vulnerat mentem Curat,* the *Wounding* of the *Flesh,* may prove the *Healing* of the *Soul.* Certainly, You ought now to be *Wiser* than you have been, and *Receive Instruction* when you have *Endured Correction.* A Learned Olevian[3] could say, *Ex hoc Morbo didici*—"By my *Sickness* I have Learned, what a *Glorious* God I have to do withal, and what an *Odious* Thing it is to *Sin* against His Holy Majesty." The Sick *Rolleck*[4] Said, "I am not ashamed to confess, that I never have reached unto so high a Pitch in the *Knowledge of God* in all my Days, as I have done since my *Sickness* has been upon me." A sick *Rivet*[5] could say, "In the Space of Ten Days that my *Sickness* has Confined me to my Bed, I have made greater Progress in *Divinity,* than in the whole Course of my Life before." O *Recovered Ones;* 'Tis to be wished, that you may now be *Recovered* out of your *Mistakes,* and more come into the *Right Thoughts of the Righteous,* than you did before.

And Since, you have tasted, what an *evil and a bitter thing it is,* to *Sin* against the Great God, you will now be more *Sick* than ever, of that which has made you *Sick:* and being *Recovered,* you will say, *Depart from me, all ye Workers of Iniquity!* Yea, Since you are *Well,* will you not be on all accounts *Better* than you were before your being *Ill?* Will you not apply your New *Strength,* to do more *Work* for God than ever you did, and *Love the Lord your God with all your Strength?* Will you not *Lead a New Life,* Since you *have* one; and make it the *Life of God?* Having your Time thus prolonged, Will you not more than formerly *Redeem the Time,* and Spend it more in *Getting* and in *Doing* of Good? Having had *This World Embittered* unto you, will you not be more *Weaned* from a World, the *Breasts* whereof have had so much *Wormwood* laid upon them? Having been under such *Cultivations,* will you not be more *Fruitful Christians,* and bring forth more of that *Fruit,* by which your *Heavenly Father may be Glorified?* It was the Custome of old, for a *Recovered* Person, to pay unto the Physician that helped him, a Gratuity which was

called, <u>Sostron</u>; or, A *Salvation-Fee*. O *Recovered* Person, I demand
thy *Salvation-Fee* to the Glorious One, who has helped thee. The
Conscience of the Person, is the *Officer* who is to *Serve the Writt* for
it. O *Thou Officer of God,* Lett him know *What* it is; Tis no less than
Himself. Require this of the Person; Say, *wilt thou be the Lords?*
Lett the Return be, *Lord, I am thine, because thou hast Saved me! I
will truly be thy Servant, because thou hast loosed the Bonds that were
upon me.*

The Roman Emperours, who exerted themselves for the *Health*
of the People, in times of Contagion, were (Even with Adoration)
called, *Apollines Salutares!* O CHRISTIAN, thou knowest no
Apollo Salutaris, but that JESUS, who is thy only SAVIOUR.

I call to Mind, the awful Words of our SAVIOUR, to a Man,
who had been Recovered of a Tedious Malady: Joh. V.14. *Behold,
Thou art made whole; Sin no more, Lest a Worse Thing come unto
thee.* I know not what Impression these Words made upon the Man.
But I know what the Words of our Judicious Dr. *Owen*[6] about him
are. "No *Outward Effects* [*writes the Doctor*] can work upon the
Hearts of Men, so that all they who are made Partakers of them,
should be brought unto *Faith,* and *Thankfulness* and *Obedience.* He
whom our Saviour cured of a Disease that he had Suffered Eight and
Thirty years, notwithstanding a following Admonition given him by
our Blessed Saviour, turned *Informer* against Him, and Endeavoured
to betray Him unto the Jews. *A Lamentable Story!*"

Be sure, If People *Recovered* from Diseases, do persist in a *State*
and *Course* of *Sin,* and if they do Refuse also to *Reform* what *Special
Sin* they may Discern God in their Affliction managing a *Controversy*
with them for; they may justly fear, that a *Worse Thing* will come
unto them. God has *Reserves* of *Arrows* in His Quiver, and He
Threatens, *If you will not be Reformed by these Things, but walk in
the Way of Chance with me* [and act as if every thing happened unto
you meerly by *Chance,* as if you were made *Sick* only by *Chance,* and
made *Well* only by *Chance!*] then *I will punish you yett Seven times
for your Sins.* Yea, anon the *Angel of Death* will have Order given
him, *Go, Cutt down that Unfruitful Tree.* And the *Sin* of the Transgressor will be found such a *Sin unto Death,* as that the Expired Patience of God will not now say, *Pray for him with hope of Speeding.*
All Entreaties from him will have no Answer but that, *I will deliver
you no more!* Yea, to be left unto *Sinning more,* This is itself a *Worse
Thing!* and will carry in it a most amazing Vengeance of God. A

Transgressor *growing worse* Every Day, with a *Spirit of Slumber* Siezing on him, is ripening for, and hastening to a *Damnation that Slumbers not.* THEN indeed a *Worse Thing* will come unto him. He *goes out of one Fire, and another Fire shall devour him:* and he falls into Torments that Surpass all Imagination!

When the Emperour *Sigismund*[7] ask'd the Bishop of *Colen,*[8] *What should he do to be Happy;* He answered, *Live, as in your Last Fitt of Sickness, you thought you would do.* I need say no more.

CAP. LXV. *Liberatus.*

or,

The Thanksgiving

of One

Advanced in Years,

and

præserved from grievous and painful Diseases.

IT is a just Observation of an Eminent Philosopher and Physician, "Such is the Surprizing Minuteness, and nice Adjustment of the Numberless Springs and Movements, on which Life depends; and so many are the Irregularities, to which Every One of them is Liable; that the Præservation of this curious Peece of Machinery, and the Continuance of its Operations and Functions for Three or Four Score years together is little less than a *Miracle.* At least, Every one must allow it, as a convincing Proof of the Inimitable Wisdome, and Contrivance of its Author and Former." A Servant of God arrived unto some *Age* in the World, and præserved all this While from those *Dolorous Diseases,* wherewith Hundreds of Thousands are cruciated, thought it but a *Reasonable Service,* to sett apart some *Time Extraordinary,* for Solemn THANKSGIVING to the Glorious God, for so Distinguishing a Favour of Heaven to Him, [yea, Among the Jews, a Man arrived unto *Threescore,* made a *Feast,* unto which he invited his Friends to give Thanks with him, in that he was come to *Old Age,* and Past the Danger of *Dying before his Time.*] I will comprise into as Little Room as I can, the *Sentiments of a Thankful Soul,* produced before the Lord, on this Occasion.

"O my God, why am I not *feeble and Sore broken, and roaring by reason of the Disquietness of my Heart,* under those *Terrible Dis-*

tempers, which Defy the *Physicians,* and which Torture the *Patients,* and under which *all the Days of the Afflicted are Evil Days? Lord,* It is not because I have *deserved* any such Exemption, any such Immunity. No, If I had my Desert, I should be *delivered up unto the Tormentors;* and *broken sore in the place of Dragons.*—It is thy *Free-Grace* that has Released me. My SAVIOUR who suffered Exquisite *Anguish* for me, has also pleaded for my Release from Deserved Anguish. And, O my SAVIOUR, Thou art *the Keeper of my Soul!*

But, *What shall I Render to the Lord?*

Oh! Lett a *Life* thus at Liberty for the *Service* of God, be industriously Employ'd in it; and be fill'd with *Devotions* and *Benignities,* from which I have not Such Things as many miserables have, to take me off.

Oh! Lett me be full of Compassion for Such as I see Languishing in the dreadful Circumstances, which I who have *Sinned as much as they,* have never tasted of. With a Bleeding *Heart,* and an Ardent *Prayer* for them, Lett me Look upon them. And Lett me study all the Ways I can, to Releeve and Comfort them.

For more particular Maladies:—

Am I free from the STONE? *Lord,* Lett there be nothing allowed in the *Lower Parts of the Earth* with me, which thou mayst be offended at.

Am I free from the GOUT? *Lord,* Lett my *Feet* carry me cheerfully to the Places of my Duty, and *go about still doing of Good.* And Lett my *Hands* be full of *Good Works,* and never be applied unto any Evil Purposes.

Am I free from the CANCER? *Lord,* Lett my Spirit be kept clear from all the Corrosions of *Envy,* and *Malice,* and Every Evil Frame towards my Neighbour. And Lett a *Sweetness of Temper* be always Conspicuous in me.

Am I free from the *PALSEY? Lord,* Lett me be Ready and Nimble in all the *Motions* of PIETY. And Lett me be One of Suitable *Activities,* in what I have to do for God, and His Kingdome, and my Neighbour.

Have I never felt the Anguish of *Broken Bones? All my Bones now shall Say, O Lord, who is like unto thee, which deliverest the poor from the Accidents, which I have been times without Number Expos'd unto!* And, oh! Lett me beware of those *Falls into Sin,* which may bring the Anguish of *Broken Bones* upon me."

Psal. CIII. 1, 2, 3, 4, 10.

"*O my* awakened *Soul, Do thou* // *Bless the ETERNAL GOD:* // *And all my Inward Powers the Name* // *of His pure Holiness.* //

O my awakened *Soul, Do thou* // *Bless the ETERNAL GOD; And O forget not any One* // *of all His Benefits.* //

Tis He who gives a Pardon to // *all thy Iniquities;* // *Tis He who gives an Healing to* // *all thy Infirmities.* //

Tis He who doth Redeem thy Life // *from the Corrupting Pitt;* // *Tis He who thee with Mercy doth* // *and with Compassions Crown.* //

His Dealings have not been with us // *according to our Sins:* // *Nor has He recompensed us* // *according to our Crimes.*

The Jews, from the Numeral Powers of the Letters in the Word תופעות[1] Issues *of Death* [Psal. LXVIII. 20.] reckon the *Diseases* in the World, *Nine-hundred and three.* I Suppose the Number of *Diseases* has never yett been Exactly *Stated:* And if it were, I suppose it would be soon *Broken,* by the Appearance of New Ones. This I am Sure of, There are *Moriendi mille Figurae.*[2] And certainly, They that have *out-lived* all these, and are gott on towards a *Good Old Age,* have cause to Sing the Praises of God their SAVIOUR: unto whom *there Belong the Issues of Death.*

Cap. LXVI.
EUTHANASIA.
or,
A DEATH Happy and Easy.

AFTER all, we See, DEATH unavoidable. There is a *Statute of Heaven* for it: *Statutum est.* My *Angel of Bethesda,* that has express'd so much Concern to arm his Readers against the *Approaches of Death,* yett confesses, *I cannot by any means Redeem thee; nor find out a Remedy for thee, that thou shouldest Live forever, and not see Corruption.* The Prophet, who had in him a *Double Portion of the Spirit* in a Master and a Father, that Escaped the *Common Lott of Dying,* yett must anon Come to That: *He fell Sick of his Sickness, whereof he died.* Yea, You may not only Say, *I know that God will bring me to Death;* while at the same time you may say, *I know not the Day of my Death;* but I will suppose you now arrived, unto that Period, in which it may be said of you, *The Time draws nigh in which he is to dy.* The *Angel* therefore will not leave you, until he has acquainted you with the *Dispositions* that should be found in a *Dying Man,* who would propose to *Dy Comfortably:* Which are indeed those *Dispositions* of, *An Healed Soul,* which all your *Sickness,* as well as this *Treatise,* has come to bring you to.

My *Dying Friend;* I Suppose Thou hast been so Wise and so Just as to have made all the Necessary Provision that should be made about thy Temporal Interest, by thy *Last Will and Testament.* And now, *Entreat me not to Leave thee, or to Return from following after thee,* until thou find those *Dispositions* wrought in thee, which will be the most Necessary and Reasonable *Præparations* for a *Dying Hour,* and will fitt thee for a *Reception* into the *Everlasting Habitations.*

O Souls just *upon the Wing;* are you able to Say?—

"I have Seriously *Considered my Ways,* and Examined the Conduct of my Life; and what I have done *Foolishly* in my *Departure* from God, so far as I have Discovered it, I have bitterly *Confess'd and Bewayl'd* unto Him: And I have above all, *Beheld* and *Abhorr'd* the *Evil Heart* in me, which has always been a *Fountain of Sin,* and inclin'd me in *Dead Works,* to *Depart from the Living God.* Unto a God *Ready to Pardon,* I have cried for the *Pardon* of all my Offences; And with a most high Esteem for the *Blood* of my SAVIOUR, as being the *Blood* of a Person who is no less than the Infinite God, I have in much *Agony* pleaded that *Alsufficient Sacrifice,* that I may be released from the *Punishment* of my Sin, because my *Surety* has with His Allowance undergone it for me. This I have done, till the *Comforter* that *Releeves my Soul,* has Irradiated my Darkened and my Distressed Mind, with a *Good Hope thro' Grace,* that, *My God has heard me;* and that, *My Sins which are many are forgiven me.* And this my *Repentance* is now come so far towards its *Perfect Work,* that I had rather *Dy* than Live as I did, when I was *alienated from the Life of God;* yea, rather Suffer *Death* itself, than deliberately do any One Wicked Thing in the World. I know no *Way of Wickedness* followed or indulged with me."

Verily, To Dy *Impoenitent,* will be to Dy *Miserable!*

Are you able to Say!—

"In the *Eternal Covenant* Established between GOD the FATHER, and God the SON, with the Concurrence of God the Holy SPIRIT, my SAVIOUR coming into the Quality of a *Mediator* took the Charge of a *Chosen People,* becoming the *Head* of that Happy Body; and Engaged, That He would yield Such a *Perfect Obedience* to the *Law* of God, as would Ransome them from the *Penalty* whereto our Sins make obnoxious, and purchase for them all the *Blessedness* of the Righteous; And, That He would Quicken them to *Turn* and *Live* unto God, and imprint His *Holy Image* upon them, and incline and strengthen them in *every Good Work to do His Will,* and fitt them for, and bring them to, the *Spiritual Blessings in the Heavenly Places.* This *Covenant* I have sincerely *Consented* unto, Entirely Acquiescing in the *Methods of Grace,* which are *Ordered* in it, and *sure;* and I have Entreated that I may find myself *comprehended in it,* and I have requested my SAVIOUR, that He would graciously take me under the *Shadow of His Wings,* and *fulfil* for me and in me *all the good Pleasure of His Goodness:* and *be* to me, all that He is, *do* for me all that He *does,* for His Redeemed Ones. I now Venture myself and my All in His Glorious Hands; *I know whom I have Beleeved;* and I am verily *Perswaded,* that He will *not cast me off.* With Satisfaction I see my *Debts* to the Divine Justice all paid by my SAVIOUR discharging of them: I see myself in what my SAVIOUR has done for me, a *Righteousness* reckoned mine, wherein I may stand with Safety before the Judgment-Seat of God: I feel my SAVIOUR possessing of me, and Beginning those *Frames* and *Acts* of *Godliness* in me, which assure me, that He will *never leave me nor forsake me."*

Soul thus in CHRIST, Thou art a *Dove in the Clifts of the Rock,* where no Harm can ever come unto thee!

Can you say?

"I have that *Root of the Righteous,* the LOVE of God, sensibly Planted in my Soul. And from this *Principle,* I aim at nothing so much, as the *Serving* and the *Pleasing* of the Glorious God; Yea, I have Embraced *This* as the *Chief End of my Life.* GOD has resumed His *Throne* in my Soul; The *Scope* of what I *Do* is, That God may have an *Homage* paid unto Him. The *Sweet* of what I *Have* is, That it helps in *knowing* of God, and in *working* for Him. I have my SAVIOUR by His Good SPIRIT acting as a *Living Principle in me.* This *Principle* causes me, to Remember and Realize the *Eye of God* upon me in all my Ways. Oh! If I may be a *Spectacle* which the Glorious God may with a *Gratified Eye* look down upon! Tis the very Top of my Ambition! Welcome, Welcome, Every thing that helps to make me so! This *Principle* causes me to desire a *Conformity* to my Lovely JESUS, and Study an *Imitation* of Him. I often sett His *Pattern* before me, that I may be a *Follower of that Good One;* and I would fain *be as He was in the World.* Yea, the very *Sorrows,* and the most *Abasing Circumstances,* wherein my *Likeness* to Him is Carried on, I Entertain as the *Favours* of Heaven unto me. This *Principle* causes me to *Love my Neighbour;* and there is no Person whatsoever, no, not among my *Personal Enemies,* or those that have *wronged* me, but what I *wish well* unto, and would, if I had Opportunity, *Do Good* unto."

Soul thus *Living to God,* Thou mayst be certain the *Sentence of Death* which once lay upon thee is now taken off; and there is that *Life* Enkindled in thee that shall never, *never!*—be Extinguished.

Can you Say!

"I am grown *Dead* unto all the Things of *this World;* I have *Sacrificed* all *worldly Comforts;* and I am willing to leave them all, that I may go and *be with CHRIST, which is by far the best of all!* I am willing to be script of Every thing, and brought into the *Destitute Condition* of the *Dead!* My *Will,* tis *Dead:* I have no *Will* of my own left unto me. My *Will* is now Swallowed up in the *Will* of God. My *Father,* whatever *Cup* thou shalt give me, I will take it: *Not my Will but Thy Will be done!*—I have nothing but a CHRIST left *Alive* unto me. I can find in *Him* all the *Good* which was ever to be found in any Creatures. And while I Enjoy HIM, in the *Precious Thoughts,* and *Views* of Him, I have *Enough! Enough!* The LORD is *my Portion, saith my Soul,* and I can *Rejoice in Him.*"

Soul Dead with CHRIST; Thy God will *Shew Wonders to the Dead.* Here's the Way to *Dy* without *Convulsions!*

The Jews have a Notion, That the *Angel of Death* stands at the Bed-side of the Dying Man, with a naked Sword, at the End whereof is a *Drop of Gall;* and this *fatal Drop* he letts fall into the Mouth of the Expiring Person. But, O *Christian,* upon these Attainments, thy SAVIOUR will Send unto thee, in a Dying Hour, that which will abundantly Sweeten the *Gall* with which the *Angel of Death* would Visit thee. Yea, He took the *Gall* from thee, on His *Cross.* The *Bitterness* of Death is over with thee.

You may now Say;

"Oh! What a *Delectable World* am I now *upon the Wing* unto! A *Paradise,* where I shall be *Comforted!* But, oh, how *Comforted,* when *present with the Lord!* O *wretched one that I am;* when shall I be *delivered* from the *Remainders of Indwelling Sin,* which are worse to me, than *Toads* Crawling in my Bosom! O *Happy One that I am;* I am just going to be *Delivered.* The *Mercy-Stroke* is just going to be struck, that will putt an End unto all my Miseries. A Few Minutes more, and I shall never *Sin* any more! Never be molested with any *Temptation* to Sin any more. My Vexations will presently be all over forevermore. The *Cross* has done its Part; my God has made it an astonishing *Instrument of Good* unto me; But Now I am taking my Eternal Farewell of it. All the *Troubles* which have been the *Discipline* under which the *Lord* my *Healer* has most wisely kept me, [*oh! I Bless Him for them all; I could not well have been without any of them!*] They are just come unto their Period; And, HEAVEN, *Heaven will make Amends for all.* I shall quickly be, where my SAVIOUR will communicate of Himself, and His *Everlasting Love* unto me, in Ways which are unto me, as yett Incomprehensible! I shall presently be a Companion to the *Myriads* of the *Holy Angels,* and be associated with the Spirits of the *Righteous,* in their Approaches to God, with their Glorious *High-Priest* leading of them. I am Entring into those *Courts of the Lord,* where *One Day* [*And it is All Day!*] will be better than a *Thousand* here below; in a *Land of Pitts and of Droughts, and fiery flying Serpents.* Ah! Roaring and Woful Wilderness, I am not at all fond of Returning back unto thee! I shall soon be brought Near to God; yea, Into God and Find His *Favour* to be *Better than Life.* I shall *See God* so as I have never yett Seen Him; and my SAVIOUR will *Feed me and Lead me to Living Fountains* of Blessedness; will do for me, *far above all that I can Ask or Think!*—Make Haste unto me, O my SAVIOUR; *Why is thy Chariot so Long a Coming? Why tarry the Wheels of thy Chariots!*

As for my Relatives, and the Dear Ones, which I leave behind me, O my God, with an Easy Mind, I leave them under the Care of thy Fatherly and Saviourly *Providence.* Oh! Take them into thy *Gracious Hands;* yea, Thou wilt be a *Shepherd* unto them, and they *shall not want.* Yea, Thou hast said unto me, That thou wilt *surely do them Good.*

And, O my BODY, I am now *dropping* of thee. Such *Flesh and Blood* as thou art, is not fitt for the *Kingdome of God.* But thou art the *Outworks* of a *Temple,* which God in His Free and Rich *Grace* has *Chosen* for His *Habitation:* and tho' thou art now Ruin'd by Sin, the God who can and will *Raise the Dead,* will fetch thee out of the *Ruines;* and thou shalt be Rebuilt into a much more splendid Edifice. I do *not fear* to lett thee go down into the *Land of Darkness;* For my God, who has *Baptised* Thee, and *Employed* Thee, will surely bring thee up again. Go, my BODY; Thou shalt Enter into a *Chamber,* where the *Doors* will be *shut about thee,* and thou shalt *be hidden as it were for a little Moment;* But the *Resurrection* of thy SAVIOURS *Dead Body,* has assured me, that thou shalt *Rise again.* It will not be Long before thou shalt Effectually hear Him saying, *Awake and Sing, You who dwell in the Dust;* and feeling His *Dew* fall with a Quickening Efficacy on thee, thy *New Birth* of *Water* and of the *Spirit,* shall qualify thee to *Enter into the Kingdome of God.* Ah, my *Vile Body,* I now lett thee go down into the *Pitt of Corruption,* full of Assurance, that I shall shortly receive thee again, marvellously changed; Vigorous, Luminous, *Incorruptible;* My Almighty Redeemer, [*I know, that He Lives!*] will come, and *Change* thee, that thou mayst be *fashioned like to His Glorious Body, according to the Working, whereby He is able to Subdue all Things unto Himself.—* My SAVIOUR, I now come unto thee!"

But One Word more.—*My Departing Friend;* Hast thou nothing to say unto the Standers-by? The *Last Words* of Men, [the, *Apophthegmata Morientium,* whereof *Mylius*[1] has not been the only Collector,] have in all Ages, and in all Places, been Esteemed Considerable. The πυμινον επθ in *Homer;* the Speech of a *Dying Man,* tis a *Pungent* and *Potent* Speech to the Survers [Survivors]. Look up to Heaven for Direction and Assistence; and if thou find thyself able to Speak, Lett fall Some Solemn Words, useful Counsils, awful Charges, which it may be for the advantage of the Survivers, to remember all their Dayes.

This done, Say, *Return to thy Rest, O my Soul!*

Of the Christian thus nobly drawing off, it may be said, *Non moritur dum sic moritur.* There is no *Dying,* but an Entring into *Everlasting Life.*

Reader, My *Angel* which helped thee against many *Inconveniences of Life,* did not vainly propose to keep thee *always Alive.* But if he may now help thee to *Dy after this Manner,* he has done all that can be proposed, or desired. And so, he takes his Leave!

Fredericus Imperator, percontatus, Quid homini optimum possit contingere? *Respondit:* Bonus ex hac Vita Exitus.[2]

Æn. Syl.[3] 1. 4. com.

Notes

Notes to Introduction: Part I

1. Mukhtar Ali Isani, "Cotton Mather and the Orient," *New England Quarterly,* XLIII (March 1970), 46–58. Mather was intensely interested in all things Oriental. He often referred to Oriental politics, religion, society, literature in his books and sermons. He corresponded with missionaries in India.

2. There is no evidence in the Society's records of such an election, but he had so been led to believe, wrote to thank the Secretary, and apparently was never disabused of the idea. He was awarded the degree D.D. by the University of Glasgow in 1710. Amusingly, John Lowthrop in the index of his abridgement of the *Philosophical Transactions* makes Mather M.D. instead of D.D.

3. See the excellent discussion of this inoculation controversy in Otho T. Beall, Jr. and Richard H. Shryock, *Cotton Mather, First Significant Figure in American Medicine* (Baltimore, 1954), pp. 93–123. (Hereafter cited as Beall and Shryock).

Notes to Introduction: Part II

1. Lester S. King, *The Road to Medical Enlightenment, 1650–1695* (New York, 1970), p. 160.

2. See Chapter VII. Dr. Richard H. Shryock (personal communication) has been unable to find any other American reference to the germ theory until that of John Crawford in his *Lectures on the Causes, Seat, and Cure of Disease* (Baltimore, 1811).

3. See Chapter XX. John B. Blake, "The Inoculation Controversy in Boston: 1721–22," *N.E.Q.* XXV (1952) 489–506. Beall and Shryock, pp. 93–122.

4. On pages 226–304 of the 1721 edition Mather discussed man, his anatomy, and some physiology. He was well read in the whole of medical literature. The *Angel* was a sequel, really, to his *Christian Philosopher.*

5. Richard B. Davis, ed. *William Fitzhugh and his Chesapeake World* (Chapel Hill, 1963), p. 50.

6. Gordon W. Jones. "Robert Boyle as a Medical Man," *Bull. Hist. Med.* XXXVIII (1964), 139–152.

7. In this discussion I have leaned heavily on Johannes Juncker (1679–1759), *Conspectus Therapiae Generalis Cum Notis in Materiam Medicam* (Halle, 1725). It is strictly contemporary with the *Angel.* Juncker was a follower of Stahl.

8. Thomas Watson (1792–1882), *Lectures on the Principles and Practice of Physic Delivered at King's College, London* (Philadelphia, 1844), p. 512.

9. Surgeon General William Hammond, of the Union Army, lost his job in large part because of the anger of the army surgeons at his order forbidding the use of calomel.

10. John Lowthorp, *The Philosophical Transactions and Collections . . . Abridged* (London, 1731), III, 226–231.

11. *Ibid.* p. 232.

12. *Ibid.* p. 234.

13. Gordon W. Jones. "A Relic of the Golden Age of Quackery: What Read Wrote." *Bull. Hist. Med.,* XXXVII (1963) 227–238.

Notes to Introduction: Part III

1. Cotton Mather, *Magnalia Christi Americana* (New ed., New York, 1967). I, 51.

2. William Osler, *The Principles and Practice of Medicine* (3d ed., New York, 1898), p. 97. Typhus is another possibility.

3. Gordon W. Jones, "The First Epidemic in English America," *The Virginia Magazine of History and Biography,* LXXI (1963), 1–10.

4. Samuel Abbott Green, *A Centennial Address Delivered . . . Before the Massachusetts Medical Society* (Groton, 1881), p. 39.

5. Jack P. Greene, ed. *The Diary of Colonel Landon Carter* (Charlottesville, 1965). Much of medical interest.

6. *Diary,* II, 154. There is mention of a Connecticut epidemic which lasted many months: Typhoid, perhaps?

7. Cotton Mather, *Euthanasia. A Sudden Death Made Happy* (Boston, 1723).

8. Greene, *Centennial,* pp. 9, 17, 18.

9. *Ibid.,* p. 64.

10. Herbert Thoms, *Jared Eliot, Minister, Doctor, Scientist, and His Connecticut* (Hamden, Ct., 1967).

11. Zabdiel Boylston, *An Historical Account of the Smallpox Inoculated in New England* (London, 1726). Douglass published in Boston in 1736 his classical account of a scarlet fever epidemic, *The Practical History of a New Epidemical Miliary Fever . . . Which Prevailed in Boston, New England, in . . . 1735 and 1736.* This was of course a report of observational clinical medicine rather than experimental.

12. Samuel Eliot Morison, *Harvard College in the Seventeenth Century* (Cambridge, 1936), p. 282.

13. Gordon W. Jones. "Medical and Scientific Books in Colonial Virginia," *Bull. Hist. Medicine,* XL (1936), 146–157.

14. Francisco Guerra, *American Medical Bibliography, 1639–1783* (New York, 1962).

Notes to Introduction: Part IV

1. *Catalogus Librorum Bibliothecae Collegii Harvardini* (Boston, 1723). There is a copy in the American Antiquarian Society and there is a photostat in the New York Public Library.

2. Julius Herbert Tuttle, "The Libraries of the Mathers," A.A.S., *Proceedings,* New Ser. XX (1910), 269–356.

3. Thomas James Holmes, *Cotton Mather, A Bibliography of His Works,* 3 vols. (Cambridge, 1940).

Notes to Proposals

1. John 5, 2–5: Now there is at Jerusalem by the sheep market a pool which is called in the Hebrew tongue Beth-es-da, having five porches.

   In these lay a great multitude of impotent folk, of blind, halt, withered, waiting for the moving of the water.

   For an angel went down at a certain season into the pool and troubled the water: whosoever then first after the troubling of the water slipped in was made whole of whatsoever disease he had.

At least six different sites at Jerusalem have been suggested as the location of this pool.

Notes to Capsula I

1. "Happy he who was able to understand causes." (Vergil, *Georgics*.)

2. Zoroaster (Greek form of Zarathrusta, literally "old camel") was a great Persian prophet whose thousand-year religion was largely swept away by the Arabian conquest and supplanted by Islam. He lived sometime between 650 and 500 B.C. He was born in northwestern Persia. In his maturity he developed a religion out of the old Persian nature religion, retaining the old pantheon as abstractions. He hoped to influence the health and welfare of the people and domestic animals. To accomplish this, his priests, formerly the magi, became adept at purification ceremonies involving fire. From about the time of Darius this became the state religion.

3. Manichaeism was a sect founded by Mani, a third century Persian, who sought to blend the teachings of Christ with the older Persian mahism. It developed something of a Christian tinge, became very widespread despite persecution, and survived well into the middle ages. Much in Albigensianism can be traced back to Manichaeism.

4. "A healthy mind in a healthy body." The full title is: *Mens sana in corpore sano. A discourse upon recovery from sickness directing how natural health may be improved into spiritual* ... Boston in N.E. 1698.

5. "The punishment of God for the sin of the world." Here Mather seems to subscribe to the idea that all sickness is one, albeit with various manifestations.

6. Commencement, derived from the Latin incohare, to begin.

7. Asa, son of Abijam, reigned over Judah 41 years. He did "what was right in the eyes of the Lord": he prosecuted idolatry. The "wrong step" may have been his use of temple funds to bribe a potential enemy king. II *Chron.* 16, 12.

8. Jehoram or Joram, king of Israel 852–846 B.C., was apparently immoral and was punished for his transgressions. "And after all this the Lord smote him in his bowels with an incurable disease." II *Chron.* 21, 18.

9. Boils and ulcers due to the bite of the Mesopotamian fly.

10. Aretaeus of Cappadocia (a spot now in east central Turkey) lived in the early second century A.D., wrote two works, *On the causes and signs of acute and chronic diseases,* and *On the treatment of acute and chronic diseases.* (First Latin printing, Venice 1552, first Greek, Paris 1554. English translation by Francis Adams, London 1856.)

11. The long-lived ancient Hebrew prophet of civilized life whose many miracles were works of healing and kindness. He is to be distiguished from his close associate, the Prophet Elijah, the rugged and harsh, whose miracles were works of wrath.

12. The most striking of Christ's miracles was the raising of Lazarus after four days of death. This was long hotly disputed by theologians. Possibly Lazarus had been in a catatonic state.

13. Close associate of the Apostle Paul.

14. genuine. This is a survival of late middle English usage.

15. St. Augustine, 354–430 A.D. His influence on Christianity was probably second only to that of St. Paul. Mather believed his doctrine that man is corrupt and helpless.

16. In medicine, a soothing or pain-relieving drug.

17. Galen (130–200 A.D.) was the last of the great ancient physicians. He was born in Pergamon, in what is now western Turkey not far from the Aegean Sea. He was educated in that sophisticated city and at Alexandria in Egypt. He practised for a time in Rome, grew wealthy, traveled some, wrote 400 treatises of which 80-odd have survived. He wrote on all phases of medicine quite dogmatically. His utterances became the final authority in things medical, pharmacal, anatomical, and physiological for 1300 years. The "dead hand of Galen," through this authority, is supposed to have held medicine back. But awe for authority is born in the spectator. Galen was a great doctor and scientist. He would be revered as such were it not for his misfortune to have been considered almost godlike by men who would not think and observe for themselves.

18. An ulcer with a hard callus and swollen margin which is difficult to cure. It was so called because Chiron the Centaur was the first to cure it. This mythological character who lived at the foot of Mt. Pelion was a wise physician who taught many of the Greek heroes. He stood in great contrast to the rest of the unpolished ignorant Centaurs.

19. Hendrick de Roy (1598–1679) of Utrecht was one of the first physicians in the Netherlands to accept Harvey's *De motu cordis* and his proof of the circulation of the blood. His book *Explicatio mentis humanae* (Utrecht, 1668) may have been the source of the work by Lorrichini whom I have been unable to identify.

20. "Adverse health, the threat to and death of members of the body is considered rather terrible. But of all things which can happen to man, the worst is illness or loss of the mind. If we seek so diligently for medication for the sick body, why not with greater care work hard to find what cures and revives the mind?" Mather must have had a copy of Lorrichini's work.

21. This approximate translation was not in Mather's hand.

22. Phillippe de Mornay (1549–1623), a French nobleman and protestant, became a prolific religious writer, especially after Henry IV abjured Protestantism. The work quoted was probably his *Traité de la verité de la réligion Chrétienne contra les athées, epicuriens, payens* . . . Antwerp 1581.

23. Julian the Apostate (Flavius Claudius Julianus) (331–363 A.D.) was the Christian emperor who turned pagan. He was a scholarly man who did his best to revive paganism.

24. Aesculapius, Greek god of medicine corresponding to Imhotep of Egypt, was evidently, like the latter, a genius of a physician who became deified and the center of a

vast number of legends and the god-head of a great healing cult which lasted for a thousand years, well into the Christian era.

Notes to Capsula II

1. *Martial's epigrams,* book 6, epigram 70, line 14. "To be, is not call'd life, but to be well." See D. H. Woodward, Ed. *The poems and translations of Robert Fletcher.* Gainesville, 1970, p. 77.

2. "The doctor must get his rewards when he can."

3. Teachings.

4. Coolers, or refrigerants, corrected heat according to the old hypothesis. Thus, mint was considered a "cooling medicine." Baglivi, whom Mather respected, felt, on th other hand, that similar qualities were better for similar conditions. In his *Practice of physic,* London, 1723, p. 297, he noted his preference for coolants in cool diseases and hot remedies for hot diseases.

5. Correctors were medicines which were believed to reduce unpleasant effects or harshness of other medications.

6. Mather seemed to use the word "humours" generally more as a figure of speech. He does not always refer specifically to the four Hippocratic ones.

7. Cordials are tonic or excitant medicines originally believed proper for stimulating the heart. Sydenham (see Rush's edition, p. 20) felt that cordials should not be given too soon in a fever. Example: blackberry cordial.

8. Medicines which purify, or, more especially, substances which purify medicines. Alcohol is rectified spirit of wine.

9. Marcus Tullius Cicero (106–43 B.C.), the Roman politician, lawyer, writer. Quotation is from his *De senectute,* his essay on old age.

10. "Gluttony is the cause of all diseases and of death." This reflects the opinion of physicians from the time of Hippocrates that proper diet is the greatest sustainer of health.

11. Hippemolgoi is from the Greek, means to milk horses. Thus, literally, the Hippemolgians were folk who drank the milk of mares. These people were the Scythians or Tartars who lived about the mouth of the Volga. They were called the "lordly Hippemolgoi who drink the milk of mares" in the *Iliad* Book 13, line 5. Zeus was looking away to the North at a people who had no part in the war.

12. Luigi Cornaro (1467–1566) was born in Venice and died in Padua nearly 100 years later. He believed that his long life was due to his dietetic regime and wrote *Discorsi della vita sobria,* in verse. Published first in Padua in 1558, it went through a dozen or more editions in several languages (first English, 1678). His teaching was widely known and quoted in the time of Mather. Probably he owned a copy.

13. Democritus of Abdera (460–370 B.C.) is famous as the originator of the idea of the atom. He was actually a physician and left a number of medical writings which were quoted by such later writers as Pliny and Caelius Aurelianus. He was impressed by the therapeutic value of music in medical practice.

14. Sir Theodore Turquet de Mayerne (1573–1655) was a French physician who practiced in Paris until his protestantism made it wise, and King James' invitation made it attractive, to go to London. There he treated Prince Henry during his fatal

illness and left such a clear bedside description of that illness that we know the prince died of typhoid fever. Besides his *Medicinal counsels and advices,* London 1667, which Mather very likely owned, he wrote on insects, arthritis, gonorrhea, and on the use of chemicals in medicine. Mather frequently refers to him.

15. Not identified. Probably Mather was relying on memory and did not check. Galen apparently died during the reign of Emperor Septimius Severus. The tenth century Greek lexicon called Suidas did have a good deal of information about Galen.

16. Aulus Cornelius Celsus (first century A.D.) was the so-called "Cicero of medicine" because of his elegant prose. Apparently he was a gentlemanly non-physician who compiled in his leisure the greatest Latin work on medicine and surgery. It was ignored by his contemporaries and by the men of the early middle ages. It was rediscovered by Pope Nicholas V (1397–1455) who appreciated and popularised it. *De re medica* was the first general medical book to be printed, Florence 1478. The Venice 1524 was at Harvard. Mather probably owned a copy.

17. There were two "learned Hoffmans." Friedrich Hoffman the Elder (1626–1675) and Friedrich Hoffman Junior (1660–1742). Both wrote a great deal. The younger became by far the more famous. His greatest work, *Medicina rationale systematica* was not published in Mather's lifetime. The text mentioned was a French translation of his *Grundliche anweisung wie ein mensch vor dem fruhzeiten tod und allerhand arten kranckheiten durch ordentliche lebens art sich verwahren konne.* Halle, 1715–17.

18. Thomas Fincke (1561–1656) was long the professor of mathematics at Copenhagen. He left a number of medical and mathematical writings. He was father-in-law to Caspar Bartholin Sr. (1585–1629) of Malmo who started the tradition of anatomical research in Copenhagen. His son Thomas (1616–1680), to whom Mather refers, was considered the greatest anatomist of his time. Caspar Jr. (1665–1738) was also an anatomist. All these men wrote books as well as articles in such learned periodicals as the "German *Ephemerides.*" The Mathers owned works by Thomas Bartholin, only one of which, the *Acta medica hafniensis* would have been of value in this work. It was the first Scandinavian medical periodical, published 1673–1680, and contained many important contributions, not all by the many Bartholins.

19. Niccolo Leoniceno (1428–1524) of Vicenzo became one of the most famous physicians of his time, being successively professor at Padua, Bologna, Ferrara. He translated the aphorisms of Hippocrates and wrote a tract on Pliny. His only original work was one on syphilis.

20. "He abstained as much as possible from food and wine, had minimal sleep, and was especially continent sexually, nor did he seek anything from fortune."

21. Arnold Manlius of Ghent (d. 1607) was professor of medicine at Cologne for thirty years.

22. "I avoid many dangerous diseases and bodily miseries by this one method, by consistently going to bed."

23. Amusing remark since Mather had a great habit of sleeping late.

24. "If doctors fail you, let these doctors work for you, these three, a happy spirit, rest, and a moderate diet." This is one of the aphorisms of the *Regimen sanitatis Salerni* (see page 3 of the Holland translation, London, 1649.) Salerno, beginning in the ninth century, was the first great European medical school. Its most popular book was this long poem of medical advice based on the Salernitan treatments, which

student physicians committed to memory for many centuries. Mather probably owned a Latin edition.

25. "Let the feasts be joyful and brief"

26. This is somewhat paraphrased from a passage in Francis Bacon's *Historia vitae et mortis,* London 1623, Leyden 1636. Though not listed. this was probably owned by Mather.

27. Antoine Galland (1671–1715) was the French orientalist who first translated the *Arabian nights* into a European language.

28. George Cheyne (1671–1743) was a Scot who became a successful London practitioner. He had learned from bitter personal experience the value of temperate living and promoted temperance in a time when it was not popular notion. The book mentioned went through many editions in several languages. The first edition is supposed to be that of 1724. However, Harvard had a copy listed in its 1723 catalog, and Mather used it in his *Angel* which he finished in 1724. Since there is no evidence of a late revision of the manuscript here, there must have been an earlier edition.

29. Robert Boyle in his *Of the reconcileableness of specific medicines to the corpuscular philosophy,* London, 1685, a book owned by Mather, was interested in the fluidity of the blood. He felt that many stubborn diseases proceed from certain tough humours which obstruct the passage of the blood, i.e., decrease its fluidity. He believed that a specific medicine may act by varying the viscosity of the blood. The modern anti-coagulants would have interested him greatly.

30. Thomas Morgan (d. 1743) was a Welsh deist turned physician. He claimed an M.D. but never disclosed the source. He wrote *Philosophical principles of medicine,* published 1725. Evidently this as well as Cheyne's book were published earlier than has been realized. In fact, the *Angel* has pushed back the published dates of several books and tracts.

31. "Safe way to a long life." The "t" of vita is in the manuscript.

32. Nechunjah Ben-Ha-Kanah was a once-famous rabbin of Jamnia (Jabneh) a town south of Jaffa which was the center of Judaism from 70 A.D. to 135 A.D. He was a mild devout man who ran his own school.

33. "What man is he that desireth life, and loveth many days that he may see good?

   Keep thy tongue from evil and thy lips from speaking guile."

34. "Life was long but he lived little."

35. "The other things are of death."

36. "Mortals live not in years but in deeds." This was Mather's sincere belief.

37. "Life is long enough if you know how to use it."

Notes to Capsula III

1. "It is better to hear Socrates discuss moral issues than to hear Hippocrates tell of the humours (of the body)." This is hardly a medical chapter. Mather was, of course, primarily a minister. Worship of, repentance before, and prayers to God and Christ were the essential first steps in the treatment of any illness. In the majority of the chapters of this book the religious tone is set before there is any reference to practical medicine.

2. The Essenes were an ascetic sect of Hebrews devoted to communal life. They

began their existence as a group or groups about 200 B.C. They avoided marriage and had many characteristics of the later Christian monks. Interest in them was largely marginal until the recent discovery of the famous "Dead Sea Scrolls" left by them. One translation of their name is "Healers." Josephus reported that they studied the medicinal properties of herbs and stones. They are thought to have been to some extent physicians to the poor. The "Therapeutae" were a group of Essenes who lived in Egypt on the shore of Lake Mareotis, in the Delta not far from Alexandria.

3. "Holy men are infirm; those who are strong are holy only with difficulty." Salvian was a fifth century Christian monk who preached and who taught rhetoric. He lived in Gaul. He wrote *De gubernatione Dei* and *Contra avaritium* and a few letters.

4. Dr. Henry More (1614–1687) was an English theologian of Calvinist persuasion, a graduate of Christ's College, Cambridge. He wrote as a Christian Platonist first a number of poems and then a large number of mostly theological prose works. He was much opposed to Descartes' philosophy.

5. Pythagoras of Croton, a once-important Greek city in the "heel" of Italy was a sixth century B.C. philosopher and mystic. He and his followers, called Pythagoreans, believed in re-incarnation. He was fascinated by numbers and may have been the inspiration of Euclid, the third century mathematician of Alexandria. Pythagoras discovered the numerical relationships of musical tones. His numerology influenced some of the Hippocratic (medical) writings.

Notes to Capsula IV

1. Addition or appendix. The original sense was "worthless addition."

2. Julip, or julep, derives from the Persian juleb. Often it was merely a sweet drink used as a vehicle for medicine. Originally it was any acidulous, mucilaginous, soothing liquid mixture with a demulcent effect which was thought to correct sharp ("acrid") conditions of the humours. Not all demulcents were julips, of course: olive oil, for instance, is a demulcent but not a julip.

3. Diodorus Siculus died shortly before the birth of Christ. He was a Sicilian who wrote in Greek what he considered to be history. Much that he wrote has been lost, but what he wrote about Egypt, which he visited 60–57 B.C., about 400 years later than Herodotus, has survived. He is the chief authority for the "sacred book of Egypt." We must remember that people of Mather's time knew little about Egyptian medicine. We know infinitely more because of the discovery of the medical papyri in the nineteenth century and because of modern paleopathological research.

4. Aurelius Antoninus (86–161 A.D.) was the able successor to the Emperor Hadrian.

5. Originally a Sabine goddess of welfare. She later became identified with the Greek Hygeia and thus became the goddess of health. Apparently she was never a healing divinity as was Aesculapius.

6. The Philosopher's Stone, the long sought quintessence of the alchemists was the catalyst which was thought able to change baser metals into gold. It was also the "universal medicine" which promoted good health and longevity. There was the vague idea, it will be recalled, that disease is essentially one condition with many

manifestations. Thus, the Philosopher's Stone, if discovered, could prevent or cure all disease(s).

7. "He who lives well always prays."

8. "The most effective prayer is based on alms and quickly a prayer made on such a basis rises to the divine ears."

Notes to Capsula V

1. Jean Baptiste van Helmont (1577–1644) of Brussels was a Capuchin friar. He became a mystic and the founder of the iatrochemical "school." (See introduction.) Paracelsus influenced him. He believed that each bodily process has its governing archaeus or spirit ("Blas"), and that each such physiological process is promoted by "gas," a special ferment. The Blas is controlled by its anima sensitiva motivaque (sensitive and motive spirit) which Helmont believed to reside in the stomach. He is generally credited with the discovery of carbon dioxide. Most of his ideas are of simply historic value. He was respected in his day, however, and was fairly typical of the early seventeenth century. He was denounced to the Inquisition for his mysticism, but was not prosecuted.

2. Probably Franz Oswald Grembs of Salzburg who lived in the second half of the seventeenth century and was a devoted disciple of van Helmont. He was noted for his *Arbor integra et ruinosa hominis* in which he tried to blend the teachings of Helmont with those of Galen. I have not been able to identify *"De Ortu Rerum."* It may have been a chapter in the above book.

3. The "old Platonists" would simply be the followers of Plato who taught that the mind is the cause of all things, that the soul is the place of ideas. The Neoplatonists tried to reconcile his teachings with Hebrew religious teachings and with Christian theology. They fine-spun Plato's teachings into a belief in a Transcendant Soul apart and separate from material things but from which all comes by emanation. These people were suppressed by Justinian in the fifth century, but some of their ideas influenced medieval church thinkers.

4. Jean Fernel (1497–1558) was professor of medicine at Paris. He wrote there his famous *Medicina* (Paris, 1554), a book which has a rather modern sound in that it was divided into physiology, pathology, and therapeutics. He made the first description of appendicitis. He helped break down the authority of Galen and so was one of the great antitraditionalists who helped pave the way for modern medicine. His works were still influential in Mather's time.

5. Another word for the pneuma.

6. Jan van Heurne (1543–1601), born at Utrecht, became professor of medicine at Leyden. He was noted for his *Institutiones medicae* (Leyden, 1592), but he does not now have Fernel's reputation. He deserves better since he introduced the bedside medical teaching method which made the Leyden medical school so famous under Boerhaave.

7. In seventeenth century usage this means belief.

8. This is the preformation theory which maintained that each organ is present in the fertilized egg in minute form and that the whole being just grows or unfolds. The opposite, epigenesis, is a process in which there is a gradual building up of parts

from early undifferentiated cells. Proponents of this latter process, among the first of whom was William Harvey, proved to be correct but the preformation theory was the more popular in Mather's time.

9. He refers to the iatro-mechanical theory.

10. Even now this is a fairly popular notion, though less so than twenty years ago. Hardly a month goes by that some maternity patient does not bring up this worry.

11. Palaephatus (perhaps a pseudonym) wrote, in the late fourth century B.C. a tract in which myths are rationalized. It is only partially extant.

12. Traducianism, a venerable Christian theological position, holds that the parents in begetting the child beget the soul also.

13. St. Justinus Martyr (second century A.D.) was a samaritan who converted to Christianity. He wrote two apologies and a few other brief tracts. He was beaten to death and beheaded in Rome.

14. Irenaeus (about 125–202 A.D.) became Bishop of Lyons in Gaul. He was born in Asia Minor. He was one of the early expositors of orthodox Christianity. He emphasized the Holy Eucharist, the Incarnation, and Resurrection. He defended the Montanists. See the next note.

15. Tertullian (150–230 A.D.) was a Roman theologian who had been born a pagan in Carthage, the son of a centurion. Some of his disciples were a branch of the Montanists. Montanists believed that a Christian fallen from grace could never be redeemed. They sought persecution. They claimed superiority over other Christians. Thus, they were more repugnant to the latter than they were to the pagans. Neither Irenaeus or Tertullian could save them and they disappeared in the third century.

16. Thespesius, or Thespis (sixth century B.C.) was the first of the known Greek tragic poets. He may have been born in Icaria in Attica.

17. Madame Anne Lefèvre Dacier (1654–1720) was a scholarly French woman who translated the *Iliad* and the *Odyssey*. She married Andre Dacier (1651–1722). They abjured protestantism in 1690.

18. Cold in the sense of one of the four qualities. Organs were considered hot, cold, moist, or dry in varying degrees and combinations.

19. Herophilus (around 300 B.C.) was a great Greek anatomist who worked in Alexandria. He was of the next generation after Aristotle who believed that the heart is the center of intelligence. Herophilus placed it correctly in the brain.

20. Hippocrates (460–370 B.C.) was the "Father of Medicine." As a keen observer of disease at the bedside he discarded priestcraft and magic from his system and made medicine an observational science. A great number of writings have been attributed to him. Some were highly respected and used as references into the nineteenth century. His general principles are still valid.

21. That liquid which was supposed to give flexibility and proper consistence to bodily structures. It was carried by the blood. Radicale is used in the sense of "root," that is, fundamental.

22. Otto Tachenius (d. 1670) was born in Westphalia. He was educated as an apothecary but finally went to Padua for his M.D. He practiced in Venice, became rather noted as an iatrochemist. He wrote a book on gout in 1662.

23. Lucian (second century A.D.) was a satirist who wrote a great number of prose works. He satirized the ancient Olympic gods. Some of his writings, as the fantastic *True History* influenced Rabelais.

24. The Sadducees denied the existence of demons. They were in the opposite pole from the Pharisees, the strict constructionists. The Sadducees tended to waver, to conform to neighboring gentiles. They were actually rated by other Jews as traitors and hypocrites.

25. Recall the fact that the circulation of the blood as proven by Harvey became accepted generally only a few years before the birth of Mather.

26. *Iliad,* Book 11, line 14: "For a leech is of the worth of many other men." (For the cutting out of arrows and giving of soothing simples.)

27. "Indeed more men are found to die from sadness and pain of the mind than by violent death." Auerbach, better known as Heinrich Stromer (1482–1542) was professor of medicine at Leipzig. He wrote a tract concerning the plague, *Saluberrime adversus pestilentiam observationes,* Leipzig, 1516.

28. See Introduction. This discussion of what we call psychosomatic medicine is sound.

29. Probably St. Boniface (675–754), the English missionary bishop to Friesland where he was eventually murdered by the pagans. There were many popes named Boniface.

30. Hysteria (pertaining to the womb) in women was once thought to be due to the wanderings of the uterus about the body. The spleen was considered the source of black bile. Thus, neurotic complainers are hypochondriac, bilious people are depressed or melancholy. One vents his spleen when he is irritated.

31. See Introduction.

32. Chalybeates are medicines containing iron.

33. A corroborant was any medicine thought to strengthen the body and improve the "tone" of the tissues. Dogwood and cinchona barks were considered examples of plant sources of corroborants.

34. Treacle (theriac, mithradaticum) was surely the most venerable medicine ever forced down a gullible gullet. It was originally prepared perhaps by Mithradates VI of Pontus (114–63 B.C.) as an antidote to poison. It was improved and embellished. Galen liked it. For centuries it was made in many places. The most famous was Venice Treacle which became so profitable an export that to prevent the sale of a spurious article it had to be prepared publicly by pharmacists under the supervision of physicians. There were as many as 64 components, many with opposite properties, some simple drug plant remedies, and some less simple, like powdered viper's flesh. Its distribution was world-wide in Mather's time. Gilbert Watson's *Theriac and mithradatium,* London 1966 is a worthy and interesting study of this phenomenal preparation.

35. See Introduction.

Notes to Capsula VI

1. Herodicus (Fifth century B.C.) was a Greek gymnast who combined exercise and diet in a system of therapeutics. He believed that all ailments arise from lack of exercise. He used walking, bathing, wrestling, friction, etc., for all conditions, even febrile diseases. He may have been a teacher of Hippocrates, but the latter opposed his strenuous treatment of fevers.

2. Plato opposed gymnastics only in excess. Herodicus used them excessively.

3. Vestricius Spurinna was a capable Roman general who defended Piacenza for the very short-reigning Emperor Otho (69 A.D.) He was especially praised by Pliny the Younger for his lyrics in Greek and Latin.

4. Pliny the Elder (23–79 A.D.) wrote the famous *Naturalis historia* which established him as perhaps the first encyclopedist. Birds, animals, plants, medicine were all discussed, often uncritically. Pliny the Younger (61–113 A.D.), nephew of the former, was a cultivated Roman statesman who left us in his *Letters* a splendid picture of Rome under the Empire.

5. *De parvae pilae exercitio,* first printed Paris, 1544 dealt with exercise by playing games with small balls.

6. An instrument, usually of metal, used to scarify the skin of athletes.

7. Gerolamo Mercuriale (1530–1606) was a native of Forli, a graduate of Padua. He became much interested in the medicine of the Ancients, especially their use of exercise in the treatment of nervous conditions. He wrote the first physical education text, *Libri VI de re gymnastica veterum,* Venice, 1569. He also wrote a number of other works on such subjects as skin disease, children's diseases.

8. Oribasius (325–403 A.D.) was, like Galen, born in Pergamon. He studied at Alexandria, became palace physician to Emperor Julian, and also dabbled some in the public administration of Constantinople. He compiled his huge *Synagogae medicae* which, quoting many authors, was an attempt to preserve all ancient medical knowledge. He also wrote *Euporiston,* a small handbook for laymen first printed in 1529 in Basel.

9. Asclepiades (born 124 B.C.) of Prusa in Bythynia was educated at Alexandria and then went to Rome where he introduced the superior Greek medicine. He adhered to the atomic theories of Democritus and Epicurus.

10. There were no public games of that name. Literally "hanging games" they probably were private gymnastics involving the use of expensive equipment.

11. Marcus Tullius Cicero. *Brutus seu de claris oratoribus* was a history of Roman eloquence by one of its all-time masters.

12. Plutarch (46–120 A.D.) was the famous Greek biographer.

13. Francis Fuller (1670–1706) was born in Bristol, son of a non-conformist divine, and was educated at Cambridge. He was not a physician, but after he cured his own hypochondriasis with exercise he wrote the book Mather mentions (London, 1704). It was fairly widely owned in the Colonies and probably Mather had a copy.

14. Christopher Bennett (1617–1655) received his M.D. at Cambridge. He evidently died of tuberculosis, the subject of his book. The edition nearest Mather's lifetime was in English (*Theatrum tabidorum or nature and cure of consumption, London 1720.*) The known Latin editions had the title reversed: *Tabidorum theatrum.* Mather may have owned an edition now unknown. The quotation loosely translated reads, "This deadly and powerful ailment among the English may yield to proper treatment if given in time."

15. Prescription: the English saddle.

16. Generalized edema.

17. Refers to a teaching of the old Hippocratic medical school on the Island of Cos off the coast of present Turkey.

18. The last three terms in this paragraph have only appproximate modern equivalents.

19. Cripples.

20. All this sounds remarkably twentieth century, with all the dire daily warnings about our lack of exercise because of our excessive use of cars.

21. Oribasius quoted Antyllus to this effect in his compendium noted above. Antyllus was a celebrated physician and surgeon who practiced probably in Rome in the second century A.D.

22. "If the horse is forced to go faster, willy-nilly the whole body goes also with the benefit, more than in any other exercise, of firming the body and especially the stomach and rendering the senses more acute."

23. See Introduction.

24. "He might easily accumulate riches."

25. "Galen gives the riches."

26. Darby Dawne was the pseudonym of Dr. Edward Baynard (1641–1719?) who was a London and Bath practitioner, who wrote *Health, a poem,* London, 1719. It was very popular, was reprinted in Boston in 1724. Mather most certainly had a copy.

27. Edward Strother (1675–1737) was a London physician who received his M.D. from Utrecht at age 45. He wrote many fairly popular treatises. His *Criticon febrium or critical essay on fevers,* London 1716, was at Harvard.

28. A people rigid in self-denial, self-discipline, and devotions.

29. The Greek goddess of justice. She was the last of the old divinities to leave the earth at the end of the Golden Age.

Notes to Capsula VII

1. "Fortunate is he who can know the causes of things."

2. Benjamin Marten (dates unknown) wrote *A new theory of consumption,* London, 1720. He stated his belief that every creature must be produced from an ovum or egg. He also believed in the animalicular cause of disease. See C. Singer, "Benjamin Marten, a neglected predecessor of Pasteur," *Janus* 16 (1911) s. 81–98. Mather's chapter follows Marten's references and train of thought so well that the latter's book must have been Mather's inspiration. Thus, Mather must have owned a copy. No other American, according to Doctor Shryock, discussed the germ theory until John Crawford did so in 1807. And, Crawford was neither native-born or educated.

3. This usage of the word "cell" was first employed by Robert Hooke (1635–1703) in his great *Micrographia,* London, 1665. Mather could have learned the word from reading the *Philosophical Transactions.*

4. Congenital syphilis, for instance.

5. Murraine was a term applied to almost any pestilence or plague affecting cattle.

6. Frederick Slare (1647–1727) was a physician and chemist (M.D., Oxford) who reported many of his experiments and observations in the *Philosophical Transactions.* He had a large practice in London, retired to Bath.

7. Ross is anticipated by two centuries.

8. Athanasius Kircher (1602–80) was a German microscopist who fled Germany during the Thirty Years War. Much that he wrote was tainted with mysticism, but he did believe that plague is due to an infestation of the body by minute organisms as shown

in his *Scrutinum physico-medicum*, Rome, 1658. Mather owned a copy of the Leipzig 1659 edition.

9. August Hauptman (1607–1674) was a German physician whose studies of parasites led him to the idea that diseases are often caused by microscopic worms.

10. Steven Blankaart, spelled Blancard in England lived (1650–1702) at Middelburg in The Netherlands. He wrote *The physical dictionary* which became very popular. On page 136 of the 1702 London edition there is to be found Mather's quotation. Mather thus undoubtedly had a copy. What the early microscopists saw was rouleaux of red corpuscles.

11. Michael Ettmuller (1644–1683), of Leipzig, was a noted teacher and medical writer. An edition in three volumes of his collected works was published in Frankfurt in 1708.

12. Through the years there have been many such observations. One J. F. Reigert, writing in 1855, observed that in Pennsylvania in three different years enormous swarms of yellow "plague" flies preceded outbreaks of Asiatic cholera. This fly is now rare if not extinct.

13. This is still a disputed point despite Sudhof's conviction that syphilis was present in the Old World before Columbus' voyage. It has been suggested that his sailors may have brought back the somewhat similar yaws, which ravages fresh nonimmunes.

14. Martin Lister (1638–1712) was a physician who was noted for his writings on natural history and on his travels in France. He made many contributions to the *Transactions*. He discussed smallpox in his medical work *Octo exercitationes medicinales*, Amsterdam, 1698.

15. William Oliver (1659–1716), physician, Monmouth conspirator, and supporter of William of Orange, found time to write a long treatise on fever, published in 1704.

16. The epidermis.

17. Nicholas Hartsoeker (1656–1725) was a Dutch naturalist, physician, and microscopist who lived variously in Leyden, Paris, Dusseldorf, and Utrecht. He wrote *Principes de physique* (Paris, 1696), *Conjectures physiques* (Amsterdam, 1706), *Essai de dioptrique* (Paris, 1684).

18. Giovanni Alfonso Borelli (1608–1679) of Naples was a leader of the iatromechanical school.

19. Mayerne.

20. Nicholas Andry (1658–1742), professor of medicine at Paris, was famous for his widely translated and often reprinted *Traité de la génération des vers dans le corps de l'homme*, Paris 1700. It was widely owned in the colonies and undoubtedly on Mather's shelves.

21. A fistula involving the lacrymal gland or duct resulting from injury or infection. Every conceivable pathological condition was easy to find in the seventeenth century. Those "worms" may have been large spirochaetes.

22. Richard Bradley (1688–1732) was a botanist and diligent author of many horticultural works. The book mentioned was published in London in 1717. It was very popular. We may assume that Mather had a copy.

23. Antony van Leeuwenhoek.

24. A Richard Ball wrote *Astrology improved*, second edition London, 1723.

25. Running the gauntlet? A corruption of the Swedish gantlope or gatlope meaning lane.

26. We worry about organic mercurial pollutants. As a medicine the family of mercurials is now little used. But it was greatly respected by our forefathers. The pure metal was used as an inunction externally and mercurous chloride (calomel) internally as a "specific" in the treatment of syphilis. As an "alterative" calomel was used, to the point of salivation and the loosening of teeth, until the time of our Civil War. Mather was wiser in his fear of mercury than many in the nineteenth century.

27. A deobstruent is a medicine capable of opening all orifices of the body, salivary, intestinal, urinary, etc. Paracelsus used calomel as a diuretic. It is a cathartic and also a salivant.

28. Aethiops mineral is black sulfuret of mercury, an insoluble black powder which is fairly safe because of its insolubility. Cinnabar is red sulfuret of mercury and was often used as a fumigant for venereal sore throats. The powder was thrown on a red hot iron to create fumes. Mather is in error in listing cinnabar of antimony.

29. Antihectic of Poterius is white oxide of antimony, which was used as a purgative, emetic, and diaphoretic in the treatment of fever. It was introduced by Pierre de la Poterie who died early in the seventeenth century. He was an ardent Paracelsian who promoted his preceptor's chemical therapeutic ideas. Before we laugh at the use of violent chemicals let us remember Ehrlich and his salvarsan. Paracelsus' spirit finally bore effective fruit.

30. Richard Mead (1673–1754) was an extremely successful London physician, writer and bibliophile. He was famous for his *Mechanical account of poisons*, London, 1702. He early mastered Newton's theories and wrote a not important work on the influence of heavenly bodies on human bodies, *De imperio solis ac lunae in corpora humanae* . . . London, 1704. This Newton interest is doubtless in Mather's mind. Mead was an iatromechanist.

Notes to Capsula VIII

1. Raphael was an angel whose duty was to control evil spirits and who taught men how to use simple medicines. He furnished information for the Book of Noah, an early Jewish treatise on the materia medica.

2. The great and often successful ancient method of psychotherapy. After being thoroughly awed by the rites and bathing and the presence of harmless serpents in the temple, the patients finally were allowed to sleep in the innermost part of the temple with the expectation that in their dreams they would have healing visions.

3. The legend states that during the terrible epidemic of 293 B.C. the desperate Romans sent an embassy to the temple of Aesculapius at Epidaurus. While they were negotiating there a great snake boarded the vessel, was recognized as the god, and was taken to Rome. The snake slithered off the vessel, landed on Isola Tiburina where a temple was soon built in gratitude for the prompt abatement of the epidemic.

4. It was the custom for grateful patients to leave testimonials at the temples where they found health.

5. Not a personal name, but the title of an encyclopedia of Greek history and literature compiled in the tenth century. It gives thumbnail sketches of a large number of men and historical incidents.

6. A very ancient Egyptian goddess, wife of Osiris. She was the beloved protectress of women and a healing divinity of great repute.

7. An important element in treacle was viper's flesh, dried and powdered.

8. Richard Napier or Napper (1559–1634) was an astrologer and medical practitioner and rector at Great Linford, Buckinghamshire. The seventeenth century Elias Ashmole who founded the Ashmolean Museum acquired the papers of Napier and deposited them in his museum late in the century. The *Responsa Raphaelis* was a manuscript of Napier's in which there is a collection of prayers and religious ceremonies used before invoking the help of the Angel Raphael in curing disease. For this information I am grateful to Mr. P. R. S. Morley of the Ashmolean and Miss Molly Barratt of the Bodleian. It is not clear how Mather knew about these papers.

9. Published in 1678.

10. Marcus Antoninus (121–180 A.D.) was a great Roman emperor and author of *Meditations*.

11. Approximately, "who aided him through dreams (or visions)"

12. Samuel Clarke (1599–1683) was a divine and biographer who wrote *A collection of the lives of ten eminent divines*, London, 1662.

13. *Essay for the recording of illustrious providences*, Boston, 1684.

14. A "hectic" is an illness accompanied by extreme emaciation.

15. Johann Rhode (1587–1659) was a Danish physician who studied at Padua. He wrote *Libellus de natura medicinae*, Padua, 1625.

16. "Behold the old man dressed in white who promises help by Divine aid."

17. Not identified.

18. Arnold Manlius (d. 1607) was professor at Cologne. Mather may have read about him in the writings of his pupil Fabricius Hildanus or he may have read the letters of Manlius in Lorenz Scholtz' *Epistolarum philosophicarum*, Frankfurt, 1598.

19. Robert Boyle.

20. *Acta medica et philosophica* was published in five volumes in Copenhagen between 1673 and 1680. Mather quotes this so often that it is reasonable to assume he owned a set.

21. "Conceding a supernatural cause, brought on by the offices of an angel of God."

Notes to Capsula IX

1. "In the theater he deserves applause who offers suitable rather than miscellaneous ideas."

2. Repellants were medicines which when applied to a tumefied part were believed to cause the fluids of the tumor to recede from it. Cold water and ice were viewed in this manner. Mather is saying that in many cases it is better to draw out the pain than to drive its cause inward into the body.

3. Baize, a coarse woolen cloth.

4. Sal ammoniac received its name from having been first extracted from dried camels' dung before the temple of Ammon in Egypt. It is ammonium chloride. It was usually administered in wine for "stimulant" purposes.

5. Oleum amygdalarum was once much employed as a demulcent (soothing compound) and emollient (softening substance) in liniments, etc. Oils of sweet and bitter almonds were used interchangeably.

6. "Opium" is derived from the Greek word for juice. Opium is, of course, obtained from the juice of the poppy capsule. It has been known for millennia but it was first mentioned by Theophrastus in the fourth century B.C. Apparently its medical use did not become widespread in Europe until the sixteenth century when Paracelsus praised it highly. Helmont used it for nearly every ailment and was called "Doctor Opiatus." Laudanum is an alcoholic solution of opium, contains about 10 per cent opium.

7. It is sometimes difficult to understand just what the older physicians meant by the "fibres" and the "solids." Sometimes they referred to the nerves. At other times they included all firm tissues as distinguished from the body fluids.

8. That is, dilute further in wine for patient acceptance.

9. Tincture of senna. Senna is the powdered leaf of various species of Cassia, a low shrub of Africa and India. Senna is still much used as a laxative.

10. Syrup made from the berry of the buckthorn, a small European shrub. The black and shiny berries contain a very active laxative principle.

11. Rhubarb was for centuries one of the great laxative favorites. It is a yellowish powder made from the roots of various species of Rheum, found originally in the Caspian Sea region. It is a plant with large roots and stems. Rhubarb colors the urine yellow. Because of its yellow color it was once widely used in the treatment of jaundice: similars cure similars some thought.

12. Derived from vola of Sanscrit, Gola of Egyptian languages. It meant myrrh, much used for centuries for its bitter aromatic property which presumably made it useful in the treatment of nervous conditions. Myrrh is the gum resin of Balsamodendron myrrha, a small tree with a whitish bark found in the Mid-east.

13. Spirit of ammonia, asafoetida, myrrh, for instance.

14. Medicines which augment the fluidity of the humours. Calomel might be an example.

Notes to Capsula X

1. A seventeenth century word meaning to pluck or tear or irritate small areas.

2. Burning.

3. "You will see how with light and delicate medicine you can safeguard your health in a short time."

4. Joannes Manlius (fl. 1548–1563) published in his *Libellus medicus variorum experimentorum* in Basel in 1563.

5. Substances which promote sneezing, powdered tobacco, for instance. Supposedly this clears the head of blocked-up phlegm and thus helps the headache.

6. To open a vein.

7. Enemas.

8. Guajacum is of great antiquarian interest. It is the resin of a small evergreen tree of Cuba, Jamaica, and Haiti. Early in the sixteenth century the Spaniards got the idea that it is a specific for syphilis. Great quantities of the wood, also called lignum vitae, were sent to Europe. A decoction of this wood was made and given in huge doses to the patient. Later, and this was not in the *London pharmacopeia* until 1677, the resin was used for treating syphilis and as a diaphoretic and alterative. Apparently oil of guajacum was a solution of the resin in oil of cloves, since no other oils dissolve it. It was absolutely worthless in the treatment of syphilis.

9. Thomas Willis. See introduction.

10. The harmless vegetation-eating millipede, otherwise known as the wood louse or sowbug, was in great demand in the dried and powdered state. Its use died out in the eighteenth century.

11. Caffeine is a component of most headache remedies even today.

12. Oil expressed from the aromatic seed of Myristica moschata, a large East Indian tree similar to an orange tree.

13. The bitter tasting useless root of Verbena, a European odorless weed. Even until the last century the root was often suspended from the neck as a charm because the Ancients considered it sacred.

14. Publius Terentius Afer was a great Roman playwriter of the second century A.D.

15. Pieter van Foreest (1522–1597) was a prominent Dutch physician who wrote a great deal. At Harvard in 1723 there was a copy of his *Opera omnia*.

16. Presumably yeast.

17. Oil of the damask rose of Turkey.

18. Pulvis de gummi gutta is the pulverized gum of a handsome Siamese tree called gamboge. It is a very drastic purgative. Adding the cinnabar (red sulfuret of mercury) surely compounded the misery.

19. Thomas Fuller (1654–1734) practised medicine in Kent. He published three collections of prescriptions or pharmacopeias in the eighteenth century.

20. A biennial American plant, widespread, tall, with yellow flowers. The infusion has a warm pleasant taste.

21. A European perennial herb with a feeble pleasant odor. Much used by the Ancients.

22. A 3–4 foot evergreen shrub of Mediterranean origin. It has a pleasant balsamic odor. An infusion of this was much used for headache until a century ago.

23. A pharmaceutical preparation of soft consistence, rather thicker than honey, and composed of various powders, pulps, extracts, syrup, honey, etc.

24. The powdered root of Gentiana lutea, a large plant of the mountains of Europe which has beautiful yellow flowers. The powder is bitter, mildly emetic and laxative in small doses.

25. The root of Inula helenium, a European plant which has perennial roots but an annual stem bearing large leaves and large yellow flowers. Medicinally, it was thought to have diuretic, expectorant, diaphoretic, and emmenogogue (property to encourage menstrual flow) properties. Thus, an almost universal relaxant.

26. "Being knowledgeable I wish to succor the wretched victim of the condition." Rather medieval than classical Latin.

27. Quintus Septimus Florens Tertullianus (155–220 A.D.) was the earliest great writer of the Christian church. He created Christian Latin literature.

28. In II Corinthians 12, 7, Paul spoke of the thorn in the flesh.

29. A liniment which is to be rubbed on the affected part.

30. All of the mints have pleasing volatile oils. That of the peppermint, Mentha piperita, was probably then as now the most widely used.

31. A medicine in the form of a thick pap which was applied externally with ingredients variously designed to make it anodyne, irritating, soothing, etc. It was a poultis with medicaments added. The volatile oil in the common black mustard, Sinapis

nigra, is very rubefacient; it creates local heat by dilating the skin capillaries beneath the cataplasm.

32. The powdered root of any member of the genus Zingiber, most commonly the black ginger, is also rubefacient. Mather should have used the word "cataplasm."

33. A biennial plant, Verbascum thapsus, having a 3–6 foot woody stem, large woolly leaves, and yellow flowers on a long spike. The powdered leaves were considered mildly anodyne.

34. Almost any conceivable combination of vegetable laxatives, mild or strong: rhubarb, betony, senna, rosemary, etc. Probably each physician had his favorite.

35. Freely, "If you believe in anything, my friend, this will work."

Notes to Capsula XI

1. Johann Jacob Rau (1668–1719) was a Dutch anatomist.

2. I.e., twenty "milk" or deciduous and thirty-two adult or "permanent" teeth.

3. "There are as many remedies for toothache as there are men."

4. St. Apollonia of Alexandria was venerated as the patroness of dental patients and dentists because her teeth were broken out before she suffered martyrdom in the fire. Mather is indulging in a Protestant witticism.

5. Millepede.

6. Johann Valentin Wille (d. 1676) was a German physician who became a Danish military surgeon. His noted book on camp diseases, *Tractatus medicus de morbis castrensibus internis* was first published in Copenhagen in 1676.

7. The leaves of Ruta graveolens, a 2–3 foot perennial plant with a coarse bark and yellow flowers. It is a native of southern Europe. It has a rather strong disagreeable odor.

8. A double salt consisting of aluminum sulfate and potassium sulfate.

9. Sambucus canadensis or nigra. It is a common shrub in America, a small tree in Europe. It has purple berries. The white flowers were used in cataplasms, the berry juice as a diaphoretic, and an infusion of the bark as cathartic and emetic.

10. Paul Dube (seventeenth century) was a French physician who wrote several books, among them *Le medecin et le chirurgien des pauvres,* Paris, 1672.

11. Literally, a falling down of humours from a superior to an inferior part. Actually often used synonymously with inflammation.

12. Gargle.

13. Any topical application which is neither an ointment or a plaster. Rather a general term which includes fomentations, ice bags, cataplasms. Mather is not strictly correct.

14. The resin of the Norway spruce.

15. Perennial European plant with a large root which was used for its mucilaginous properties after drying.

16. Rather, shepherd's purse, a plant of the genus Thlapsus, a small common weed with a four-petalled flower. A sort of cress. It yields a bitter, rather irritating volatile oil.

17. Feverfew, a cultivated 2 foot plant with pinnate leaves, whitish or yellowish flowers, and a strong not unpleasant odor due to a volatile oil.

18. Rose hips, fruit of any of several species roses.

19. Root of Anthemis pyrethrum, a North African perennial plant with a daisy-like flower. The root has a pungent taste and promotes the flow of saliva. It was used in Europe to combat toothache as early as the thirteenth century.

20. The unexpanded bud of the Indian tree Eugenia caryophyllata. The oil has the essence of the clove. Often a single clove was bitten into the affected tooth.

21. Origanum is marjoram. Origanum vulgare is a perennial herb with pinkish flowers, native to Europe and America. It has an agreeable odor and a pungent taste. Its volatile oil was long used in toothache.

22. Cloth impregnated with wax or some other gummy material. Used as a plaster.

Notes to Capsula XII

1. Sieved, referring to the "Achilles heel."

2. "Lord of diseases" . . . "disease of the lords."

3. Johann Doläus (1651–1707) was a German physician and writer who moved frequently from one German town to another. He contributed many essays to the Nuremberg *Ephemerides* to which Mather had access. He based his writings not only on such Ancients as Hippocrates and Galen but also on Descartes, Paracelsus, Helmont, and Willis. See his *Encyclopedia medica dogmatica,* Frankfort, 1691.

4. Daniel Sennert (1572–1637), a German iatrochemist, wrote many books. The Mathers owned his *Opera, Institutes, Practicae medicinae, Eius epitome,* and *Institutionum compendium,* editions not noted, according to Tuttle. Sennert was highly regarded in the Colonies.

5. Lazare Riviere (1589–1655) taught chemistry at the Montpellier Medical School. Mather owned what was probably the Nicholas Culpeper translation of his *Practice of physick,* London, 1655 (many later printings).

6. Theophilus Bonetus (1620–1689) was a Genevan physician who wrote *Sepulchretum sive anatomica practica,* Geneva 1679, which was one of the very first treatises on pathology.

7. Tophus, a mineral concretion in a joint.

8. Charles Drelincourt (1633–1697), professor of the practice of medicine at Leyden, was much interested in anatomy and used the microscope to some extent.

9. Mather is explaining clearly the etymology of the word "gout" and the contemporary medical theories.

10. The old idea of the importance of counter-irritants.

11. Jerome Cardan (1501–1576) was a sort of wandering medical adventurer whose life somewhat resembles that of Paracelsus. He wrote much, but little that is of lasting worth. He did describe syphilis. He invented a sort of Braille. He was a keen student of nature.

12. Beating the feet with a cudgel.

13. Aaron Hill (1685–1576) was an eccentric English author, poet, and dramatist. He published the work mentioned in 1709.

14. Asa (word means physician in Hebrew) was King of Judah about 910–870 B.C.

15. "We the living are lowered lest we be lowered dying." Passive of descendo was a rare usage.

16. Infernal.

17. Theophil (Gottlieb) Budaeus (1664–1734) was a prolific but unimportant

German medical writer. He wrote on ergotism in 1715 and a *Consilium medicum* in 1714. He contributed occasionally to the Nuremberg *Ephemerides.*

18. "Hardening in the joints."

19. Legend has it that Abgar V wrote from Edessa his capital begging Jesus to come to his aid and cure his leprosy—or, as Mather believed, his gout. Jesus is said to have refused.

20. "Medical problems." It has been suggested that lead poisoning from drinking wine stored in lead-lined containers raised the level of uric acid in the blood and accounted for the tremendous incidence of gout in those days, especially among the wealthy gourmets.

21. "Medicine does not know how to relieve the tophi of gout."

22. "She so battered the author himself that nothing was left of him."

23. Powder of the Spanish Fly, Musca hispanica. As a poultice it raises blisters on the skin. Taken internally it acts violently on the mucosa of the urinary tract, causing an extreme urgency to void. This is due to the active poison, cantharidine. It was much used externally until this century as a vesicant. It was used in the seventeenth century internally also in the hope that its violence might expel urinary stones. It soon became evident that this was dangerous.

24. Urine was often looked upon as a sort of distillation of the humours and thus good for many conditions.

25. Not identified.

26. See introduction. There had been Western contact with Japan since 1542.

27. Willem Ten Rhyne (1647–1700) was a Dutch physician and naturalist. He wrote *Dissertatio de arthritide,* Leyden, 1669.

28. "Why is it that only recently have we used the milk bath for the treatment of those seized by the pains of arthritis and gout?"

29. See chapter on scurvy.

30. Spermaceti is a substance which can be separated out from the whale oil obtained from the head of the huge spermaceti whale. It was used as a demulcent. The whole idea was, of course, that if an oil or a grease will cure a creaking wheel then perhaps it will lubricate a gouty joint.

31. *Miscellanea Berolinensia ad incrementum scientierum,* Berlin, 1710. The Berlin Academy existed for the first decade of the eighteenth century. Mather had access to this volume, if he did not own it. The New Englanders were much impressed by German medicine.

32. The powdered root, or decoction of it, of almost any member of the genus Smilax, a fairly widespread group of plants with large roots and large shining leaves. It was especially imported from Central and South America. For a time it was thought efficacious in the treatment if syphilis. Its reputation waxed and waned. It was used as a demulcent in joint diseases. Medically it is inert. In solution it has a rather peculiar and bitter taste.

33. Most likely a mispelling of Ipecacuanha, the emetic root of a small Brazilian shrub. The powder is bitter and nauseating. In very small doses it is expectorant and was considered stimulating to the stomach. The Brazilian Indians used it in cases of dysentery and Pierre Pomet (1658–1699) in his very popular *Compleat history of druggs* (third English Ed. 1737, p. 25) noted its great value in the bloody flux. The active principle, emetine, is specific for amoebic dysentery and a great drug. But the

physicians of the time were blinded by their proclivity to judge drugs by their emetic, cathartic, or expectorant powers (which we consider highly undesirable side effects) to recognize other values, (with the exception of cinchona).

34. Root of the fairly widespread male fern. It has a peculiar nauseating taste. It is medically inert but was once thought effective as a purgative and a cough medicine.

35. Hermadactyls were apparently identifiable as the bulbs of Colchicum, a native of Southern Europe and Egypt. The bulb is about the size of a walnut. Pomet quoted Lemery as identifying it with Colchicum. This makes Mather's prescription very interesting since it has been until recently the greatest of all gout medicines. Probably this was a potent prescription because of this one great ingredient. It took genius, patience, and luck to isolate the few valuable plant drugs out of the hundreds offered by tradition and folk lore.

36. John Quincy (d. 1722) was a London physician who prepared the *Dispensatory of the Royal College of Physicians*, 1721, *Lexicon*, 1717, *Medico-physical essays*, 1720, and a translation of Sanctorius. He was more a pharmacist than a physician. His works were widely owned in Virginia. Yale had a copy of the *Dispensatory* in 1743. Mather must have owned one or more of his works.

37. Hermann van der Heyden (1572–1650) was a practitioner in Ghent who was mainly noted for his advocacy of hydrotherapy, especially cold water hydrotherapy.

38. Althea officinalis is a large perennial found in salt marshes. It has a mild sweetish taste. The root was used, boiled or bruised, as a poultice and as a decoction for soothing irritated mucous membranes.

39. Part of the flower (the stigma) of Crocus sativus, a perennial plant rising from a bulb, with large lilac or purple flowers which bloom in the fall. It has three long orange, very odoriferous, stigmas. From ancient times until a century ago it was in great favor as a stimulant and antispasmodic. It is poisonous in large doses.

40. Samuel Fuller (1580–1633) practised in Plymouth, Massachusetts from the early days of the colony till his death.

41. A secretion, having a rather pungent odor, which is found in the glands near the sex organs and anus of beavers. It was often used internally as a "stimulant." Mather does not say castor *oil* which is expressed from the bean of the East Indian plant.

42. Olive oil.

43. Petroleum.

44. Contraction of the early English word pannikell, meaning membrane of the brain? On the other hand "panel" is an obsolete term for the lower end of a bird's intestine.

45. Lucian (115–200 A.D.), Athenian satirist of the "silver age of Greek literature," wrote such things as *Dialogues of the Gods*.

46. Fools.

47. Fourth century A.D. physician of Bordeaux who wrote *De medicamentis empiricis*, which is to a large extent a collection of folk medicine.

48. Scribonius Largus, a Roman physician of the first century A.D., left a collection of prescriptions, *Compositiones medicorum*. It too is of value in studying the folk medicine of the time.

49. Robert Boyle. *Medicinal experiments*, London, 1692 and several later edi-

tions. It is full of folk medicine and strange remedies. It was very popular both in England and the colonies, probably because of the great reputation of the author. Mather undoubtedly owned a copy.

50. Moistened flour of the flaxseed has long been considered a soothing poultice.

51. Mustard plaster.

52. Magic.

53. Sulfur. In this and the next paragraph, as occasionally elsewhere, Mather seems a little suspicious of magic.

54. Francois Valleriola (1504–1580), a native of Montpellier, died in Turin. He wrote several books which were largely commentaries on Galen.

55. Van der Heyden.

56. Antoine de la Faye (d. 1615). Swiss? He published in Geneva in 1610 a collection of the sayings of the peripatetic philosophers (in Latin).

57. That which is assuaging or palliative.

58. Quintus Curtius Rufus (probably first century A.D.) was the biographer of Alexander the Great.

59. Titus Livius (59 B.C.–17 A.D.) was the historian of Rome.

60. Desiderius Erasmus (1466–1536) "of Rotterdam" was a Dutch scholar who lived for a time in London, but died in Basel. One of the most learned men of the Renaissance.

61. Johann Valentin Wille (see above) wrote an article on the cure of gout through stimulation by pleasure for the *Acta Hafniens,* in which Bartholin published so much and which Mather owned.

62. Willibald Pirckheimer (1470–1530) was a German historian and philologist, a correspondent of Erasmus.

63. Everyone "is dissolved in laughter, mills about, jokes, and he is almost seen to be congratulated."

64. "With debility of the body, health of the mind, with flesh afflicted, spirit strengthened, with earthly affairs thrust out and things heavenly introduced, when circumstances of the times are at their lowest, that which is immortal is brought in."

65. "And very easily extinguishes the vital spirit."

66. "You will unanimously condemn my accusors by your common vote."

67. "What sort of man gout makes! Just, guiltless, continent, prudent, wakeful. No one is so mindful of God as one who is racked by gout. He who suffers gout cannot ever forget that he is mortal."

68. Philander Misaurus (misery lover). *The honour of the gout, or a rational discourse by way of a letter to an eminent citizen,* London. Mather's manuscript proves that the copy in the National Library of Medicine, dated 1735, is not the first edition as assumed.

Notes to Capsula XIII

1. This sentence is not in Mather's hand.

2. An uncastrated stallion.

3. Containing calcium carbonate.

4. The common small American tree of which the bark of the root was once considered a sovereign remedy. Large quantities were once shipped to England. Very fragrant, it makes a refreshing drink which was once thought to be a great diaphoretic.

5. Not identified.

6. Mercurous chloride or calomel.

7. The gum or hardened juice of the huge root of Convolvulus scammonia, found in Asia Minor. It is a mild cathartic.

8. A preparation of senna.

9. A very widespread evergreen tree varying in size from a shrub to a tree. The pleasant-smelling oil comes from the berries. It was considered a diuretic.

Notes to Capsula XIV

1. "The mind shudders at the memory, flees from the grief."

2. "If there were no sins there would be no punishments."

3. Joshua, 4:20, "And those twelve stones which they took out of Jordan did Joshua pitch in Gilgal." Gilgal was the first encampment of the Israelites west of Jordan.

4. A brattice was a wooden tower or parapet. "Bratts" was an old English term for coarse clothing.

5. Richard Mather (1596–1669) died of stone.

6. Kidneys.

7. Jan Groeneveldt was a seventeenth century Dutch physician and lithotomist who moved to London, anglicised his name to Greenfield, and won some notoriety. He wrote *A compleet treatise on the stone and gravel,* London, 1710. Previously, in 1698, he had published a tract on the use of cantharides internally to aid the expulsion of stone. Some patients died and the author got into moderate trouble. "Honest" was perhaps not the best choice of adjectives.

8. Not identified.

9. Johann Hartmann (1568–1631) was professor of chemiatry (iatrochemistry) at the University of Marburg. He wrote *Praxis chymiatrica,* Leipzig 1633.

10. Fabricius Hildanus (Wilhelm Fabry) (1560–1634) was a famous wandering German physician and surgeon who graduated from no school. He wrote *Lithotomia vesicae,* Basel 1626.

11. Pierre Franco in the mid-sixteenth century invented two operations for stone. One, the high, was to be employed where there were large bladder stones: a finger in the rectum pushed the stone upward and it was then removed through an incision in the lower abdomen, *i.e.,* the suprapublic approach. In the other an incision was made in the perineum (anterior to the rectum) and the prostate and bladder were cut laterally and the stone removed intact or fragmented. Good operators attained incredible speed. Collot was the name of a distinguished line of Parisian physicians. Francois Callot, who died in 1706, wrote a book on the subject. Apparently, according to the bibliographies, this was not published either in the lifetime of the author or in that of Mather. However, Mather's manuscript offers proof that many books were actually published at earlier dates than the printed records show.

12. Diaz (died about 1500) of Portugal, in the service of his King, John II, was the first European to round Africa. He called the promontory Cabo Tormentoso because of the terrible storm he encountered near it.

13. Not identified.

14. Penis.

15. Ptisan, or tisane, was an aqueous preparation, like barley water, for instance, containing little if any drug.

16. Probably the hip.

17. Arsesmart, smartweed, or water pepper, Polygonum punctatum, is a common weed of moist places. An alcoholic solution of whatever principle there is in the plant was once used for stone and to promote menses. It gives a "pleasant sense of warmth in the pelvic area."

18. In the seventeenth century claret was a light red wine. Sack (originally "dry" wine) was any white wine imported into England from southern Europe.

19. The expressed oil of the walnut achieved considerable repute as a laxative in the eighteenth century. It was much used in our Revolutionary Army.

20. Elkron was a sanctuary of Baal (2 Kings 1: 6 ". . . Baalzebub the god of Ekron . . ."). Acheron was the river of Hades in Greek mythology. Another name for Ekron was Accaron. Mather is playing with words.

21. Württemberg.

22. Various species of Nepeta, a rather rank-growing spreading strongly aromatic group of plants which prefer shade. An infusion of the plant was an old remedy for pulmonary diseases.

23. Coarse corn meal porridge. Samp is a New England word derived from the Algonkian Indian word nasamp.

24. The "doctrine of similars" which held that similar things cure similar diseases.

25. Common nettle, Urtica dioica, a weed with inconspicuous flowers but very irritant when applied to the skin because of the formic acid content. Roman soldiers used to scour their flesh with it as a defense against the cold. A decoction of the plant was once much used for urinary complaints, hemorrhage, and jaundice.

26. The root of this common garden plant was considered diuretic. The seeds were often thought to be a substitute for quinine.

27. A biennial weed with large leaves and burrs which were the bane of sheepmen since they spoil the wool. The seeds were considered diuretic.

28. Johann Philipp Hoechstetter (d. 1635) was a German physician who wrote *Rararum observationum medicinalium,* Augsburg, 1624.

29. Ysbrand van Diemerbroeck (1609–1674) was professor of anatomy at Utrecht. He wrote *Anatome corporis humanae* Utrecht 1672 and *Disputationes practicae in . . . capitis thoracis et infimi ventris,* Utrecht 1664.

30. Mather should have known better than to make this statement.

31. Potassium nitrate in alcoholic solution.

32. Sulfur dissolved in turpentine. It was used as a diuretic. A linctus is a syrupy medicine.

33. A thin turpentine obtained from the larch, Pinus larix.

34. Root of Glycyrrhiza glabra, a south European plant (leguminous). It is a demulcent and was considered excellent for soothing the mucous membranes of the respiratory and digestive tracts.

35. Alkalinize the water. Actually a large dose of baking soda will often give temporary relief from a mild strangury by alkalinizing the urine.

36. Potassium nitrate and sulfate.

37. Potassium nitrate.

38. The mucilaginous gum of the acacia, a type of Egyptian mimosa.

39. A gentle laxative, especially for children, made from the flowers of the common violet. Also a cough medicine.

40. It is interesting to note that there is no mention of the sweetness of diabetic urine, a fact so recently described by Thomas Willis, whose works were certainly available.

41. Iron was given in the form of filings of steel, iron steeped in vinegar, sulfuric acid, or alcohol, simple rust, and the water from the forge (water in which iron had been cooled). They were compounded variously with other substances. The value of iron has been recognized for many centuries. It is not, of course, a treatment for diabetes.

Notes to Capsula XX

1. "Was this odious disease known to the Ancients?" . . . "I should not dare doubt it."

2. Aetius of Amida, sixth century (A.D.) physician who lived in a city on the Tigris River. He wrote the *Tetrabiblus,* a large compilation from several authorities besides himself. He was held in great esteem by the men of Mather's day. He described an epidemic of what we now know as diphtheria.

3. "The egg may not be more similar to the egg."

4. The Plague of Cyprian (he was a third century bishop of Carthage) of 255–6 A.D. is now thought to have been the first definite epidemic of smallpox. Most of the great pandemics have originated in India. Mather mentions fascinating mysteries in this chapter. Great diseases lie dormant for centuries. Virulence waxes and wanes. Only speculations explain the highly mortal sixteenth century "English sweat." The 1918–type influenza has not been virulent since. Bubonic plague is widespread among the rodents of western America, but we have not had an epidemic. No one has explained why plague apparently never was present in eastern America despite its constant presence in seventeenth century England.

5. Blank line in manuscript. Apparently no one else in that period is known to have suggested that smallpox is caused by germs.

6. Bernard Nieuwentijdt (1654–1718) was a Dutch physician and eager microscopist. His writings, in Dutch, were theological.

7. "My flesh is clothed with worms and clods of dust . . ."

8. "These are not its places."

9. "It makes scepters no better than hoes."

10. Immunity is a fundamental fact of which man has long been aware. Its true significance was not generally appreciated until the late nineteenth century, after the marvellous structure of microbiology had been created. But, Fracastorius (1483–1553) had clearly proposed the germ theory. Men of the seventeenth century first *saw* germs and theorized. Many much more fanciful theories than the germ theory had long been popular and accepted. Why did not the germ theory take hold sooner? Mather was in a select group of believers.

11. As a constantly visiting minister and eager medical observer Mather must have had smallpox in his youth, though I can find no mention of it in his writings.

12. Fermentation is the approximate meaning.

13. Such as diaphoretics and sudorifics. Ipecac, antimony, hot drinks, sassafras, friction, would have been considered expellers.

14. An electuary containing water germander or diascordium (Teucrium scordium), a small fragrantly aromatic European plant. However, the effectiveness of the electuary depended upon the small amount of opium which it contained. Actually, often the germander was lacking and other herbs such as cinnamon, gentian, gum acacia were used to make the opium more palatable. Primarily used in the treatment of diarrhea and dysentery.

15. Ammonium carbonate. Doubtless the large amount of water helped.

16. Diascordium. See above.

17. Properly, the small European spring-blooming plant with yellow flowers. Sometimes the lovely Virginia bluebells (Mertensia virginica) was called cowslip, and a decoction of it may have been an Indian treatment. At any rate, "cowslip water" is not mentioned in any contemporary or later European or American pharmacopeia at my disposal. It must have been of local Massachusetts use, probably Indian, and probably bluebells decoction.

18. Putrefaction was a vague term signifying the presence of "putrid" or decaying animal matter in the body, especially the blood. This was detected by noticing the odor of the patient's breath and bodily secretions.

19. Sulfuric acid.

20. It will be recalled that Archimedes of third century B.C. Syracuse was so excited by the significance of the amount of water displaced by his body during a bath that he jumped out and ran naked into the street shouting in happy transport, "Eureka."

21. Loosely, "should be carefully considered."

22. Irritants which when applied to the skin cause redness, pain, and blistering of the skin: mustard plaster, cantharides, for example. The blisters burst and weep.

23. "If you have treated wisely." This detailed course of treatment of course was largely Sydenham's. Since we never see smallpox today, for all we know this is a sensible regimen except for the heroics of blistering, purging, bloodletting. Possibly physicians of today would have to turn to the old books if they were in the presence of a smallpox epidemic. Historical medicine might come to life!

24. Cinnamon, from a small evergreen tree of Ceylon, has always been in great demand as seasoning. The bark yields an oil on distillation. We use the powdered bark as a condiment.

25. Anyone who has seen an asthmatic relieved after spontaneous vomiting will realize why emetics were so much favored of old.

26. Hyssopus officinalis, a perennial herb native to Europe. The flowering heads and leaves have an agreeable aromatic odor and were used especially for catarrhs.

27. Tussilago farfara is a perennial herb with a creeping root which sends up leafless flower stems in the spring. The leaves come after the blooms. The leaves and roots were used medicinally, but are inert.

28. The dried ripe capsule of the poppy as grown in European and American gardens then. Of very low opium centent.

29. Archibald Pitcairne (1652–1713) was a distinguished professor of medicine at the University of Edinburgh. He was a good teacher and a fervent exponent of the iatromechanical school.

30. The idea was that if the pox did not vesiculate enough and discharge material, the attendant must artificially create vesiculation to promote discharge of the putrid humour of the disease.

31. In the days before the acceptance of the germ theory of disease dung, like urine, was considered a sort of distillation of bodily processes and humours and thus of some value in the treatment of illness.

32. That is, you shall not be afraid of "the pestilence that walketh in the darkness" (6) ... "neither shall any plague come nigh thy dwelling." (10)

33. Seventeenth century word for "small tastes," that is short extracts.

34. John Woodward (1665–1728) was a rather cantankerous London physician who was more interested in rocks and fossils than in medicine. He did publish, in 1718, the medical work noted by and probably owned by Mather. In it he rather violently attacked one of his London colleagues, John Freind. According to his son, Mather and he corresponded.

35. Medicines which "absorb," neutralize stomach acids.

36. "You perform a work full of dangerous hazard and you advance through fires hidden under deceitful ashes."

37. Coromantee. The Coromantees were a rather brave and warlike people of the African Gold Coast. Because of their spirit they did not make good slaves. In the late seventeenth century a number of them revolted in Jamaica, and were never really suppressed. It is interesting to speculate on how the knowledge of inoculation spread across Africa from the Mideast to these people of the Gold Coast.

38. One of the earliest examples of African-slave English.

39. Emanuel Timoni or Timone was a Greek physician whose dates are unknown. He studied in Padua and Oxford, was elected Fellow of the Royal Society in 1703. In 1713 he wrote to various people in Europe about his observation of smallpox inoculation in Constantinople. By then smallpox had been of consequence in England only about a century. In the Middle East it had been a problem for more than a millennium.

40. Narrow strips of bandage.

41. Serum.

42. Scars. From the Latin, caecare, to conceal, because it conceals the wound.

43. More or less synonymous with abscess.

44. That is, they always go to a patient naturally infected to obtain matter for the next person to be immunized.

45. Giacomo Pilarino (b. in Kephalonia 1659, died in Padua 1718) was a Greek doctor who traveled much over the Middle East and apparently became a Venetian citizen, and as such became Venetian consul at Smyrna. Padua was under the control of Venice. His small book was published in Venice in 1715. The title translates, "A new and safe method of causing smallpox by transplantation."

46. Excess of black bile. Actually this term meant different things to different physicians.

47. An emunctory organ is one with the purpose of draining off or cleansing secretions which should be discarded. The nose was believed by the Ancients to be the emunctory organ of the brain.

48. Peter Kennedy (dates unknown) was a London surgeon who observed inoculation during a trip to Turkey and wrote about it in *An essay on external remedies,*

London 1715. Mather probably owned a copy since he was so much interested in the subject.

49. Then synonymous with contagious substance. Later the word became more or less restricted in usage to mean the "dangerous malarial effluvia" of swamps.

50. Zabdiel Boylston (1679–1766) was one of the courageous physicans in American history. Mather gave him the stimulus and the great Mather backing but he performed the actual treatments. He had been educated by his father and a Doctor Cutter in Boston.

51. The chief of these was William Douglass M.D. (1691–1752), a Scottish physician educated at Leyden and Edinburgh. He was the only practitioner in Boston with a formal medical education. It was not until mid-century that Douglass became convinced of the value of inoculation, after having rather viciously fought Boylston and Mather. See Beall and Shryock, *Cotton Mather,* Baltimore 1968, p. 93–126 for an excellent account of the controversy.

52. "Behold how when I glimpse a natural cure he should become its enemy."

53. Six lines obliterated here.

54. There is little wonder that Mather should confide to his diary his supreme disgust with Boston as a "terrible town."

55. "Constant" was first used here and "vast" substituted. Six persons did die out of the 242 inoculated. Inoculation was not the direct cause of death in all cases, apparently.

56. Probably a plaster made of a resinous gummy substance.

57. To relieve the headache by irritating the opposite end of the body.

58. Bread boiled in water to the consistency of pap.

59. Today even the immensely safer vaccination for smallpox is considered unwise during pregnancy.

60. It has recently been observed that vaccine applied to warts often promotes their disappearance.

61. These two sentences were crossed out in the manuscript.

62. The corrected mortality from inoculation was evidently a little less than one percent. As a medical-historical essay on experimental smallpox by an eye-witness this section is extremely important. It describes something which will never be seen again.

Notes to Capsula XXI

1. Seventeenth century word for pollution.

2. Guy Patin (1601–1672) was a dominant figure in Parisian medicine in his century. He was an unusually quarrelsome man who opposed all progress. The *Lettres de Gui Patin* recreates the medical world of the seventeenth century.

3. William Becket (1684–1738) contributed three papers on the antiquity of venereal disease to the Royal Society. These Mather saw in the *Transactions.* Becket was a surgeon by profession, an antiquarian by hobby.

4. Gonorrhea ("clap") and syphilis were not proven to be two separate diseases until 1793 (Benjamin Bell of Edinburgh receives the credit).

5. Brothels.

6. "Women having an execrable disease."

7. Fairly typical seventeenth century English slur at the Roman Church.

8. Burned brutes.

9. French pox = morbus gallicus, so named by Fracastorius in his famous poem *Syphilis sive morbus gallicus,* Verona, 1530. Each nation tended to name syphilis after its chief enemy.

10. Chiliad means millennium. Mather is saying that disease was unknown before the fall of Adam.

11. The "Bills of Mortality" were weekly lists of deaths in London especially, more or less accurately done, which were published during the seventeenth century and were digested by John Graunt (1620–1674) in his pioneering work, *Natural and political observations upon the bills of mortality,* London 1662. Mather may have had a copy or may have known of its contents through reading the *Philosophical transactions.* Death from "French pox" was listed as being at the rate of 40–80 cases a year.

12. Mather was correct of course. It is often very difficult to interpret the old diagnoses and listings.

13. A disease caused by a treponeme similar to the one which causes syphilis. Yaws is a tropical disease characterized by much destruction of skin and subcutaneous tissues. In fact, some believe that it was yaws which Columbus' sailors brought back to Europe and was confused with syphilis. Possibly a combination of the two in a given patient gave the alarming symptoms. Syphilis and/or yaws raged in the sixteenth century.

14. "The despair after sinful pleasure."

15. Not identified.

16. The Citrullus colocynthis, a very common plant in Egypt and the Near East. It produces a gourd-like fruit the pulp of which is violently cathartic.

Notes to Capsula XXII

1. "Northern ailment." Scurvy in modern times first became most seriously manifest during the great voyages of discovery. Da Gama lost 55 sailors from it. Orange and lemon juices were used in its treatment in the late sixteenth century. Citrus was first recommended in print by John Woodall in his *Surgeon's mate,* London 1636. But this was ignored for a century to a large extent until James Lind proved the value of citrus fruit experimentally in 1753.

2. Refers to the bloody bowel movements. In our usage volvulus is a twist of the bowel which results in great pain and ultimately in gangrene due to interference with the circulation.

3. Vitiligro nigra is literally "black leprosy." But Mather is here referring to the dark purpuric spots on the skins of scurvy patients.

4. Soft bleeding gums.

5. Alopecia areata? (Spotty baldness).

6. A Roman general (15 B.C.–19 A.D.) and provincial governor during the reign of Tiberius.

7. A prophetic sea-god in the service of Neptune. When caught he would assume different shapes to avoid detention. Thus, the term protean is applied to any disease of many different appearances or signs and symptoms. Scurvy is protean.

8. Severinus Eugalenus (1535– ?) was a practitioner in Hamburg and Emden who published his *De scorbuto* in Bremen in 1588. It was many times republished.

9. Georg Wolfgang Wedel (1645–1721) was a noted German physician and teacher who lived principally at Jena and wrote a great many pamphlets and books. Mather probably knew of his work through his writings published in the *Ephemerides*.

10. Not confirmed, but doubtless Mather is correct. At any rate, the term is no longer used.

11. A small herb of the genus Rumex. It has a rather sour taste because of its oxalic acid content. As late as 1860 it was recommended for scorbutic patients.

12. Another plant long popular, Cochlearia officinalis, a native of Europe and cultivated as a salad. It has heart-shaped dark green leaves and clusters of white cruciform flowers.

13. Lepidum sativum, nasturtium. Most fresh vegetables have at least a modicum of vitamin C.

14. A kind of clover.

15. An infusion of malt, germinated barley.

16. Clarified.

17. Potassium bitartrate. Useless, of course.

18. Water trefoil, again.

Notes to Capsula XXIII

1. "The more you drink the more you thirst."

2. "Abstain and you will accomplish what medicine will not."

3. Probably ferrous sulfate.

4. A fossil resin found in many places. It is usually a yellow brittle solid susceptible of a high polish. It was highly favored by the Ancients as a medicine.

5. An annual European plant, cultivated as an herb, which has a strong agreeable odor due to its volatile oil. Once thought to be a cure-all. Of no value.

6. Probably one "doctor" Ponteus who in 1676 wrote *Man and woman their own doctor; or a salve for every sore, a book full of rare receipts for the most dangerous distempers. . . .* Published in London?

7. Scabiosa succisa, a variety of field scabious, a plant with a bitter, astringent quality. It was seldom used even in the seventeenth century. Quacks were attracted to preparations with strange names, of course.

8. Either Edward Hulse (1631–1711), who received his M.D. at Leyden, or Sir Edward Hulse (1682–1759) who received his from Cambridge. Neither wrote much.

9. Producers of sweat.

10. Chamomile. The flowers of Anthemis nobilis, a trailing plant with a perennial root, are solitary with a yellow disc and white petals. They have a bitter aromatic taste. The plant is a European one. In small doses chamomile is pleasant, in large, emetic. It was sometimes used externally as a fomentation (bathing with a hot concoction) for intestinal troubles.

11. Tympanites. Abdominal swelling due to an accumulation of gas in the intestines, as in peritonitis, obstruction, etc.

12. Carminatives supposedly allayed pain and helped in the discharge of flatus. Usually aromatics like anise and fennel were used.

13. The resin of several plants found in equatorial regions, particularly Siam. It is a drastic cathartic, was even known to cause death.

14. Brandy.

15. The product of Pimpinella anisum, a native of Egypt. It is a small annual plant with white flowers. Seeds are sweet and aromatic and were considered soothing to mucous membranes.

16. Not identified.

17. "Upward and downward." All of these remedies were tried on, but none helped, Dr. Hermann Boerhaave, the medical light of the age, in his last illness: cardiac failure with marked edema of the legs. In some cases incisions were made to drain off the dropsical fluid. In Boerhaave's case this was not necessary because the skin of his legs burst spontaneously. All this was before the discovery of digitalis.

Notes to Capsula XXIV

1. Refers to St. Mary of Bethlehem, a London monastery founded in 1246 A.D., which in the mid-sixteenth century was converted into a hospital for the insane. The name became "Bedlam" in popular speech.

2. Nebuchadnezzar.

3. "Wines affect the mind and make it prone to rage."

4. He means swallow-wort, Cynanchum vincetoxicum, a European perennial the root of which in small doses causes vomiting, in large, very great distress. It was once considered an antidote to poisons.

5. Potassium nitrate and sulfate fused.

6. Anagallis arvensis is a small annual plant of Europe which bears small scarlet rather than purple flowers. It was considered an antidote to poison by the Ancients. It causes vomiting.

7. Hypericum perforatum, a perennial herb, almost a ground cover, with pretty yellow flowers. It once enjoyed a great reputation in the treatment of demoniacs. It has a balsamic odor and a bitter taste. It was used in cases of hysteria, worms, and jaundice.

8. Helleborus niger, a perennial with dark green leaves and rose-like flowers and a large blackish root. A decoction or powder of the root was used. It is a drastic cathartic. It was highly esteemed by the Ancients in the treatment of mania and melancholy. It is obvious from their interest in all these anti-poisons and violent cathartics that physicians of old believed insanity to be due to some poison, best eliminated violently.

9. Camphor. The volatile oil from a large evergreen tree, of the laurel family of plants, which grows in the Far East. It was not known to the Ancients. It was considered anodyne for nervous conditions and was often combined with laudanum. It is in our paregoric of today.

10. Meconin is poppy juice. Meconic acid is an inert component of opium. Meconium is a word obscurely derived from meconin and is the greenish black first bowel movement of a baby. Whether Mather meant meconin or meconium is problematical. Certainly fecal matter was much used in medicine.

11. Here Mather obviously means the living bird. Often "swallows" was used interchangably with swallow-wort.

12. Mather does not finish this sentence. The root of the Nymphaea alba, or European white water-lily, was once thought to have sedative value. It does not.

13. Probably Johann Jacob Waldschmidt, German seventeenth century physician who contributed many papers to the *Ephemerides*. Little else is known of him. Or the

reference may be to Wilhelm Ulrich Waldschmidt (1669–1731) who wrote *Dissertatio medica de ignorantia et nequita empiricorum,* in 1692. ("Medical essay on the ignorance and malpractices of quacks." There was a great polemical literature in that century opposing quacks.)

14. Hysteria.

Notes to Capsula XXV

1. "Remarkable master of treating minds."
2. Epicurus (342–270 B.C.), the Greek philosopher who believed that pleasure is the only good.
3. "Bathing place of the Devil."
4. "Bear up the spirits." Mather refers to the medieval medical school of Salerno.
5. John Smith, C.M. (1607–1673) wrote on a variety of subjects besides clocks. His *The curiosities of common water,* London 1722, reprinted Boston 1723, was very popular. It was a compilation from many medical writers. It was translated into French, German, Italian, and Dutch. Mather surely had a copy of the Boston edition.
6. Extensively used until fairly recently, this is an aquatic worm 2–4 inches long found abundantly in marshes in Europe. They were popular because they afforded the least painful method of blood letting. They suck blood until gorged and then drop off. A single European leech might suck off as much as an ounce of blood.
7. Usually made by dissolving ferrous sulfate in Gentian water and a large amount of apple syrup.
8. Dodder, a plant resembling a brush of hair, grows on various plants. The epithymum of medicine grew on thyme and other herbs and has a pleasant aromatic odor. It is no longer common.
9. Tincture of quinine. I was unable to find it in the available copies of Quincy's *Dispensatory* or his *Dictionary,* however.
10. Oluf Borch (1626–1690) was a Danish physician, botanist, and chemist.
11. "Cured melancholics hate their doctors and all others concerned with their illness and recovery."

Notes to Capsula XXVI

1. Exactly backwards, of course.
2. Hedeoma pulegioides of America (Mentha pulegium if the European plant of the name) is a tiny herb with a strong aromatic odor. It is found in dry places all over Eastern America. Mather refers to the essential oil obtained by distillation. It has been used as an emmenogogue and a cordial. Pennyroyal is not even mentioned by most English seventeenth century pharmacopeias. Dodoens in his herbal does, but does not refer to its use. Junkens, the German quoted in the introduction, does mention its use.
3. The root of the common peony was much used by the Ancients in the treatment of epilepsy and as a charm. Its use died out in the nineteenth century. No one else seems to mention the use of the fragrant oil of the flowers.
4. The blessed thistle, Centaurea benedicta, is a large annual plant with barbed rough leaves. At flowering time the leaves are plucked and dried. In small quantities

it is mildly "tonic," but in large it produces vomiting, and in very large doses profuse perspiration.

5. Prepared by heating antimony with potassium nitrate. Depending on the proportions and the exact method of preparation used, diaphoretic antimony had varying amounts of antimonic acid, antimoniate of potassium, and other minor compounds. It is quite useless.

6. The "greases" of many birds and animals have been thought to be excellent as ointments and rubs: bear's grease, goose grease, and of course, fox grease or oil.

7. The berries of the well-known mistletoe are quite poisonous. Because of its Druidical, and thus magical, association it was used in small doses even until the nineteenth century for the treatment of epilepsy and palsy. It is a bitter nauseating dose.

8. The squill or sea onion is a member of the lily family. Its bulb is bitter, nauseating, diuretic, and purgative. Most often its principle was dissolved in vinegar and then mixed with honey to make oxymel of squill. It was most often used as an expectorant. Squill is most irritating to the skin and so you can imagine its intestinal effect.

Notes to Capsula XXVII

1. A figure of speech, probably referring to the burnable sulfur of Paracelsus who considered sulfur one of the three elements. Apparently no one has considered sulfur a true narcotic.

2. That is, the normal channels for the discharge of phlegm have been blocked. Now we complain of lack of sinus drainage.

3. Wine with antimony tartrate added.

4. Where the skullbones of the newborn fuse together.

5. The alcohol-soluble portion, or resin, of the smoke of burning wood. Obviously, it contained many organic compounds, each preparation being different to some extent from all others. Powdered soot was much used in various chronic skin diseases. Spirit of soot was also used in the treatment of intestinal worms.

Notes to Capsula XXVIII

1. The "sacred disease," the very ancient name of epilepsy. Hippocrates was perhaps the first to dispute the term.

2. Paul Barbette (seventeenth century) practised in Amsterdam. After having been tutored by his surgeon father in Strasburg he attended medical school at Montpellier and Paris. He was highly respected and wrote much on anatomy, surgery, and on medicine in general.

3. The same thing, apparently, as Toulon soap, a very dry bluish white, glossy, pleasant-smelling soap.

4. Remedy. This was the name of a medical work by Oribasius (325–403 A.D.).

5. This sentence was inserted in small writing, evidently as an afterthought.

6. Oak bark, noted for its bitter taste, was long used in the treatment of diarrhea. Supposedly its astringent properties would help in cases of epilepsy.

7. Fern, more properly male-fern, carried its supposed great astringent and worm-killing powers in the root. Any plant of the genus Aspidium.

8. Many species of Aristolochia have been employed as tonics and stimulants. They have contorted roots, brown in color, with a bitter disagreeable odor. They are widely distributed over Eastern United States. They were once a great article of commerce. They are very poisonous in large doses.

9. Cannibals.

10. "Heap up a sepulchral mound for the reception of the bones." Fuller was a little in advance of his times! Most of his contemporaries were much impressed by the value of pulverized human skull and by the "moss from a dead man's skull," Boyle among them.

11. Sir John Colbatch (d. 1729) was an apothecary turned physician. He was knighted by George I in 1716 for some obscure reason. He wrote many tracts, one of which was *Dissertation upon misteltoe, a remedy in convulsive distemper.* It was published some years before the *Angel* was finished. He did not rate as highly as Mather thought. It will be obvious from the text which follows that Mather had a copy available.

12. A play with words. Boyle's social state was that of "Honourable" since he was the son of an earl. He repeatedly declined elevation to the peerage.

13. Abdiah Cole (1610–1670) may or may not have been a physician, but he did produce, translate, or edit, sometimes in association with Nicholas Culpeper, a great many medical tracts and texts. Mather probably refers to his *Experimental physick,* 1662, which is a compendium of a thousand cures.

14. Assafoetida is the gum-resin of the root of Narthex assafoetida, a plant with large leaves rising directly from a perennial foot-long fleshy root, native to Persia. The value of assafoetida lies in its stench. Even in this century it has been used to treat hysterical women.

15. Syrup of poppy. The very words in this phrase are to be found in Quincy's *Dispensatory,* making it obvious that Mather owned a copy.

16. The dried sap of a number of trees, European larch, European flowering ash (that of Sicily was considered best), and a Eucalyptus. It is a gentle laxative.

17. "Frailty of the lung." Mather evidently means severe asthma. We may doubt the efficacy of mistletoe in the cure of the case described, but asthma is still such a mysterious disease in many cases that we cannot categorically deny it. A placebo given with Colbatch's assurance might have done as well.

Notes to Capsula XXIX

1. Lorenzo Bellini (1643–1704) of Florence was a brilliant anatomist, physiologist (he studied the kidney) and physician. He became professor of medicine at Pisa at twenty-six.

2. Simple dizziness is most likely to be due to some disturbance of the inner ear. True vertigo is due to a disorder of the eighth cranial nerve. In this paragraph Mather may be referring to petit mal epilepsy, a quite different matter.

3. Olibanum was the frankincense of the Ancients. It is thought to have been the gum resin of a fairly tall tree which grows in dry rocky areas on the African coast of the Red Sea. Another kind comes from a large tree, Boswellia serrata, which grows in northern India. It has a balsamic smell, is bitter. It was often used in plasters, seldom internally.

Notes to Capsula XXX

1. With us coma denotes the profound condition. In the older terminology "coma" was divided into four progressive stages: sopor, coma, lethargia, and carus, the last being the most profound and what we today understand as coma.

2. When lettuce "goes to seed" the flowering stalk provides a juice of a slightly sweetish taste which was once thought to have narcotic properties. It does not.

3. Spirit of Rosemary was known as Hungary water.

4. Actually, opiates are more likely to constipate.

5. Oil of roses is the oil expressed from petals of the damask rose. Rosewater is an infusion of eight pounds of rose flowers in two gallons of water, boiled down to one gallon. Rose cake is what is left after distillation to get the oil. Oil of roses, syrup of roses, were considered great cordials. Now merely used as an elegant vehicle and occasionally as a cough syrup for children.

Notes to Capsula XXXI

1. "To sleep in both ears."

2. The demon was female: the spirit of evil among the Hindus, the demon of the nightmare among the early Germans.

3. In the sense of mean or wretched.

4. Edmund Dickinson (1624–1707) received his M.D. from Oxford. Because of his great love of chemistry he became a favorite of Charles II. He retired after the accession of William and Mary and wrote some rather obscure books.

5. Inuus was identified with the god Pan who gave fruitfulness to the flocks and herds of Greece. But he was a rather complicated little god in that he was also dangerous to women. If offended, he could cause mental aberrations and panic. In fact, another name for him was Incubus. He was also something of a healing god through the means of hallucinations (halucinogens?) at his favorite springs. Ephialtes is a synonym for incubus or nightmare. Artemidorus was a noted second century A.D. interpreter of dreams. His work is a mine of information on ancient superstitions.

6. "Thus may he lay hold of me!"

7. Struggle.

8. A small shrub with a woody stem, native to southern Europe. The flowers are very fragrant. The oil upon which the fragrance depends was often a component in prescriptions for nervous disability.

Notes to Capsula XXXII

1. John Ray (1627–1705) was one of England's greatest naturalists. Harvard owned three of his works. His *Wisdom of God manifested in the works of creation,* first published in London in 1691, went through many editions and was widely owned in the colonies. Certainly Mather had a copy. It was one of his tools in preparing his *Christian philosopher.*

2. William Derham (1657–1735) was a divine who was especially interested in natural history. He edited Ray's *Wisdom* after the latter's death. Mather quotes him often in the *Christian philosopher,* especially his *Astro-theology,* London 1715, which Mather certainly owned.

3. Probably Johannes Sturm (1507–1589), the German scholar who founded the Strasburg gymnasium and promoted his own system of education.

4. Cheyne.

5. Possibly Johann Gottfried Tympe (1699–1768), professor of theology at Jena. There was another Tympe or Timpe who was a Roman Catholic preacher of Munster in the early seventeenth century. Because of the dates the latter would seem to be the more likely possibility.

6. Alfonso V (1396–1458), the magnanimous and cultured King of Naples 1443–1458 and Sicily 1416–1458. At Naples he was noted for his patronage of the arts and letters.

7. It is possible that Nero watched the Roman sports through a crude magnifying instrument of emerald (Pliny, Book 37, chapter 5). Possibly spectacles were invented by Roger Bacon (1240–1292). More likely, they were invented in Italy in the early fourteenth century. In a fresco in Modena, dated 1352, a monk is shown wearing primitive spectacles.

8. An alloy of gold, silver, and copper, much appreciated by the Ancients.

9. Euphasia officinalis, a small annual weed once common in Europe and America. It has bitter-tasting leaves. Of no value.

10. Birds.

11. Swallows will lead you to swallow-wort or celandine. See Chapter 24, note 4.

12. Probably rain-water, next to distilled water the purest obtainable.

13. Copperas. Ferrous sulfate or green vitriol.

14. A friable red clay containing much iron oxide, found in Armenia.

15. Nutmeg.

16. Bartolommeo Montagna (d. 1460) was professor of medicine at Padua 1422–61. He wrote a tract on composing prescriptions which gave dosage details.

17. Watery discharge from the eyes.

18. Foeniculum vulgare, an herb with a perennial root out of which there grows a tall stem with flowers in flat terminal umbrels. It is a carminative and an aromatic condiment. The seeds and roots were used.

19. Sir William Temple (1628–1699) was an English statesman of better character than many of his day. At various times of retirement from public office he wrote a great deal on various subjects. He made an important contribution to English prose style. In this he may have been a model for Mather.

20. A term for eye-water.

21. Lady Fitz-Harding not identified. "My Lady Fitz-Harding's eye water" is #94 in the third edition of Boyle's *Medicinal experiments*. Mather copied it almost word for word.

22. Sugar of lead, lead acetate.

23. Zinc oxide.

24. William Jameson (d. 1720) was an outspoken Presbyterian as well as lecturer in history.

25. Abu Bakr Muhammed ibn Zakaria, usually known as Rhazes (865–925) is said to have been blinded when his royal master Al-Mansur hit him in a rage. He was a great Persian physician, a keen observer, and a true innovator. He left three books which were widely translated and respected in the West, his *Liber continens, Liber medicinalis,* and his *Aphorisms.*

Notes to Capsula XXXIII

1. One whose ears have been boxed, literally.

2. "Considered the worst of all."

3. William Salmon (1644–1713) was a self-educated physician who practised irregularly and wrote or translated many books, including one on domestic medicine. He is thought to have visited New England late in the seventeenth century. If so, he probably met Mather.

4. Simon Paulli (1603–1680), born in Rostock, a German Baltic city, spent much of his life in Denmark as an anatomist and botanist and gained a considerable reputation.

5. From 1566 until 1702 there were at least four Fabers in Germany, each of whom made contributions to the medical literature. From the context one would assume that Mather did not have a Faber book at hand, but was quoting someone else.

6. Martin Martin (d. 1719) was born on Skye. His *Description of the western islands of Scotland* (1703) inspired Samuel Johnson's more famous tour.

7. Salvia officinalis, the still commonly used herb.

8. Alcohol.

9. Sir Kenelm Digby (1603–1665) was a flamboyant "man of the Renaissance," a Catholic nobleman who on one hand could write a fairly sensible philosophical work like *Of bodies,* first published in Paris in 1644, but frequently reprinted, and on the other fervently advise his powder of sympathy which, if placed on the sword would heal the wound it had caused. His "Receits" (*Choice and experimental receipts in physick and chirurgery,* London 1668 was possibly a false attribution. It was published posthumously) is a collection of folk-lore remedies much like that of Boyle. Mather definitely owned the Boyle piece, perhaps the Digby one.

10. Probably Philipp Jacob Hartmann (1648–1707) a German medical professor who wrote many papers for the *Ephemerides.*

Notes to Capsula XXXIV

1. A word of Greek origin meaning astringents.

2. Incautious, a seventeenth century word.

3. A common perennial herb found in fields and lawns. The leaves and roots have a salty taste and are astringent. The Ancients thought highly of the herb in hemorrhagic conditions.

4. Hematite, an iron ore of a lovely reddish color when found in crystalline form. It is sesquioxide of iron. Use of this was essentially treatment by similars originally, probably, but iron salts do have styptic qualities.

5 Copper sulfate.

6. Freed from acidity, purified.

7. Sulfuric acid.

8. The residue after distillation, usually considered worthless.

9. Possibly Charles II was the monarch in question.

10. Substances which were credited with closing over wounds.

11. Submitted to strong heat to drive out the water. Copper sulfate was Digby's "powder of sympathy."

Notes to Capsula XXXV

1. Acute suppurative tonsilitis.

2. The roots, leaves, and flowers of this ornamental plant, Aquilegia vulgaris, have a disagreeable odor and a bitter taste. Columbine was once considered diuretic and diaphoretic. Actually, it is merely poisonous.

3. A grayish-yellow aluminous earth originally found in Lemnos, an island in the northern Aegean Sea.

4. Curdled milk.

5. A perennial European succulent plant which grows on rocks and old walls. The leaves have a cool sour taste and were often used as poultices for burns and insect stings.

6. Hezekiah was King of Judah for about thirty years ca. 700 B.C. He was something of a religious reformer.

7. A first century Greek who served as a surgeon in the Roman army and studied plants from the point of view of the materia medica and wrote a book, *De materia medica,* better known simply as "Dioscorides," which remained a standard text for fifteen hundred years.

8. "Figs disperse indurations about the ears and soften boils."

9. A woody perennial European plant with a strong odor and a bitter nauseating taste due to its essential oil. It was long considered a great tonic, a vermifuge, and an antiseptic.

10. The much swollen tonsils of childhood.

Notes to Capsula XXXVI

1. "Aids for a cattarrh."

2. "Catarrhal nonsense."

3. Distilling apparatus.

4. Most people at that time believed that the secretions of glands were merely extracts from the blood, not products manufactured by the glands themselves.

5. Francois Duport (1540–1624) was a Parisian physician who wrote *De signis morborum,* Paris, 1584.

6. "When the phlegm produces an unhealthy catarrh there is coldness in the head; the face is pallid; the voice croaks; there is a taste; the urine is more crude; the mind is dull; there is torpor."

7. He probably means enrouer, to make hoarse.

8. Jonathan Mitchell (1624–1668) was a prominent New England divine. Mather wrote of him at considerable length in his *Magnalia* (Vol. II, p. 66–113).

9. James Keill (1673–1719) was a physician, brother to John Keill (1671–1721), the astronomer and mathematician. James was also an anatomist. He is best known for his *An account of animal secretions,* London 1708.

10. Not identified.

11. That is, if they do not cause constipation.

Notes to Capsula XXXVII

1. Hugh Latimer (1485–1555) was one of the martyrs burned in the reign of Queen Mary. He was a hero to the Puritans, and his sermons were long popular.

2. Copaiba is the resin obtained from Copaifera officinalis, an elegant Venezuelan and West Indian tree. In the smallest doses it is laxative, in large ones a violent purgative.

3. Discharge, in the sense of a filthy discharge.

4. Marrubium vulgare, a twelve- to eighteen-inch annual herb with a perennial root. It has a strong pleasant odor and thus was considered a tonic for debilitated persons. Until recently it was used in hard candy.

5. A kind of hard pea used in baking.

6. "Of each a sufficient quantity." A standard old prescription abbreviation.

7. Sulfur is soluble in alcohol.

8. Sulfur heated in volatile oils to make a foul-smelling substance.

9. Possibly the minister grandfather of John Hancock the patriot.

10. Mead, or fermented honey.

11. "By good authority."

12. Mixture of beer and spirit, sweetened, and heated with a hot iron.

13. Barley made to germinate for the purpose of forming beer.

Notes to Capsula XXXVIII

1. To the dismay of most asthmatics physicians still maintain that there is a large psychosomatic element in the disease.

2. Though it is occasionally effective in stopping an attack of asthma, vomiting is no longer induced as a treatment.

3. The resinous milky juice of the ammoniac plant of Persia, a shrub about seven feet high which exudes its juice freely at the slightest wound. Probably it derives its name as a corruption of armeniacum which stems from the fact that the drug was originally imported to Europe through Armenia. The resin is very bitter and was chiefly used as an expectorant.

4. Suspension of the insoluble ammoniac in water.

5. Balthasar Brunner (1533–1604) was a physician who practised in a great many different cities. He was interested in chemistry and alchemy.

6. Tobacco is very effective in producing secretions: Sniffed as snuff it causes sneezing and a copious nasal secretion, chewed it is a salivant, injected rectally it is a cathartic. The vinous solution of course contained nicotine and tar and was used as a salivant. Thus it was assumed to be an expectorant or producer of bronchial secretions.

Notes to Capsula XXXIX

1. "They are wasted and they do not enjoy food."

2. The famous "Hippocratic facies" which signifies impending death, first described by Hippocrates.

3. "From the candelsmoke consumed everywhere in shut-in studies."

4. Josue de la Place (1606–1665) was a famous French protestant divine, born in Brittany.

5. Probably this term refers to the calcifications found in tuberculous lungs. On very rare occasions these calculi have been expectorated by patients.

6. Several different antimony compounds heated together for two hours and then ground to a fine gray powder.

7. The milk of mares and jennies is remarkably like that of women. A stable of milking mares was actually maintained by a foundling hospital in Paris in the nineteenth century.

8. Avicenna (980–1037) was an illustrious Persian physician who left a great number of writings which were highly regarded in the West well into the eighteenth century.

9. "The water of life is the water of death."

10. Restorative medicine, or food, which restores health during convalescence.

11. This came to be greatly in vogue by the nineteenth century when mountain fresh air was considered especially beneficial to consumptives.

12. The root of Smilax china, actually identical with sarsaparilla. China root enjoyed great vogue in the sixteenth century as a treatment for venereal disease.

13. This and the preceding sentence not in the hand of Mather.

14. Richard Lower (1631–1691) was a London physician who was famous for his *Tractatus de corde* (1669), one of the classical works in cardiology. His biographies seem to ignore the fact, but in 1700 there was published *Dr. Lowers and other eminent physicians receipts*. Apparently Mather had a copy. Probably Lower's famous name was merely used posthumously to help sell the book.

15. Adiantum pedatum, the maidenhair fern. It has bitter leaves and was once much used in chronic catarrhs.

16. Dianthus caryophyllus, the carnation.

17. Pilulae Rufi, a prescription in which aloes and myrrh are compounded as a cathartic.

Notes to Capsula XL

1. Gideon Harvey (about 1640–1700) was a London physican of rather poor repute who wrote many works. One, against physicians entitled *The conclave of physicians,* London 1683, was owned in Virginia at least. He also wrote *The family physician,* 1676.

2. Lohochs = looch = eclectos, a thick syrupy medicine used to allay coughs. It was usually sucked from the end of a liquorice stick.

3. Girolamo Capivaccio (d. 1589) was professor of medicine at Padua.

4. Another synonym for eclectos, above.

5. Felix Plater (1536–1614) was an anatomist and physician at Basel. He had a great contemporary reputation. Harvard owned his *Praxeos medicae,* Basel 1602–6.

6. Franz de le Boë (1614–1672), known as Sylvius, was a Dutch physician who was a founder of the iatrochemical "school" of medical thought.

7. Frederick Dekkers (1648–1720) was a student of Sylvius who became famous himself and finally taught medicine at Leyden.

8. Johann Michaelis (1606–1667) was professor of pathology and therapeutics at Leipzig.

9. Snails, raw or in a syrup, were once considered almost specific as nourishment for consumptives.

10. Hugues de Salins (1632–1710) was a French physician who was especially noted for his promotion of wine as a cure-all.

11. Richard Morton (1637–1689) was a London physician who was pioneered in the study of tuberculosis. He wrote *Phthisiologia*, London 1689.

12. Arnold Weickhard (1578–1645) of Frankfurt-am-Main wrote *Thesaurus pharmaceuticus galeno-chemicus*, Frankfurt 1626.

13. Cathartics containing aloes.

14. Tincture of aloes and myrrh.

15. Michele Mercati (1541–1593) was a physician, botanist, and mineralogist. He did write a book on the plague but I can find no listing of a general work by him.

16. Adriaan van den Spieghel (1578–1625) was born in Brussels but studied and settled in Padua as professor of anatomy and surgery. He wrote much on anatomy, something on malaria and on worms, but in his *Opera omnia* of 1645 I find nothing by him on consumption. Mather may be passing on second-hand information.

17. Johann Crato von Kraftheim (1519–1585) was a distinguished Protestant physician whose collection of consilia (written consultations) was published posthumously in 1589.

18. Giovanni Battista Monte (1498–1552) was a distinguished Paduan physician, author of several original works and of many commentaries on the writings of the Ancients.

19. Vincent Alsario della Croce (1570–1632?) was a Genoese who practised in Bologna and Ravenna. As a phthisiologist he ranks with Morton because of his *De haemoptysi seu sanguinis sputo*, Rome 1663.

20. Of Juan de dios Huarte (1535–1600?) little is known. He was a Spanish physician who wrote *Examen de ingenios para las sciencias*, Baeza, 1575.

21. Fifth century Roman writer and commentator on Virgil, Cicero, and other ancient writers.

22. "Never known either to deceive or be deceived."

23. "He was so full of goodness that he wrote nothing which he did not wish us to know. Such was his skill and knowledge that no one after him presented anything which he did not know."

24. "The art of medicine received hardly any precepts."

25. Marchmont Nedham (1620–1678), journalist and part-time physician, wrote this attack on the College of Physicians. This book, incidentally, published in 1665, is apparently the first to mention the germ theory of disease in English.

26. Andreas Vesalius (1514–1564) was a Belgian who became professor of anatomy at Padua and while there wrote the first great modern anatomy book and thus is credited with having started modern medicine. He began the questioning of previously sacro-sanct pronouncements of Galen.

27. "Certain it is that the number of sick cured by doctors does not approach the number of those sent to the hereafter with their pompous Latin phrases."

28. "The divine art of medicine is held in check by the fear that it may become criminal or homicidal, an opinion shared by the Romans with regard to the ancient physician."

29. Giovanni Argenterio (1513–1572) was an Italian physician of some note who sojourned in many different cities. He wrote a number of books on the errors of the ancient physicians, on disease in general, on fever, on urine, etc. Perhaps Mather's comment accounts for his short stays in so many cities.

Notes to Capsula XLI

1. St. John Chrysostom (347–407) was a great Greek father of the Church. His name in Greek means "golden-mouthed."

2. Hardly anything escaped being used as a treatment by someone.

3. Probably Franz Joël (1595–1631), the last of three German physicians of the name. He wrote *Praxis medica,* Lauenberg 1622.

4. Root of Curcuma longa, a Southeast Asian plant. The root is of a deep yellow color. It tinges the saliva yellow. It is something of a condiment. Note that most of the drugs used in the treatment of jaundice are yellow or turn bodily secretions yellow: similars cure similars, according to the old doctrine of similars.

5. Chironia centaurium, a small annual herb having lovely rose-colored flowers. Obviously, it was named after Chiron the Centaur. It has a very bitter taste and thus was considered a tonic.

Notes to Capsula XLII

1. Anorexia.

2. "A badly affected stomach is the origin of nearly all ailments."

3. A clear exposition of the notion, held by many, that the efficacy of cinchona is due to its bitterness.

4. "Pitch upon" was a common seventeenth century usage. Boyle was very fond of it.

5. Artemisia absinthum, a low perennial plant, native of Europe, the leaves and flowers of which are very bitter, and thus tonic. It is very interesting to note that it was used in the treatment of malaria before cinchona was discovered. Possibly this was the occasion for the first use of the very bitter cinchona: the more bitter the medicine the better its action on intermittent fevers. Malaria was apparently unknown in the Americas before the Discovery. Thus, the Indians would hardly have discovered a specific for a non-existent disease.

6. Ligusticum levisticum is a wild plant of southern Europe which has a yellowish juice. It is aromatic.

7. Mugwort is another species of Artemisia, thus is related to wormwood. It was long used in Germany in the treatment of epilepsy.

8. The fragrant aromatic gum of a small Near-Eastern tree. Styrax officinale, which is a component of the still-used compound tincture of benzoin. It was once used for a great variety of conditions.

9. Sea weed.

10. Refers to a distinguished family of ancient Rome, one member of which was father-in-law of Julius Caesar.

11. Bitters.

12. This is an obscure reference. There were two men of the Spon name in the seventeenth century, father and son, who were scholars of ancient medicine, Carolus Spon (1609–1684) and Jacobus Spon (1647–?). They were French protestants.

13. Berberis vulgare, a once commonly used shrub, esteemed for its pretty berries which are pleasant tasting.

14. "Cholera infantum," a bacterial enteritis which was once a great cause of infant mortality.

15. A vague term which included all debilitating diarrheas and dysenteries.

16. Mostly composed of calcium carbonate with a small amount of gelatin. The more exotic the source the better the effect of the medicine.

17. Aqua mirabilis or spiritus pimento is a delicious decoction of Jamaica pimento or pepper.

Notes to Capsula XLIII

1. Rose syrup or candy. I have not found this term in any book more recent than the seventeenth century.

2. A plaster which was made of a mixture of equal parts of sulfur, antimony, and arsenic melted together. It disappeared from use in the eighteenth century.

3. Powder to counteract heartburn.

Notes to Capsula XLIV

1. Intestinal worms were astonishingly prevalent in colonial America. See Jack Green, Ed. *The diary of Landon Carter,* Charlottesville 1965. Usually these were either round worms or flat worms. Infestations were often so overwhelming as to be fatal, especially in children. The sources were usually bad water and poorly cooked infected meats. Possibly worms are more prevalent today than realized. It has been claimed that round worm infestation may be a factor in many cases of asthma; eliminating the former may relieve the latter in such cases. This may account for some of the worm mortality in colonial times.

2. Thomas Moffett (1553–1604) was a physician who wrote on both medical and natural history subjects. He was especially interested in insects.

3. Edward Tyson (1650–1708) was a physician and a distinguished comparative anatomist. He wrote on the tape worm in # 146 of the *Philosophical Transactions.*

4. Maggots, of course.

5. Charles Leigh (1662–1705) was a physician, naturalist, and member of the Royal Society. He practised in London and Manchester but did not achieve a great reputation.

6. "Sea moss" or Corallina officinalis, an animal related to the coral. It grows about an inch high on rocks and shells in the Mediterranean Sea. It was once in great favor as a vermifuge.

7. Giovanni Battista Zapatha (1520–1586), a Roman physician, wrote *Maravigliosi secreti di medicina e cerurgia,* Rome 1586.

8. Probably Arnold Weickhard. See Chapter 40, note 12.

9. Johann Wittich (1537–1598), a physician of Arnstadt, wrote many treatises. Probably Mather's source refers to his work on children's diseases, *Libellus de infantilium aegritudinum medicatione* . . . . Leipzig 1596.

10. A heavy, sweet, red wine from Spain.

11. Andry greatly favored the use of tobacco.

12. A southern European perennial herb, Gratiola officinalis, which has a bitter nauseating taste. It is a violent emetic and cathartic.

13. The dried tops of Juniperus sabina, an evergreen shrub of southern Europe. Often in the Colonies common American red cedar was used instead.

14. Cyclamen europaeum, the wild cyclamen. The fresh root was considered anthelmintic.

15. The fruit of Chenopodium anthelminticum, also called Jerusalem oak, a rather common American plant. The seeds are toxic, but effective. The expressed oil was more often used.

16. "The doctor should always keep them in mind."

17. "A wasting unfortunate."

18. "With the expulsion of innumerable worms."

19. Tanacretum vulgare is a European herb naturalized in America. It is tall with serrated leaves and yellow flowers in dense terminal corymbs. It is warm, fragrant, and bitter. It was used both for hysteria and as a vermifuge. It is poisonous in large doses.

20. Anthemis cotula, an annual plant with a fibrous root, hairy leaves, and yellow flowers, is common in America and Europe. It has a strong disagreeable smell and thus also was used in the treatment of hysteria.

Notes to Capsula XLV

1. Lienteria, "smooth intestine," refers to frequent liquid evacuations. In "coeliaca" the food is passed "undigested." Both terms have been abandoned and diarrhea is used as the term for all loose bowel actions. In older times dysentery was the term used for painful diarrhea. Now, diarrhea is the symptom while dysentery refers usually to certain specific bacterial and parasitic conditions.

2. "Bad things will prevail because of long delays."

3. He refers to tuberculous enteritis. Lienteria was a term often used for the diarrhea of that condition.

4. Potentilla tormentilla, the septfoil, is a small perennial plant, common in Europe. It has a woody root which was used as an astringent.

5. Malva sylvestris, common mallow, is a large perennial plant with large purple flowers. It is a common weed in Europe. Because of its slimy taste it was considered emollient.

6. The wood of Haematoxylon campechianum, a small tree of Central America. The wood, dark red in color, has a sweet astringent taste, and was long considered soothing to the bowel.

7. Medicines used to prevent the bad effects of poisons, or, more especially, medicines thought capable of expelling from the body poisonous substances. Note the now obsolete spelling.

Notes to Capsula XLVI

1. Jehoram. See Chapter 1.

2. Tartrate of antimony and potassium, made by various methods, was extremely popular until late in the nineteenth century. It was considered a superb emetic, diaphoretic, and laxative, according to the dose given. Antimony is very toxic, but is effective in the treatment of certain protozoal infections. The emetic action of the large dose

recommended by Mather is evidently central rather than due to the local irritation of the stomach.

3. Secret remedy. A favorite word of the iatrochemists.

4. Perhaps the tannic acid content of the walnut helped a little.

5. Citrus medica. It is related to the lemon, and like it is anti-scorbutic. The thick rind is used in preserves today.

Notes to Capsula XLVII

1. Mather's spelling is confusing. Cholic referred to the bile and chola was a name for the gall bladder in the seventeenth century. And, then as now, the word for the large bowel was colon.

2. Appendicitis.

3. Tiberius Caesar (42 b.c.–37 a.d.), Roman Emperor, was unpopular because of his autocratic ways and because he tried to eliminate governmental waste. To Mather he was a monster because it was during his reign that Christ was crucified.

4. Contemporary term for an earthy mineral.

5. A gun from Pistacia lentiscus, a small shrub which is said to produce the gum only in certain spots, the island of Scio, for instance. It was once thought to have the same virtues as turpentine in diarrhea. It was also once used to fill carious teeth.

6. Fruit of Tamarindus indica, a huge, beautiful tree having a rough bark, pinnate leaves, and yellowish flowers. The fruit is a large pod with a pulpy interior which has laxative properties.

7. A mixture of beer and spirit sweetened with sugar and heated with a hot iron.

8. "With this mildest remedy."

9. Decoction or infusion.

10. Thomas Daffy (d. 1680) was an English clergyman who invented the Elixir Salutatis (elixir of health). It was sold by his son and after his death by other relatives for a time. It was what was later known as compound tincture of senna. It was composed usually of senna, bruised carroway seeds, bruised cardamon, raisins, and alcohol steeped together for seven days and then drained. The liquor thus resulting was a cathartic. Caraway is a biennial European plant about two feet tall. Its roots are used as food, its seed in medicine as a carminative. Cardamon is the seed of Elettaria cardamomum, a small plant found in the forests of Malabar. The seeds are very aromatic; they were considered cordial. The formula Mather advises is a little different from the more standard. Perhaps his was a New England version.

11. An annual plant native to Italy. The seeds are pleasantly aromatic. They were used for the same purpose as liquorice.

12. Guaiac.

13. Cajacia = caacica, a Brazilian plant once thought to be effective in the treatment of snakebite.

14. Willem Piso (1611–1678) was a Dutch physician who in 1637 went as personal physician to Count Moritz, the commander of an expedition to Brazil. He gained and retained an interest in tropical medicine after his return to the Netherlands. He wrote *Historia naturalis Brasiliae* (1648) and *De Indiae utriusque naturali et medica,* 1658. Both were published in Amsterdam.

15. Apparently here Mather refers to a plant of the genus Polygonum. It is fairly

widely distributed. It has roots which are so folded upon themselves as to give a snake-like appearance. Taken internally the powdered root gives a "sense of warmth" and acts as a diuretic. Snakeroot is a different plant. It also has contorted roots. It is a stately plant having a perennial root and small white flowers in a raceme. It is widely distributed in America. It is poisonous in large doses, but in tiny doses it was much used in the eighteenth and nineteenth centuries in treating rheumatism, consumption, and hysteria.

16. Paracelsus had a secret, expensive remedy which he called "laudanum" because he thought it so praiseworthy. Even in his day physicians thought it was a preparation of opium.

17. An obscure reference. Opium seems to have been used in Virginia no more or less than elsewhere.

Notes to Capsula XLVIII

1. Ashdod was an ancient city of the Philistines on the Mediterranean coast near Gaza. 1 Samuel 5 : 6 "But the hand of the Lord was heavy upon them of Ashdod and he destroyed them, and smote them with emerods . . ." Emerods was an occasional seventeenth century spelling of hemorrhoids.

2. Achillea millefolium, or yarrow, is a perennial herb or weed about a foot high, bearing finely divided leaves and a dense corymb of whitish flowers. The whole plant has an agreeable aromatic odor. Because of its content of a volatile oil, tannic acid, and "achilleic acid" it is rather astringent and was once much used to control hemorrhage as a decoction by mouth or by rectum as an enema.

3. Purified.

4. Oil of box was apparently extracted from mistletoe.

5. Properly olibanum. Mather's may have been merely the yellowish tears from a sort of pine and thus actually an impure raw turpentine.

6. Sulfur vivum, the dregs found when sulfur is purified by melting.

7. Milk curdled with yarrow.

8. Allium porrum is an onion-like biennial bulbous plant native to Switzerland. It has a most offensive odor.

9. The white dung of a dog. It is largely calcium phosphate originating in the bones in the dogs' food.

Notes to Capsula XLIX

1. "The itch to argue is the scabies of the Church."

2. Raw mercury applied to the skin is, of course, highly toxic if used in any quantity.

3. Sulfur.

4. Made with olive oil and potash, or, more primitively, with rendered lard and wood ashes. Sodium hydroxide makes hard soap.

5. This paragraph not in Mather's hand.

6. Oil from the berries of Laurus nobilis, an evergreen tree native to Mediterranean countries. The oil has a pleasant odor and has had its greatest use in the improving of the scent of external remedies.

7. Rumex obtusifolius, a large plant with large leaves. The root was used as an astringent both internally and externally.

8. Impure soap, with the soot of the wood ashes not removed.

Notes to Capsula LI

1. The reader will recall that Mather himself was so badly afflicted with stammering in his youth that he almost missed the ministry. He managed to cure himself.

2. Hezekiah Woodward (1590–1675), non-conformist divine and educator, like Mather overcame a speech impediment. In Woodward's case it was possibly caused by an unhappy childhood. He wrote of his unhappiness in *Of a child's portion*, London, 1640. Doubtless Mather owned a copy.

3. Dervishes are the Islamic equavalents of monks or friars. Their variety is great. Only a few have been "whirling" or "howling."

4. "Stupid sounds."

5. A silentiarius was a Roman court official sworn to keep secret all affairs of state.

6. A seventeenth century word for tottering or unsteadiness.

7. Henry Gellibrand (1597–1636) was an English divine.

8. Marcellinus Comes (d. 534 in Constantinople) was chancellor to Justinian I. He wrote his *Annales,* a chronicle of Byzantine history.

9. Arianism, started by Arius, probably of Alexandria, in the fourth century, in brief seemed to make Christ less than a Son of God and more just a divine creature.

10. "Emitted true voices."

11. Not identified.

12. Justinian I (483–565). Arianism lived long, was last found among the Vandals and Lombards.

13. Aeneas Gazaeus was a late fifth century Platonic philosopher who turned Christian.

14. Procopius was a sixth century Byzantine historian who wrote a classic and valuable historical source.

15. Jacques Cujos (1522–1590) was a French jurist who studied Roman law as an historian.

16. Herman Wits (1636–1708) was a Dutch theologian and writer.

17. Isaiah 32:4.

18. Autobiographical.

19. "Comfort to the wretched."

20. Michael II, The Stammerer (d. 829) was a Byzantine emperor. He was indifferent to religion during most of his reign, and thus was tolerant. Toward the last of his life he became anti-religious.

21. Origanum vulgare is a perennial herb with erect purplish downy stems and pinkish flowers. It is native to Europe and America. It has an agreeable aromatic odor and a warm pungent taste.

22. A lixivium is the result of a percolation which removes the potash from ashes.

23. Martin Ruland (1533–1602) was a German physician who wrote many minor medical works on such subjects as practical medicine, cures at baths, phlebotomy, etc.

Notes to Capsula LII

1. Jean Varandé (d. 1617), known as Johannes Varandaeus, was a very popular and famous teacher of medicine at Montpellier. He wrote *De morbis et affectibus mulierum libri tres,* Lyon 1619.

2. Eclampsia, a dangerous condition of late pregnancy, of still unknown etiology, characterized by hypertension, albuminuria, and convulsions. Often there is edema. It is far less common now than formerly.

3. A resinous substance from a large tree of the East Indies, Calophyllum inophyllum. It is of a pale yellowish green color, soft to the touch, and agreeable in odor. It was used much like turpentine.

4. Inert medically.

5. The Aquilegia vulgaris of our gardens is poisonous. All parts of it were once used for their presumed diaphoretic and diuretic actions. Thus, presumably, the edema of eclampsia would be reduced.

6. Dried human blood was once considered anti-epileptic.

7. The resinous part of a Persian plant. It is no longer used. Just what its plant of origin was is unknown. It had much the same use as assafoetida. It has a disagreeable odor and bitter taste.

8. Chlorosis, an iron-deficiency anemia.

9. Elixir proprietatis of Paracelsus. Essentially it consisted of tincture of aloes and myrrh. It is amazing how long Paracelsian prescriptions, only slightly modified, remained popular. This one was used until late in the eighteenth century.

10. Luke 8:43 and 44: And a woman having an issue of blood twelve years, which had spent all her living upon physicians, neither could be healed by any, came behind *Him* and touched the border of his garment and immediately her issue of blood was stanched.

Notes to Capsula LIII

1. Boston, 1710. This long sermonizing chapter should be read with understanding, not impatience. It was about the best that Mather, or anyone else, could offer a woman faced with the terrors of pregnancy in 1724. Hemorrhage, eclampsia, malpresentations, disproportions, and infection caused their fearful toll then and for many generations. Women had to put up with great pain and with the terror of that pain. The forceps had been invented but it was still a Chamberlen family secret until about 1732. So, even that benison was denied the women of Mather's Massachusetts. A pregnant woman's fearful reading of Mather's exhortations may have been of some help. After all, this compassionate man had seen fifteen children of his own born under his roof.

2. Exodus 15:23. "And when they came to Marah they could not drink of the waters of Marah for they were bitter, therefore the name of it was called Marah." The daughters of bitter sorrow.

3. Michal, wife of David, daughter of Saul. By a strategem she saved David's life from the wrath of Saul. Later, II Samuel 6:16, she came to despise David.

4. Father of Samson. See Judges 13. His wife was barren until an angel of the Lord told her to avoid wine and strong drink.

5. Wife of Abraham, mother of Isaac. Long barren, she bore the latter at ninety years of age, according to the Scripture.

6. Even then ergot was used by the midwives, in Europe at least, though not by physicians to any extent until after 1800. John Stearns of New York is credited with having first noted it in print, in the *Medical repository* of 1808. Probably Morgan was opposing ergot rather than the inert preparation described by Mather.

7. Cuminum cyminum is a small Egyptian annual plant which has dark leaves, white flowers, and elliptical seeds. The last were considered stimulant.

8. Small earthen pot.

9. "It is rather often found."

10. "No griping pain at all." Apparently, lubrication by the oral roote seemed logical.

11. Magnetic oxide of iron.

12. A rather acidulous mineral water from Bristol Hot Wells, unlikely to have been obtainable in Massachusetts.

13. Hernia plaster.

14. Three ounces of opium to two pints of alcohol, and filtered after seven days.

15. Scrofula is tuberculosis of the cervical lymph nodes, with ulceration. Scrofula was considered hereditary. By "latent scrofula" Mather probably meant debility.

16. Breast abscess. It is always accompanied by chills and fever.

17. "This my expert wife taught me."

Notes to Capsula LIV

1. "Good strength often lies in mean things."

2. Published in 1690, this was the collection of the prescriptions of court physician George Bate (1608–1669). He deserves some recognition because he managed to become successively physician to Charles I, Cromwell, and Charles II.

3. Perhaps the equivalent of a million dollars today. Quacks have always done well financially, but never better than they did in the seventeenth century.

4. Xenocrates of Aphrodisias (fl. about 75 A.D.) was the source of much of the pharmaceutical lore of Pliny.

5. "Dung and urine are of prime importance to doctors."

6. "Western civet," comparing it to the pungent odor of the Indian civet. It is hard for us to understand the rationale of the use of solid and liquid offal in medicine. But, as I have remarked before, such material was considered to be a sort of distillation of food and humours.

7. Johann Joachim Becher (1635–1682) was a German chemist and physician.

8. "Internal use is not really nice."

9. John of Gaddesden lived in the late thirteenth and early fourteenth centuries. He wrote *Rosa Anglica,* an interesting medieval English medical text. This was printed twice in the sixteenth century but apparently not, in England at least, in the seventeenth century. Mather's information was probably second-hand.

10. Jean Baptiste Tavernier (1605–1688) was a French traveler and merchant.

11. Probably this was Raymund Minderer (1570–1621), a German physician who wrote *De pestilentia liber unus* . . . Augsburg, 1608. In this there was found

Mather's reference. He was the discoverer of ammonium acetate, known as spirit of Minderer.

12. Nicholas de La Roche (fl. 1542), Parisian (?) physician, wrote on women's diseases. No reference has been found to a plague tract by him, but he may well have written one. Most literary physicians of the day seem to have done so.

13. Herman Corbejus of Nuremberg, born at the end of the sixteenth century, also was mainly interested in women's diseases.

14. From ancient times physicians and quacks alike have looked learnedly at urine and pontificated. We still do, with more reason.

15. "Uncouth remedy."

16. Antoine Mizauld (d. 1578) wrote on astrology in medicine and on medical botany. Probably he was a Parisian.

17. Martin Pansa (sixteenth century) was a German physician who practised in various German cities. He wrote on peripneumonia and phlebotomy.

18. Johann Jacob Wecker (1528–1586) was a Swiss German physician who wrote a number of books, none of any originality, an antidotarium, Basel 1576, and a general medical work, Basel 1585, for instance.

19. Suckerus or Stockerus was probably Johann Stockar, a German sixteenth century physician. He published a "regimen" or general health book in Augsburg in 1538.

20. Probably Hieronymus Reusner, a seventeenth century German physician of little note who wrote a book on his cures and observations, Augsburg 1668.

21. Guillaume Rondelet (1507–1566) practised in Montpellier. He wrote two general medical books and a work on fishes.

22. Esteban Rodrigo de Castro (1550–1627) was a Portuguese Jewish physician who wrote voluminously but contributed nothing really new.

23. Probably this was Matthew Backmeister (1580–1626), a German physician of Rostock who wrote several tracts, one of them a general treatise on the practice of medicine, Rostock 1614.

24. Johann Theodor Schenck (1619–1671) was a German physician who wrote on plants, anatomy, and general medicine.

25. "Maintainer of strength."

26. "With strength intact, with sense and speech strong, he lived healthy from that day onward."

27. "Let no one consider this a fiction. I the writer saw it and what is more certain than what is seen?"

Notes to Capsula LV

1. In the National Library of Medicine there is a copy of *Warme beere, a treatise wherein is declared that beere so qualified is more wholesome . . . than cold,* Cambridge 1641, by an unidentified "F.W." Mather gives evidence that the tract was published at least seventeen years earlier.

2. The serous and purulent discharge from a wound in the skin which is intentionally held open by a pea or a string.

3. See Introduction. It is not certain what Mather meant by "cupping without fire." The air in the cup had to be heated to create suction.

4. Not identified certainly. Franz von Zeigler (1700–1761), a Swiss, would seem to have been too young.

5. Johann Jacob Wepfer (1620–1695), was a distinguished Swiss physician and anatomist. He was a student of apoplexy and convulsive diseases.

6. Stroking "with a dead hand" was literally practiced.

7. Valentine Greatrakes (b. 1628) was a famous seventeenth century English quack who won fame and fortune for a time largely by "the laying on of hands," that is, stroking his patients.

Notes to Capsula LVI

1. Hagar, mistress of Abraham, mother of Ishmael, was sent into the desert because of Sarah's jealousy. There an angel comforted her.

2. Samuel Hartlib (d. 1670), descendant of a Polish family, was a merchant and writer on educational and agricultural subjects. He is a prime source of information on conditions in seventeenth century England. The work mentioned is *Samuel Hartlib, his legacie, or an enlargement of the discourse of husbandry used in Brabant and Flaunders,* London 1651.

3. Medicine composed of five ingredients.

4. In Mather's opinion "punch" is an abbreviation of "panchayat" an East Indian word for a council of five persons.

5. "There is an English drink which they call bola puncha."

6. "Country folk who drink nothing but cold water are the healthiest of people and attain great age."

7. Sextus Pompeius Festus (? fourth century A.D.) was a Roman writer who left as his sole surviving work *On the meaning of words.* He was referring to the fact that the Roman temple to Aesculapius was on an island in the Tiber.

8. Probably Thomas Curteis who wrote *Essays on the preservation and recovery of health,* London 1704.

9. Apparently his *Discursus quinque . . . in quibus clare et compendiose deducuntur seri lactis in fluxu torminale et maxime dysenterico, aquae frigidae . . effectus . . ,* Leyden 1752, evidently a Latin translation of his *Discours et advis sur les flus de ventre,* Ghent 1643.

10. William Cockburn (1669–1739) practiced in that vague seventeenth century professional realm of part physician and part quack. He made a fortune on his secret remedy for dysentery. No one knows just what this marvel contained. He is most noted for the work Mather cites, published in London in 1696. It was based on what he learned in two years as a naval surgeon.

11. Jerry Wainwright (late seventeenth and early eighteenth centuries) practiced medicine in London and became noted for his *Mechanical account of the non-naturals,* London 1707. The "non-naturals" of the ancients were air, meat and drink, sleep and watching, motion and rest, retention and secretion, and the affections of the mind. They were called the non-naturals because they are not naturally causes of disease.

12. Hermann Boerhaave (1668–1738) was the most noted figure in world medicine in Mather's time. He was professor at Leyden and a great teacher and prolific writer. It seems strange that Mather did not quote him more often. Probably he simply did not own any of his publications.

13. Edward Baynard. See above.

14. From the Greek meaning literally "I wash cold."

Notes to Capsula LVII

1. A spagyrist was an iatrochemist.

2. Dabblers in natural history.

3. Cure-all.

4. A fabulous herb mentioned in the *Odyssey,* Book 10, line 305. Later writers meant garlic by the term.

5. Theophrastus (370–285 B.C.) was the favorite pupil of Aristotle and became the first botanist. He was an authority until well into our colonial times, especially because of his *Historia plantarum* which saw many editions and translations. Harvard had his *Opera omnia,* Leyden 1613.

6. "Why should man wither away?"

7. "Spirit of the lungs."

8. Ground ivy.

9. Paronychia, infection of the flesh beside the finger nail.

10. Johannes Sambucus (1531–1584) was born in Hungary, died in Vienna. Editions of the book mentioned were published in Italy, France, and Germany. He also edited Dioscorides and Vegetius.

11. Very close to the word quinine, a word seldom used in the seventeenth century.

12. "They quiet with a small compressed dose of the powder."

13. Possibly Jean de Renou, called Renodaeus, (late sixteenth century), a French physician who wrote a book on therapeutics which was first published in Paris in 1608 in Latin and finally translated into English in 1657. Mather's spelling, when the reference was not at hand, was often faulty.

14. Probably Martin Van Hille (1633–1706), a Dutch naval surgeon who wrote on surgery and on syphilis after he entered private practice.

15. Common sage, Salvia sclarea.

16. The vegetable oils all are of some value in protecting the gastric mucosa after the ingestion of corrosive substances. Otherwise, Mather's eloquent testimony is exaggerated.

17. More correctly spelled Parmaceti.

18. A Daniel Coxe (d. 1730) wrote *The interest of the patient. A discourse wherein the interest of the patient in reference to physick and physicians is soberly debated.* . . . London 1669. Evidently Mather had a copy.

19. There are several aspects of the St. Veronica legend. One view has it that she was a woman of Jerusalem who pitied Christ while He was carrying the Cross, and gave Him a handkerchief with which to wipe His face. He used it and handed it back to her with a perfect image of Himself on the cloth. Eusebius believed that she was the woman of Caesarea Philippi whom Christ cured of an issue of blood when she touched His garment. That woman erected a statue of Him outside her door. Veronica is supposed to be derived from vera icon, true image.

20. Samuel Bowden. Cataloguers at the National Library of Medicine believed that he flourished about 1733–1761 since that library has a 1754 edition of his *Poems on various subjects or a treatise on health.* Obviously, his first edition must have been

more than thirty years earlier since Mather mentions it here and probably owned a copy.

21. Robert Godfrey is another obscure writer. In London in 1674 there was published his *Various injuries and abuses in chymical and Galenical physick. Committed by physicians and apothecaries* .... Mather probably had a copy.

22. All through the middle ages prescriptions were incredibly complex polypharmacal affairs. There began to trend away from this in the seventeenth century. Robert Boyle was one of those who favored "simple medicines."

Notes to Capsula LVIII

1. "Writings on the marvels of insects."

2. Possibly John Cock (1603–1669) who was only one of a number of seventeenth century minor theologians of that surname. There were also several physicians. One, Virgil Cocchi (b. 1692) of Perugia wrote on natural historical subjects.

3. "Liberator of the world."

4. Linguistic scholars have disagreed about Beelzebub. Their interpretations of the name run from "god to whom flies are sacred," the sacred dung beetle of Egypt, another word for the Devil, to, simply, the god of Ekron, a Philistine city.

5. Arsenic.

Notes to Capsula LIX

1. A waxy, yellowish substance with a pleasant odor, found floating in the Indian Ocean. It is thought to be formed in the intestine of whales. It is used in perfume.

2. Oxycroceum was a plaster composed of saffron, pitch, yellow wax, turpentine, galbanum, gum ammoniac, myrrh, olibanum and mastic.

3. After infusing the rose flowers for hours, the pharmacist added honey and then let the mixture boil gently to a proper consistence. It was used usually as a gargle, sometimes for a cough.

4. Ring worm.

5. The oily matter obtained from boiling pitch.

6. More properly this is an American wild geranium which has very fleshy roots, the extract of which, when dried has a not unpleasant taste. It is quite astringent due to its high tannin content.

7. Convallaria polygonatum is a perennial plant having a jointed white root. It is emetic. The logic of these recommendations for hernia is obscure.

8. Possibly lime water with an excess of lime.

9. Not identified.

10. Spirit of aromatic ammonia.

11. Francis Glisson (1597–1677), physician and anatomist, was the discoverer of rickets. His *De rachitide* was first published in 1650. He published his superb *Anatomia hepatis* in 1654. It is true that Daniel Whistler had written about rickets in 1645, but he was a pupil of Glisson.

12. Osmunda regalis, royal fern, is an American swamp fern.

13. Tamarix gallica, a North African tree, exudes a sap which is of a sugary mucilaginous character.

14. Scolopendrium officinarum is another type of fern, found both in Europe and America.

15. Perversity.

16. Largely calcium phosphate.

17. Hepatica americana or triloba. The leaves are vaguely liver-shaped, the roots tough and fibrous. All parts have a slightly bitter taste, are rather mucilaginous. Once used to combat liver trouble (largely because of the shape of the leaf), it was more often used as a mild soothing tonic.

18. John Locke (1632–1704) was an English philosopher, and, briefly, physician, who is famous for his *Essay concerning humane understanding,* 1690. Harvard had a set of his works. Mather doubtless owned a copy.

Notes to Capsula LX

1. Things previously passed over but here added as a supplement.

2. Lard.

3. That is, very dilute ferrous oxide.

4. An old variety of pear.

5. A variety of apple.

6. A vague term which included all diseased conditions of the gums which were accompanied by malodor and bloody discharge.

7. Also called chicory, Cichorum intybus, a tall thin weed with lovely blue flowers. The root is a famous coffee adulterant.

8. Galls are the reaction of various kinds of oak to injury by gall wasps which lay their eggs in the wounds they cause. Usually young shoots are affected. Galls, which contain gallic acid, are very astringent. So, of course, are acorns and alum.

9. Gum arabic, the gum of several mimosa-like plants found in Africa and the East.

10. Roche alum, named from Roccha in Syria where pieces the size of an almond are found. They are covered with a reddish efflorescence.

11. Terra japonica is an astringent extract made by boiling the leaves and shoots of Uncaria gambir, an East Indian climbing shrub. The water of extract is evaporated and the dry remains cut into cubes for sale.

12. A red alum-bearing clay found in Armenia and several places in Europe.

13. Whooping cough.

14. Frequent, often vain, and painful desire to defecate.

15. Inflammatory swelling, or sore, due to exposure to cold.

16. Ulcerated chilblain of the heel.

17. A fine, soft silk.

18. A paronychia or run-around, an infection of the flesh of the finger next to the nail.

19. Erysipelas.

20. "Of these (remedies) I consider few safe and certain."

21. Fresh wounds.

22. Put in a cask.

23. "Has proven a thousand times."

24. Martin Mersenne (1588–1648) was a French philosopher and mathematician, a friend of Descartes.

25. Gonorrhea.

26. In any quantity laurel berries or leaves are poisonous. The leaves were once used externally, powdered or as a decoction for various skin ailments including syphilis.

27. "As though by incantation."

28. Probably zinc silicate.

29. Copper sulfate.

30. The residuum from the gum of the pine after a distillation of the volatile oils.

31. Ferric sulfate.

32. Ranunculus bulbosus, a perennial having a solid fleshy root and rich yellow flowers. It was never used internally, but externally as a vesicant.

Notes to Capsula LXI

1. "Medicaments without any special preparation."

2. Probably a local lady with a knack for healing.

3. "Female Galens."

4. Possibly John Whitlock (1625–1709), an English nonconforming divine. In the seventeenth century there were many pamphlets published attacking various aspects of medical practice.

5. "For the sexes change."

6. "O wretched ways."

7. "An old woman imagines herself a doctor, be she as you please an ignoramus, a profane person, a distiller, an actor, a barber."

8. Daughter of a warrior whom Nestor killed. "Fair-haired Agamede" knew all the pharmaceuticals the wide earth knows. *Iliad,* 11, line 740.

9. *Odyssey,* 4, 1.228. Polydamna was a woman of Egypt, wife of Thon (a medical man?) from whom Helen had obtained an amnesic drug. The reference speaks very highly of Egyptian medicine. It is interesting to note that Herodotus, II, chapters 112–120, placed the Helen and Paris saga in Egypt. Homer rejected this for his Trojan one, but he harks back to the Egyptian story in this brief reference.

10. George Herbert (1593–1633) was a poet and divine. His chief work in prose was *A priest to the temple or the country parson.* . London 1652. Obviously, Mather had a copy.

11. The root of Valeriana officinalis was used. The plant is large and handsome, having white or rose-colored flowers with a pleasant odor. It is native to Europe. The root is large and perennial. As an infusion, or in powder for, it was used internally largely for "nervous affections."

12. Ophioglossum vulgatum is a kind of fern.

13. Melilotus officinalis is a European annual or biennial which has a very sweet odor when dried. It was often used locally in cataplasms.

14. Parsley.

15. Agnodike (third century B.C.), an Athenian, was perhaps the first woman to study and practice medicine.

16. "Healthful bitters." Remember, bitter medicines were considered especially tonic.

17. Bernardino Ramazzini (1633–1717) was an Italian, a professor at Modena, who was famous for his *De morbis artificium,* Modena 1700, one of the earliest works on industrial medicine.

18. It is a fascinating fact that although the value of lemons in the prevention and treatment of scurvy was known in the seventeenth century, was proven by a valid experiment in 1753 by James Lind, lemons were not used by the Royal Navy until very late in the eighteenth century. Nowadays a new drug has almost instantaneous acceptance.

19. Currants.

20. "When given in time are beneficial."

21. Zinc sulfate.

22. A Lionel Lockyer published in London, 1664, *An advertisement concerning those excellent pills called pillulae radiis solis extractae.*

23. James Cook of Warwick, England (c1615–1690) was a military surgeon in the Parliamentary forces. Later he won some fame as a sort of gynecologist. He wrote his popular *Mellificium chirurgiae or marrow of surgery,* London 1647 and in 1657 published his *Select observations on English bodies of eminent persons in desperate diseases first written in Latin by Mr. John Hall, physician.* That John Hall was Shakespeare's son-in-law. His widow had allowed Cook to use her husband's manuscripts in 1643.

24. A gentle laxative made with damask roses. It is still sold over the counter in many drug stores.

25. Potassium tartrate.

26. Like syrup of roses, syrup of violets is mildly laxative. It is seldom used today.

27. Probably ferrous chloride. Chalybeation meant mixing a medicine with an iron salt.

Notes to Capsula LXII

1. "The power of the Devil is not so great as to heal a lame little foot."

2. "There is something diabolical, in my opinion, in these cures or in some deal with the Devil, as anyone can see."

3. "Concerning the obscure causes of things (diseases)." The works of Fernel (1497–1558) were still being reprinted in Mather's youth.

4. Probably Niels Hemmingsen, sixteenth century Danish theologian who wrote *De lege naturae* (1572) which made him noted all over Europe as the first man to propose natural law.

5. St. Augustine?

6. Not identified.

7. Quintus Serenus Sammonicus wrote *De medicina praecepta,* a long poem with a number of popular remedies and magic formulae, including the Abracadabra, as cures for fever. It was apparently his son, however, who was the tutor of Gordian.

8. Gordian I, a Roman of great wealth, became emperor in 238 A.D., with his son, Gordian II, as co-emperor. The son was killed in an uprising and Gordian I committed suicide. They had reigned together only a few weeks.

9. "Men fearing the Trojans substituted the quartan of Lydia."

10. Sixtinus Amana, or Amama (1593–1629) was a Dutch protestant theologian.

11. St. John's wort.

12. A cabalistic word engraved on an amulet and worn, in former times, to ward off evil.

13. John Selden (1584–1654) was an English liberal politician, scholar, and legal historian. He wrote *De diis Syris,* London 1617, which established his reputation as an orientalist.

14. A mystical word used as a charm when engraved on amulets. Its Greek letters were said to add up numerically to 365. Abraxas was thus the name given by an Egyptian gnostic named Basilides to the supreme deity who ruled the 365th heaven in his philosophical system.

15. Probably Johann Hartmann Beyer (1563–1625), a German physician who was interested in mathematics as applicable to medicine.

16. Not identified.

17. Possibly Andreas Langner (b. 1548) who in 1576 published, in German, a medical book which in part dealt with the use of the Zodiac in medicine.

18. Amulets with occult signs.

19. "Cure of disease through measurement." Author not identified.

20. Jakob Wolf (1642–1695), professor of medicine at Jena published the work mentioned in 1690 at Leipzig.

21. Gottschalck (d. about 870 A.D.) was an unorthodox German priest who taught an extreme form of predestination.

22. "The Devil plucks out your eyes and fills the sockets with dung."

23. "Whence the efficacy of this unless done by a demon who was delighted by the fraud?"

24. St. Paul's *Epistles.*

25. Acts 19:14. And there were seven sons of one Sceva a Jew and chief of the priests (of Ephesus). The seventh son has long been considered lucky and gifted both with medical and occult powers.

26. Montpellier in southern France was the second oldest medical school in Europe, was very prestigious in the thirteenth and fourteenth centuries.

27. "This understanding is impressed upon the fool and he is thrust out of the city, after having been conducted through the city with great dishonor, having had rotten eggs and other putrid matter thrown at him, that he might seek another location."

28. St. Medard of Noyon was a sixth century bishop who was a patron of agriculture and horticulture and was invoked to aid in the relief of toothache and migraine.

29. There are too many possibilities here for definite identification. Through the millennia there has been a host of saints, many of whom have been forgotten, decanonized, or confused with others of the same name.

30. St. Acca was the Bishop of Huxham who encouraged Bede and promoted learning and libraries.

31. Probably St. Aventine of Troyes (fl. about 538 A.D.), an abbot, and a man who was remarkably gentle to all living things. He even nursed a sick snake. A bear came to him for the removal of a thorn in its paw.

32. This third century Christian bishop preached near the city of Saintes (western France) and lived in a hovel. He was killed by order of the governor and was burned near his hut. A church, no longer standing, was erected on the site.

33. St. Mammas was a shepherd boy of twelve who was martyred. Some authorities claim that he was another, older man.

34. St. Maen (or Maven) was a sixth century Welshman who spent much time in Brittany.

35. St. Phiacre (Fiacre) was born in Ireland, died 670. He cured blindness, polyps, and "le fic de Fiacre" (hemorrhoids) by the laying on of hands.

36. Genou, of course, refers to the knee. "St. Genou" not identified.

37. St. John the Baptist or St. John the Evangelist?

38. St. Valentine was probably a priest martyred in the third century. The medieval custom of love notes on Valentine's Day stemmed from the belief that it marked the mating season of birds. So far as his relationship to epilepsy is concerned, apparently it is a case of phonetic analogy since his name in German sounds much like the word for "fallen."

39. No one knows why epilepsy was called St. John's evil. One idea is that it derives from the fact that the head of St. John the Baptist fell to the ground when he was beheaded. See Owsei Temkin, *The falling sickness,* Baltimore 1945, p. 99–100 for a discussion of these designations.

40. Native of Milan, this Christian was martyred about 300 A.D. by being shot with arrows. There is a fifteenth century fugitive sheet against the plague, bearing a figure of St. Sebastian full of arrows and with an invocation.

41. St. Roch (1295–1327), also called Rocco, was a native of Montpellier and known as the healer of the plague-stricken because of his many cures.

42. This woman of the first century, said to have been St. Peter's daughter (spiritual?), became paralyzed but when St. Peter called to her she arose and walked and became well.

43. St. Romain was in 304 A.D. martyred by having his tongue torn out. But he miraculously retained the power of speech. He was at Antioch when the churches were destroyed on the order of Diocletian.

44. These were the patron saints of physicians, not just surgeons. Nothing is known of their lives. Tradition says these twin brothers practiced without fee. They were martyred by being beheaded. They became a very popular subject of medieval art.

45. St. Claire was a man of the ninth century who lived a life of great seclusion and severity. A woman whose advances he rejected had him beheaded. After that he went about with his head in his arms and whenever a woman appeared he covered his eyes with his hand.

46. Died in 286 A.D. after enduring incredible tortures. Finally he was beheaded and then a dove flew out of his throat to Heaven.

47. Traditionally this Greek suffered martyrdom in Asia Minor in the third century. He is particularly the patron of wayfarers because he was a powerful fellow who earned a living carrying travelers over a river.

48. Not identified.

49. St. Anthony of Padua (1195–1231) was a Franciscan friar born in Lisbon to a noble family. He was canonized in 1232. He was invoked for the return of lost property, he was patron of the poor, and was believed able to protect pregnant women.

50. Nicholas Culpeper (1616–1654) practiced medicine in London after minimal preparation. He was much interested in astrology. In addition to his medical practice he wrote, edited, or translated a great many medical works. These works were very

popular. Harvard College owned his *English physician enlarged,* London 1656. Very likely this is the work Mather refers to since in the subtitle we find, "Being an astro-logo-physical discourse of the vulgar herbs of this nation . . ." He makes arbitrary assertions as to which planet governs which herb, as Jupiter governs houseleeks, Mercury governs houndstongue, etc.

Notes to Capsula LXIII

1. "Smoke hater."
2. Philip II of Spain.
3. Plain near Babylon where Nebuchadnezzar established a golden idol.
4. Tamerlane (1336–1405) was the Mongol conqueror.
5. Sir Ralph Lane (1530–1603) was the leader of the 1585 expedition, sent out by Raleigh, which headquartered on Roanoke Island and explored eastern Carolina. The expedition left Carolina in 1586 in the ships of Sir Francis Drake who was returning home from a raid on the Spanish Indies.
6. An able Roman general, Syrian by birth, who died in 175 A.D. at the hands of his own officers after he had tried to win the imperial title from Marcus Aurelius.
7. The Indians of Haiti called the tube used in smoking a tabac. The Spanish gave the plant itself that name.
8. Jean Nicot (1530–1600), French courtier, during his embassy in Portugal in 1559 saw tobacco used and then introduced the plant and habit to France. The genus Nicotiana is named for him, as is nicotine.
9. Catherine de Medici.
10. Johann Neander (1596–?) published his *Tabaco-logia* . . . at Leyden in 1620. In 1632 he published *Sassafrasologia.* He was born in Bremen, educated at Leyden.
11. Castor Durante (d. 1590) was an Italian whose Latin epigram on tobacco was published posthumously at Utrecht in 1644.
12. Johannes Posthius (1537–1597) was a German anatomist who studied and traveled widely. Essentially, a distich is a couplet.
13. "With nothing health-promoting can tobacco be compared; it surpasses all the rest in strength." King James I in his *Counterblast,* mentioned above by Mather, heartily disagreed and took the position recently confirmed by the United States surgeon general.
14. Laurent Joubert (1529–1583) was a prolific medical writer and professor at Montpellier. Among other things, he wrote on pharmacology and the preparation of drugs and medicaments.
15. Johann Heinrich Alsted (1588–1638) was a German theologian and historian.
16. Possibly John Dryden (1631–1700) although this quotation could not be found in the Dryden concordance available.
17. Tierra del Fuego, the archipelago at the tip of South America, so named by Magellan probably because the aborigines built signal fires when they sighted him.
18. Old legends maintained that salamanders can go through flames unharmed.
19. "O ye born to slavery."
20. "I suck up smoke out of need, not desire." The "t" of sorbeto is redundant.
21. Sedative.

22. Abdu-l-Malik (646–705), the fifth Omayyad Caliph, was a very able man both as a warrior and an administrator. He quieted for a time the dissension in Islam.

23. Pieter Pauw (1564–1617), born in Amsterdam, taught botany and anatomy at Leyden. Harvard had his *Primitiae anatomicae. De humani corporis ossibus.* Leyden 1615.

24. Adrian van Valkenburg (1581–1650) was a student of Pauw who later became professor of anatomy and surgery at Leyden.

25. Francis Raphalengien was a scholarly printer of Leyden. He was a translator of Galen.

26. Johannes Chrysostomus Magnen (seventeenth century) wrote *De tabaco exercitationes . .* Pavia 1648. He had studied at Pavia. Despite his name, he is thought to have been French.

27. Probably this is Thomas Gale (1635–1702), historian and divine, and an active member of the Royal Society. He wrote a good deal on religious and historical subjects. From the context Thomas Gale (1507–1586), the surgeon, would seem unlikely.

28. Probably this was Lucius Septimus Severus (146–211), the only African emperor of Rome, who reigned from 193–211. He had been an able general.

29. Adam von Lebenwaldt was a German seventeenth century physician.

30. "I eliminate and discourage this drug as much as is in my power."

31. "To whom therefore its smoke and odor are pleasant."

32. Kaspar Schwenckfeld (1563–1609) was a botanist and physician who wrote *Thesaurus pharmaceuticus,* Basel 1586.

33. Possibly Joseph Hall, D.D. (1588–1676), Bishop of Norwich.

34. Gysbert Voet (1588–1676) was a Dutch theologian and extreme Calvinist.

35. "Although in itself the use of tobacco may not be illicit, nevertheless it very slightly becomes honest and serious men (namely ministers and candidates for the ministry) in the presence of others because the common vanity of licentious men is indicated not so much by their food as by their smoke.

The use of it is bad except for medicinal excuse, whether it be for killing time of course, or for drawing off the dregs of the humours of the body that it may be filled with meat and wine, or out of custom or conformity with the famous gormandizing effect of tobacco."

Notes to Capsula LXIV

1. "The goal of a cure made through Christ is the cure of the soul."

2. See 4 Kings 20:9–11 and Isaiah 38:4–6. Ezechia was the sick man. He was assured by Isaiah that his life would be prolonged by God. As proof of this the sun was made to retrogress as evidenced by the reversal of its shadow on a stairway.

3. Kaspar Olevianus (1536–1587) was a German church reformer. He was an ardent follower of Calvin. He became professor of theology at Heidelberg.

4. Not identified.

5. André Rivet (1572–1651) was a French Protestant theologian and firm Calvinist who in 1620 received the chair of theology at Leyden.

6. Possibly Griffith Owen (1647–1717), born in Wales, became one of the first Pennsylvania physicians. He was an ardent Quaker who visited all the colonies. Mather was friendly toward the Quakers.

7. Sigismund (1368–1437), King of Hungary 1387–1437, was crowned Holy Roman Emperor in 1433. He had an extremely turbulent career.

8. The Archbishop of Cologne had great power as one of the princes of the Holy Roman Empire.

Notes to Capsula LXV

1. The most probable reading is TOFA'OT meaning phenomenon or manifestation.

2. "A thousand ways of dying."

Notes to Capsula LXVI

1. Not identified.

2. Frederick III (1415–1493), crowned emperor in 1452, was the Hapsburg monarch who laid the foundations for the long years of power enjoyed by his family. "When the Emperor Frederick was asked what is the highest good a man can attain, he replied, 'To die well.' "

3. Aeneas Sylvius Piccolomini (1405–1464), Pope as Pius II 1458–1464, was a poet and politician who turned priest and rose to the papacy on merit. He was noted for his literary ability and left an excellent autobiography.

4. There are four prescriptions not in Mather's handwriting but included on a page in the manuscript as deposited with the American Antiquarian Society. They are in a much more legible and typical eighteenth century hand.